The Art of EKG Interpretation

A *Self-Instructional Text*

SEVENTH EDITION

with Special Sections on

- Hemodynamic Monitoring
- Diagnosis and Treatment of Acute Coronary Syndromes
- Pacemaker Basics
- Pacemaker Features and Interventions
- Pediatric EKG Interpretation
- Advanced Practice

Stephanie L. Woods, R.N., Ph.D.
Karen S. Ehrat, Ph.D.

Kendall Hunt
publishing company

Book Team

Chairman and Chief Executive Officer   Mark C. Falb
President and Chief Operating Officer   Chad M. Chandlee
Vice President, Higher Education   David L. Tart
Director of National Book Program   Paul B. Carty
Editorial Development Manager   Georgia Botsford
(Senior) Developmental Editor   Denise M. LaBudda
Vice President, Operations   Timothy J. Beitzel
Assistant Vice President, Production Services   Christine E. O'Brien
Production Editor   Abby Davis
Permissions Editor   Elizabeth Roberts
Cover Designer   Jenifer Chapman

Cover images: Bull image © Wikus Otto, 2009
EKG paper © Bruck Works, 2009
Sky and ground image © Victor Habbick, 2009. Used under license from Shutterstock Inc.

Kendall Hunt
publishing company

www.kendallhunt.com
Send all inquiries to:
4050 Westmark Drive
Dubuque, IA 52004-1840

Copyright © 1978, 1985, 1993, 1997, 2002, 2005, 2009 by Kendall Hunt Publishing Company

ISBN 978-0-7575-6401-7

Special Edition ISBN 978-0-7575-6403-1

Printed in the United States of America
10 9 8 7 6 5 4 3 2

Dedication

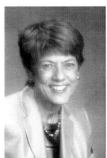

This book is dedicated to Karen S. Ehrat, R.N. Ph.D, the originator of this long running, best selling text, who passed away on February 12, 2006 at the age of 56 from a rare form of cancer. I wish you could have met her, but then of course you will as you read this book. Her personality is evident throughout. When she began the book in 1978, her intent was to teach EKGs in a low stress, fun way. Clinicians responded to her unique covers, wonderful drawings and simple explanations by using the book over many years. Karen's legacy, in part, is literally thousands of clinicians who can interpret EKGs, thereby providing improved care to patients.

Karen began her career as a diploma nurse, but ended her career with a PhD. She was a critical care nurse who ultimately became a highly successful healthcare executive who led hospitals in Arizona, Michigan, Ohio and lastly Texas. She loved Texas and the Longhorn on the cover is a nod to that.

She was so very *proud* of this book and I was greatly honored when she left it in my care. I am a nurse with thirty years of experience. I have had the privilege of practicing, teaching and managing in critical care units. I taught critical care nursing in universities and have taught hundreds of EKG courses. I have often joked that when I die they will not inscribe my birth and death dates, but rather my QRS interval. . . .

I met Karen when I moved into an administrative role. It was a delightful opportunity to work for and with her. As my Chief Executive Officer, she modeled leadership and integrity coupled with a zest for life and a great sense of humor.

This book is now edited by two nurse leaders who passionately believe in the power of knowledge and competency. But who said becoming competent couldn't be fun, and as Karen always said, "and as painless as possible!"

Brief Contents

v

Contents

(Participant Objectives Precede Each Section ⊙)

Acknowledgments

We would like to acknowledge the following individuals for their contributions in writing *The Art of EKG Interpretation:*

> Karen Corlett, R.N., M.S.N., A.P.N.
>
> Victoria A. Paparelli, M.S.N., R.N., CCNS-AC
>
> Delores D. Schultz
>
> Jane D. Werth, M.S., R.N.

About the Author

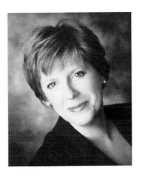

Dr. Stephanie Woods began her career in critical care nursing and has served in the roles of staff nurse, manager, faculty member and healthcare administrator. She has a Ph.D. in Nursing Administration from the University of Texas at Austin and has served on the national board of directors for the American Association of Critical-Care Nurses. She has presented at numerous national conferences including the National Teaching Institute for the American Association of Critical-Care Nurses and the American Organization for Nurse Executives National Meeting.

A Long-Winded Introduction Worth Reading

Cardiac rhythms can be *relatively* straight forward or amazingly confounding. **Not to worry!** The purpose of this text is to provide the reader with an excellent baseline understanding of both the simple and more complex rhythms, imparting terminology along the way. Importantly, a consistent methodology for evaluating and describing rhythms is emphasized throughout. Numerous illustrations and analogies serve to aid learning and demystify complex concepts. Sufficient structure has been incorporated to prevent even the novice learner from floundering! At the conclusion of the text, the reader will be *comfortable* describing simple and complex rhythm disorders and determining when action is warranted. Several Advanced Study (☞) discussions are included for the more adventurous student.

This seventh edition of *The Art of EKG Interpretation* considers rapidly expanding diagnostic and therapeutic interventions and provides additional rhythm interpretation practice exercises. Faculty and student suggestions have been incorporated into the content. The author's undergirding assumptions remain unchanged: complex material can be easily learned when it is broken into its simplest, component parts; learning technical material can be both *fun* and *painless;* and, humor aids adult learning!

One introductory point deserves *special* attention. Professionals in cardiac monitoring areas excel in the everyday use of complex, technical terminology. The new learner should consider that the use of highly technical terminology is simply a means for distinguishing one's practice specialty . . . similar to surgeons wearing green, surgical nurses displaying Kelly clamps, ICU nurses draping stethoscopes over their shoulders, etc. Rest assured, comfort with terminology will follow as a *natural* consequence of rhythm description!!

This text has been structured to allow for *self-paced learning* and utilizes a self-instructional format. Information and encouragement are provided under headings labeled **Input**. **Practice Exercises** follow Input sections. Practice Exercise answers are provided under **Feedback** headings. Practice rhythm strips are included throughout.

As a final *important* word, please be advised that diagnostic and therapeutic interventions change at rates *faster than speeding bullets!* Both technologic and pharmacologic developments, in concert with clinical research, continue to evolve the efficacy of both diagnosis and treatment of rhythm disorders and related pathology. The reader is always advised to consult the most current version of the American Heart Association's **Advanced Life Support** for treatment updates.

LEADS: Leading into Section 1

> **IMPORTANT NOTE FROM THE MANAGEMENT:** "LEADS" may be confusing to the novice learner. Later in the text, you will be directed to reread this section!

Welcome to this book! You're probably wondering who I am . . . Right? Well, this is me.

Actually, this is the back of my head. If you think it would be difficult to recognize me in a crowd . . . I'll help you out by showing you my best side. . . .

 (Cute, huh?)

If you're still uncertain about my identity, you can view me from any angle that you choose.

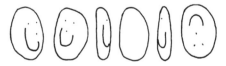

Sometimes, if one has a common face, it's necessary to look closely to determine identity!

The same thing holds true when looking at monitors tracings or electrocardiograms. Sometimes all those "peculiar" waves and bumps are *almost* **impossible** to identify. However, by looking at the various wave forms and patterns from different views or angles, identity becomes more clear.

Before you start through this book, there are several things you should know. For instance, all cell membranes in the body are charged . . .

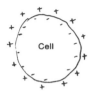

. . . and *charged* means that the cell membranes have *electrical potentials.*

When cells are in a **resting** or **polarized** state, the cell membranes carry a net positive charge.

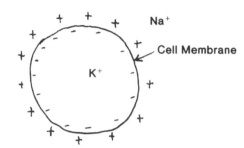

This charge or electrical potential results from the difference of intra and extracellular electrolyte concentrations. Technically speaking, the development of energy or electrical potential is dependent upon the dissipation or restitution of the ionic gradient across the cell membrane. The electrical potentials created by this charge can be measured on the EKG.

When the cells are electrically stimulated, the cells depolarize and contract. The cell membrane which is usually only slightly permeable to sodium (Na^+), allows Na^+ ions to rush into the cell while potassium (K^+) moves out of the cell.

This shift in electrolyte concentrations reverses the charge of the cell membrane and is known as **depolarization**.

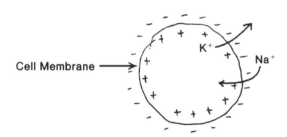

Once depolarization occurs, the cell activity transports Na^+ back to the cell membrane surface, and pumps K^+ back into the cell.

That brings us back to where we started. This returning to the resting state is called **repolarization**.

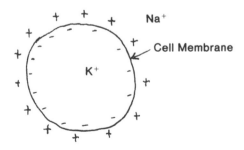

It is this process of **depolarization** and **repolarization** of the myocardial cells that produces the various wave forms observed on the EKG or cardiac monitor. The EKG or monitoring unit *measures and displays (or records) electrical potential . . . it tells one nothing about muscle contraction.*

It is well worth remembering that electrical depolarization occurs *before* cardiac muscle contraction . . . and that electrical repolarization *follows* cardiac muscle contraction!

Rather than tackling the history of electrical potential measurement, we will just accept the fact that the standard EKG machine has the capability of measuring electrical potential using a 12 lead system.

If you think of leads as simply providing different views or angles from which to view the heart's electrical activity, the subject is less confounding.

The standard 12 lead EKG system has 5 electrodes. One electrode is placed on each extremity, while the 5th electrode is used as a **floating electrode** . . . or used for recordings from 6 locations on the chest wall.

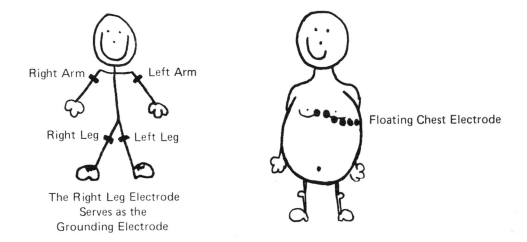

Right Arm   Left Arm

Right Leg   Left Leg

The Right Leg Electrode
Serves as the
Grounding Electrode

Floating Chest Electrode

There are actually three different types of leads . . . **standard limb leads**, **augmented leads**, and **precordial** or **chest leads**. Each lead is made up of a negative ⊖ and a positive ⊕ electrode. These electrodes sense both the magnitude and the direction of the electrical forces and record surface information from the heart borders. Because that sounds a bit confusing, each type of lead will be discussed separately. Whew!

First, however, there are a few critical points to consider. Though these points will be discussed later in the text, they will assist you in understanding the EKG presentations associated with the various leads.

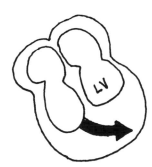

First, the major (net) direction of ventricular electrical activation is leftward (moving right to left), through the free wall of the left ventricle (LV) as noted by the arrow in the above diagram.

Secondly, ventricular depolarization or activation is recorded on the EKG as a QRS complex. QRS complexes are either positive (upright) or negative (directed downward) depending upon the placement of the electrodes and the movement of the depolarization force toward, or away from, those electrodes. Study the diagram at the top of the next page.

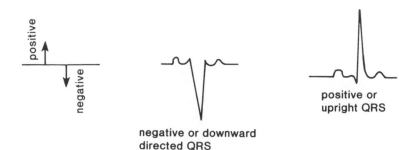

positive / negative

negative or downward directed QRS

positive or upright QRS

The QRS (usually the most easily identified wave formation) represents ventricular depolarization or activation. When the major (net) direction of ventricular depolarization spreads through the left ventricular (LV) muscle moving toward a positive ⊕ electrode, the QRS deflection on the EKG will appear upright or positive.

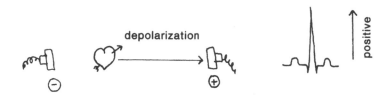

depolarization

⊖ ⊕

positive

When the major (net) direction of ventricular depolarization spreads through the LV heart muscle moving *away from* a positive ⊕ electrode or *toward* a negative ⊖ electrode, the QRS deflection will appear negative or directed downward.

depolarization

⊕ ⊖

negative

Sounds *fairly simple* . . . right?!

As we move forward, you will notice that various electrodes change their *polarity* . . . in other words, sometimes a given electrode is positive ⊕, and sometimes that same electrode is negative ⊖. ***Not to worry!*** The EKG recording machine is programmed to change the polarity when the various lead channels are selected ***Whew!***

Now . . . more about the 12 leads. . . .

The Standard Limb Leads

The **standard limb leads** are leads I, II, and III and they record frontal plane activity. These leads are *bipolar leads* . . . which means that each of these leads has two electrodes which record the electrical potential of the heart flowing toward two extremities. In other words, each lead records the difference of electrical potential between two selected electrode sites.

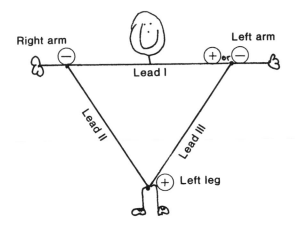

Leads I, II, and III are all electrically equidistant from the myocardial activity. The right arm is always the negative ⊖ pole, while the left leg is always the positive ⊕ pole. The left arm electrode is positive ⊕ in Lead I and negative ⊖ in Lead III.

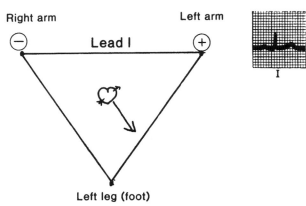

Lead I records the difference of potential between the left arm and the right arm. Specifically, in Lead I, the positive electrode is on the left arm and the negative electrode is on the right arm. The important thing to observe is that the direction of depolarization (see arrow) moves more generally toward the positive ⊕ electrode. Thus, the QRS (which represents ventricular depolarization) is predominantly positive or upright in Lead I.

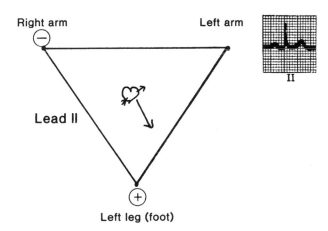

Lead II records the difference of potential between the left leg and the right arm. In Lead II, the left leg electrode is positive and the right arm electrode is negative. Notice the direction of depolarization (see arrow) moves generally toward the positive ⊕ electrode. Therefore, the QRS in Lead II is positive or upright.

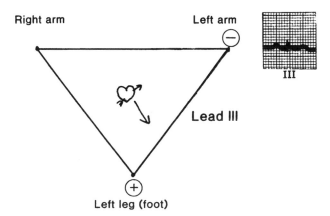

Lead III records the difference of potential between the left leg and the left arm. In Lead III, the left leg electrode is positive and the left arm electrode becomes negative. Once again, you will see that the direction of depolarization (see arrow) moves between the positive ⊕ and the negative ⊖ electrodes. Thus, we can expect that the QRS in Lead III will appear partly positive and partly negative. *Neat, huh!*

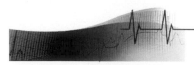

The Augmented Leads

The **augmented leads**, leads aVR, aVL, and aVF are designed to increase the amplitude of the deflections by 50% over those recorded by the standard limb leads. The augmented leads are unipolar in nature (one electrode on the body) and record electrical potential from both the right and left arms and the left leg.

P.S. aVR stands for augmented voltage right arm
aVL stands for augmented voltage left arm
aVF stands for augmented voltage foot

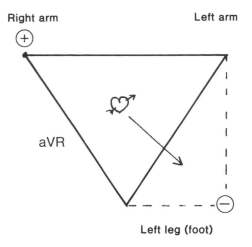

Lead aVR faces the heart from the right shoulder and is oriented to the cavity of the heart. In lead aVR, the right arm electrode extends in an imaginary direction between the left arm and left leg electrodes. The *important* thing to notice is that the direction of depolarization (see arrow) moves toward the negative ⊖ electrode. Thus, the QRS is directed negatively in lead aVR.

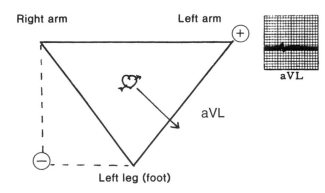

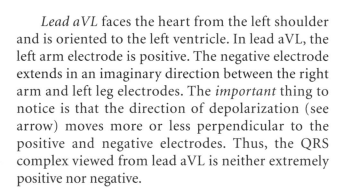

Lead aVL faces the heart from the left shoulder and is oriented to the left ventricle. In lead aVL, the left arm electrode is positive. The negative electrode extends in an imaginary direction between the right arm and left leg electrodes. The *important* thing to notice is that the direction of depolarization (see arrow) moves more or less perpendicular to the positive and negative electrodes. Thus, the QRS complex viewed from lead aVL is neither extremely positive nor negative.

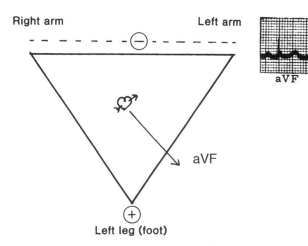

Lead aVF faces the heart from the hip and is oriented to the inferior surface of the left ventricle. In lead aVF, the left leg electrode is positive. The negative electrode extends in an imaginary direction between the right arm and left arm electrodes. The *important* point to notice here is that the direction of depolarization (see arrow) moves principally toward the positive ⊕ electrode. Thus, the QRS complex viewed from lead aVF is positive.

The Precordial Leads

There are six **chest** or **precordial leads** that are identified as V_1, V_2, V_3, V_4, V_5, and V_6. The V leads record electrical potential in the *horizontal plane* and provide six views of the heart's activity! There is a single, floating positive electrode which is moved to all six positions on the chest wall.

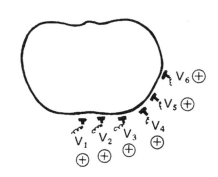

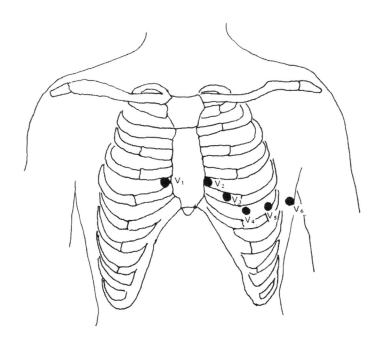

Lead V_1 is located over the 4th intercostal space to the right of the sternal border.
Lead V_2 is located over the 4th intercostal space to the left of the sternal border.
Lead V_3 is located between V_2 and V_4.
Lead V_4 is located at the 5th intercostal space on the mid-clavicular line.
Lead V_5 is located at the 5th intercostal space on the anterior axillary line.
Lead V_6 is located at the 5th intercostal space on the midaxillary line.

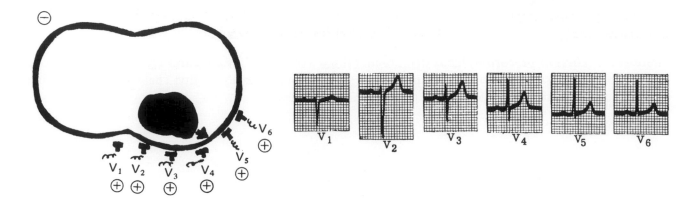

You are probably wondering where the negative electrodes are if the V leads are all positive! (You will remember that each lead is made up of both a positive ⊕ and a negative ⊖ electrode . . . remember? Well, in the precordial leads (V leads), the negative electrode extends backwards or posteriorly toward an imaginary point created by the limb leads.

Normally the *major* (net) direction of ventricular depolarization moves from *right to left* (see arrow above). Thus, the QRS deflections in the right precordial leads (V_1 and V_2) are mostly negative (the wave of depolarization is moving away from the positive chest electrode). As the positive ⊕ chest electrode is moved further left, the QRS deflections become positive (the wave of depolarization is moving toward the positive electrodes).

Now that you are no doubt **thoroughly** perplexed, let me reinforce the important points to remember about leads. . . .

When the major (net) direction of depolarization (electrical activity) spreads through the heart muscle toward a positive pole (electrode), the QRS deflection on the EKG will appear upright or positive.

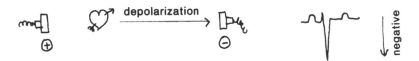

When the major (net) direction of depolarization (electrical activity) spreads through the heart muscle moving away from a positive pole (electrode) or toward a negative pole (electrode), the deflections will be inverted or negative.

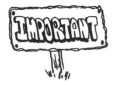

In the absence of electrical activity, there will be no wave forms to record.

Electrical inactivity or electrical silence is recorded as a straight line called an **isoelectric line**. So here's an isoelectric line ――――――― representing electrical silence.

If you think all this is confusing, you're right! It also means that you're progressing in a normal fashion. **Honest!** "LEADing into Section 1" is *purely* introductory! The content will be reviewed later in the text.

Whew!

Probably the *most* important thing to remember is that the 12 EKG leads allow one to look at the various surfaces of the left ventricle . . . or simply look at the electrical activity from different views or angles.

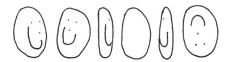

Since the left ventricle (***the pump***) is the most important heart chamber, recording leads are designed to capture electrical activity on the various left ventricular surfaces.

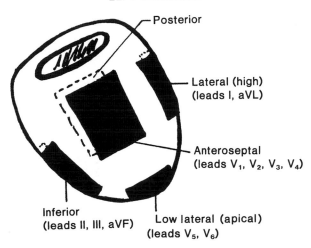

Leads I and aVL view the lateral surface of the left ventricle (high lateral).

Leads II, III, and aVF view the inferior surface of the left ventricle.

Leads V_1, V_2, V_3, and V_4 view the anteroseptal surface of the left ventricle.

Leads V_5 and V_6 view the low lateral or apical surface of the left ventricle.

There are no leads that directly view the posterior region of the left ventricle.

So, with the introduction now *under your belt,* you can proceed on to Section 1.

P.S. If the content is not securely under your belt, don't worry! "LEADing into Section 1" comes at the beginning of the text because history and tradition so dictates! It makes much more sense when you reread this section later in the text. So progress ahead without a care!

Bedside Monitoring

Besides monitoring systems provide for the ongoing observation of cardiac rhythms. It is important to recognize that monitoring technology is ever expanding. Wireless EKG monitoring is now available using Bluetooth technology. This technology provides for continuous monitoring without antennas, thus allowing both patients and staff greater degrees of freedom! 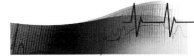 The wireless system, made up of disposable cables and a small transceiver, communicates via radio waves to a transceiver attached to the monitoring system. Most hospitals employ traditional five lead monitoring systems.

5 Lead Monitoring Systems

Most beside monitoring systems utilize a five lead arrangement which allows for the monitoring of all leads within the capability of the system. In a five lead system, four electrodes are placed in stationary positions as indicated in the diagram at the top of page 10. The fifth electrode (labeled Ⓥ) can be placed in any of the $V_1 - V_6$ positions as shown on page 7. (To monitor on a specific V lead, the V electrode will need to be moved to that position.)

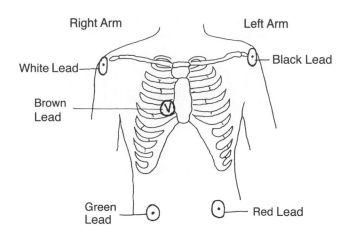

The Ⓥ lead electrode has been placed in the V_1 position.
The Ⓥ lead electrode can be repositioned to any of the precordial lead positions (V_1–V_6).

You will notice the WHITE lead attaches to the electrode positioned on the upper outer part of the right arm; the BLACK lead attaches to the electrode located in the same position on the upper outer left arm; the GREEN lead attaches to the electrode positioned on the right hip, just outside the nipple line; the red lead attaches to the electrode placed in that same position on the left hip. (**Electrode placement at points where the limbs attach to the torso assists in eliminating motion artifact and keeps the field (chest area) clear in the event that emergency procedures are necessary.**)

Expert *lead clinicians* remember correct lead placement locations by the following.

> **White on right,**
>
> **Black (smoke) over fire (Red). . . .**

. . . then all one has to remember is that the GREEN lead attaches to the electrode placed opposite the RED lead, and the Brown lead connects to the chest (precordial) electrode!

The five lead system allows one to select (using the lead selector) the preferred lead(s) to be monitored. Most five lead monitoring systems allow two leads to be simultaneously monitored.

3 Lead Monitoring Systems

Some health care institutions utilize a three lead bedside monitoring system. A three lead monitoring system is made up of a positive ⊕ electrode, a negative ⊖ electrode, and a ground Ⓖ electrode. Depending on how these three electrodes are positioned on the chest surface, the resulting monitor picture will closely resemble the standard, bipolar limb leads I, II and III.

A three lead monitoring system has lesser capabilities than a five lead system, requiring the electrodes to be repositioned in order to monitor the specific limb leads. Using a three lead system, it is not possible to obtain true V (or chest) leads; instead, the electrodes can be repositioned to obtain Modified Chest Lead (MCL) positions. A three lead system affords a single channel for EKG monitoring (only one EKG lead can be viewed on the monitor).

The following diagrams demonstrate electrode placement for obtaining leads I, II, and III and MCL_1 and MCL_6, modified chest leads.

LEAD I

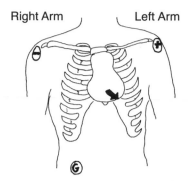

In the bedside version of lead I, the general (net) direction of ventricular depolarization (see arrow) is moving more toward the positive ⊕ electrode. Thus, the QRS in lead I will be positively deflected or directed.

Notice that the left arm electrode is positive ⊕; the right arm electrode is negative ⊖; the right leg (name, not location) electrode serves as the ground.

LEAD II

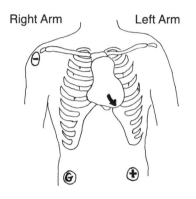

In the bedside version of lead II, the net direction of ventricular depolarization (see arrow) is moving toward the positive ⊕ electrode. Thus, the QRS in lead II is positively deflected or directed.

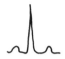

Notice that the left leg (name, not location) electrode is positive ⊕; the right arm electrode is negative ⊖; the right leg (name, not location) electrode serves as the ground.

LEAD III

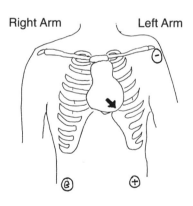

In the bedside version of lead III, the net direction of ventricular depolarization (see arrow) flows between the positive ⊕ and negative ⊖ electrodes. Thus, the QRS observed in lead III is partly positive and partly negative.

Observe that the left leg electrode (name, not location) is positive ⊕; the left arm electrode is negative ⊖; the right leg (name, not location) serves as the ground.

It is also possible to arrange the three bedside monitoring electrodes to mimic certain precordial leads, specifically leads V_1 and V_6. However, since the precordial leads are unipolar in nature (using a positive electrode on the chest wall with an imaginary negative electrode), and our bedside monitoring system is bipolar, certain modifications must be made. Thus, these leads are referred to as **modified chest leads (MCL)**!

Modified Chest Leads

As will be discussed later in the text, certain rhythm abnormalities are best viewed from leads approximating right (V_1) or left (V_6) precordial leads. By adjusting the bedside monitoring lead placement, one can achieve modified versions of these two leads.

<table>
<tr><td>Lead MCL₁ (modified V₁)</td><td>Lead MCL₆ (modified V₆)</td></tr>
</table>

Lead MCL$_1$ (modified V$_1$)   **Lead MCL$_6$** (modified V$_6$)

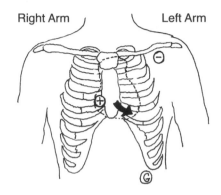 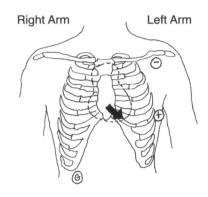

The positive ⊕ electrode is positioned as V_1 at the 4th intercostal space to the right of the sternum. The negative ⊖ electrode is placed on the left arm. The ground electrode can be placed anywhere.

Remember . . . V_1 is a right chest lead . . . so, MCL$_1$ is a modified right chest lead.

Because the net direction of ventricular depolarization (see arrow) moves between the positive ⊕ and negative ⊖ electrodes, the QRS in lead MCL$_1$ will be partly positive and partly negative.

The positive ⊕ electrode is positioned as V_6 at the 5th intercostal space on the left mid-axillary line.

The negative electrode ⊖ is placed on the left arm. The ground electrode can be placed anywhere.

Remember . . . V_6 is a left chest lead . . . so, MCL$_6$ is a modified left chest lead.

You will notice that the net direction of ventricular depolarization (see arrow) moves toward the positive ⊕ electrode. Thus, the QRS observed in lead MCL$_6$ will be positive or upright.

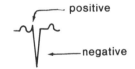 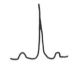

In both of the above modified systems (MCL$_1$ and MCL$_6$), the left arm electrode is the negative ⊖ electrode. The positive electrode is placed in the appropriate V lead position. If you need review, please turn back to page 7.

> **NOTE:** MCL stands for "modified chest—left arm" lead.

Let me **reassure** you once again! If you are uncertain or confused, please understand that this is a **normal** state. It will all begin to fall into place as we move along. **Trust me!** And, be assured that manufacturers of monitoring equipment include diagrams for lead placement.

Notes

Notes

The Conduction System and Related Matters

Objectives

When you have completed Section 1, you will be able to describe, identify or calculate

1. normal electric impulse transmission across the myocardium
2. P, Q, R, S, T intervals
3. heart rate
4. paper time
5. sinus rhythm
6. the conduction system
7. a method for interpreting dysrhythmias

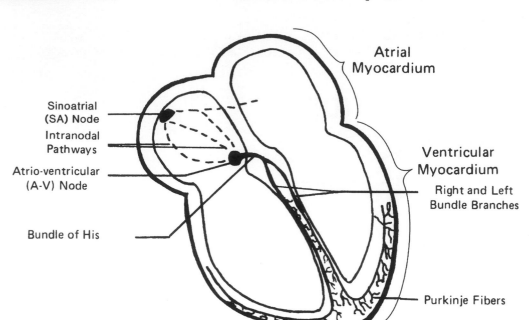

Each normal heart beat is the result of an electrical impulse that originates in the sinoatrial (SA) node. The SA node lies at the junction of the superior vena cava and the right atrium. *The SA node is the normal heart's physiologic pacemaker, initiating impulses at a rate between 60–100 times per minute. From the SA node, the impulse travels across intranodal pathways activating the atria. The activation (or depolarization) of the atria is recorded as a P wave on the EKG. The intranodal pathways connect the SA node and the AV (atrio-ventricular) node. The intranodal pathways are preferential or semi-specialized pathways consisting of concentrations of normal myocardial cells and Purkinje cells. (The tissues between these cells consist mainly of collagen and fat which have high electrical resistance.) The AV node lies on the floor of the right atrium. Conduction through the intranodal pathways is rapid; conduction is then slowed in the AV node itself. The AV node serves only to transmit the impulse. Impulse conduction speeds up as it leaves the AV node passing to the bundle of His. From the bundle of His, the impulse passes rapidly down both the right and left bundle branches to the terminal Purkinje fibers. Ventricular depolarization or activation then occurs, producing the QRS complex on EKG. Following depolarization, the mechanical activity of muscle contraction occurs, producing a pulse. Cellular recovery (repolarization) follows depolarization and is evidenced on the EKG as a T wave. It is during the repolarization phase that the ventricles fill with blood. The next electrical impulse arrives when filling is completed and ventricular depolarization again occurs. *Each cardiac cycle consists of depolarization and recovery (repolarization).*

> ***IMPORTANT NOTE:** The SA node is the normal pacemaker of the heart because it has the *fastest* rate of impulse formation and discharge. The SA impulse reaches slower potential pacemakers and discharges their immature impulses before they have the opportunity to discharge spontaneously. Sounds complicated, right? The important thing to remember is that the *fastest* pacemaker always controls the heart rate . . . just like the *fastest* runner controls the race! It's also helpful to know that the SA node is influenced by both the sympathetic and parasympathetic nervous system . . . thus, the sinus rate of discharge fluctuates with nervous stimulation.

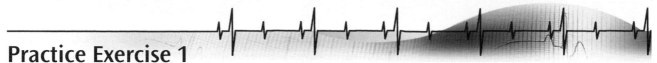

Practice Exercise 1

Now it's your turn.

The electrical impulse normally originates in the sinoatrial node and travels across the heart to initiate myocardial muscle depolarization. Trace and label the parts of the conduction system on this diagram.

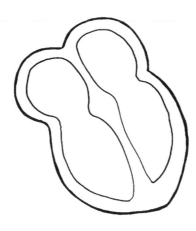

The activation phase of the cardiac cycle is known as _____.

The recovery phase of the cardiac cycle is known as _____.

Normally, the SA (sinoatrial) node fires _____ to _____ times per minute.

 For Feedback 1, refer to page 35.

For Feedback 1, refer to page 35.

input section ## 1.2   The P Wave and P-R Interval

All electrical activity can be recorded. As an electrical impulse travels across the myocardium initiating depolarization, a monitoring device will display various wave forms.

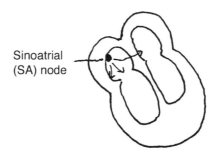

Sinoatrial
(SA) node

Atrial excitation begins in the sinoatrial (SA) node, spreading through specialized conducting pathways to activate the right and left atria. The monitor will display a wave form that usually looks like this.

P

For reasons unknown to me, this is called a P wave! Owing to the direction of electrical activation, P waves are *normally upright* in leads I, II, aVF, and V_3–V_6. P waves are normally inverted in leads aVR and may be inverted in leads V_1 and V_2. P waves may be upright, flat, biphasic, or inverted in leads III and aVL.

The P wave represents depolarization of both the right and left atria. Remember, muscle contraction follows electrical depolarization.

So, whenever a P wave is observed, the "monitor observer" will know that depolarization of the atria has occurred.

Since the impulse originates in the sinoatrial node and since the SA node is the heart's natural pacemaker, the P wave should be the *first* wave form one sees in each cardiac cycle.

$$\text{Atrial Depolarization} = \quad \overset{\text{P}}{\underline{\quad\frown\quad}}$$

We now have a P wave, telling the monitor observer that atrial depolarization has occurred. Not unlike other muscles, after activation there must be a rest or recovery (repolarization) period. And, just as you might suspect, during this rest period no work is done. No work presents on the monitor as a straight line known as the P-R segment.

Atrial depolarization (the P wave) is followed by a straight line (the P-R segment) which represents both atrial recovery time and transmission of the impulse through the AV junction, to the ventricles. Taken together, the P wave and the P-R segment, make up the P-R interval. The P-R interval (the combined P wave and straight line) thus represents atrial activation and recovery and, the further conduction of the impulse through the AV node. The P-R interval begins at the initial P wave deflection and terminates at the beginning of the QRS.

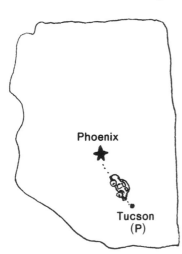

Phoenix ★

Tucson
(P)

A number of factors influence the P-R interval. Though they will be discussed in a later section, for now, a simple analogy will be used. Suppose that I live and work in Tucson, but must also drive to Phoenix because I have a second job there. My work in Tucson corresponds to atrial work, so I'll call my Tucson work "P." Then, I jump in my VW and drive to Phoenix. The time it takes me to both do my work in Tucson and then drive to Phoenix could be called my Tucson-Phoenix interval. This corresponds to the "P-R interval" which is the time it takes for the sinus impulse to activate (do work in) the atria, for the atria to recover, and for the impulse to travel through the A-V node.

Using this analogy further, it's easy to understand that my Tucson-Phoenix interval could vary depending on how fast I work, how fast I drive—or, if there is highway construction. Similarly, the P-R interval could vary depending on the rate of impulse conduction or pathway obstruction.

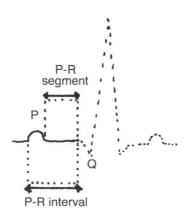

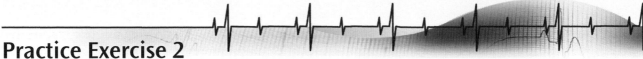

Practice Exercise 2

Let's review!

A. Atrial excitation (in the healthy heart) begins in the _____ .

B. As this impulse spreads across the atria, atrial muscle contraction follows atrial _____

_____ .

C. The monitor picture associated with atrial depolarization is the _____ wave.

D. Okay, now draw a P wave.

E. In the healthy heart, the _____ will note the beginning of each cardiac cycle.

F. The P-R interval looks like this: (draw one 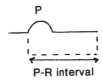)

G. The P-R interval represents the time it takes the impulse to depolarize the atria and travel from the atria,

through the _____ to the ventricles.

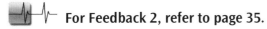 **For Feedback 2, refer to page 35.**

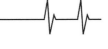 **input section 1.3 The QRS Complex**

So, now what??
    So far, our EKG complex looks like this.

P

P-R interval

The sinoatrial-generated impulse has traveled to the ventricles.

The next major event in the cardiac cycle is ventricular depolarization (the traveling impulse reaches and activates the ventricles). Ventricular depolarization is identified on the monitor as a QRS complex, a Q wave, an R wave and an S wave. The QRS complex is predominantly upright in leads, I, II, III, aVL, aVF, V_4, V_5, and V_6. (Refer back to pages 5, 6, and 7.)

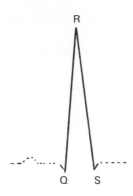

These waves (QRS) represent depolarization of the ventricular muscle. When present, the first downward (negative) deflection is the Q wave. Not all QRS complexes have a Q wave. Some begin with an R wave.

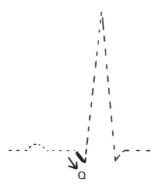

The R wave is the first upward (positive) wave or deflection following the P wave . . .

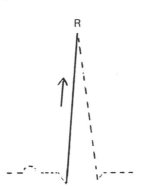

. . . and, if a negative deflection (below the baseline) follows an R wave, it is labeled an S wave.

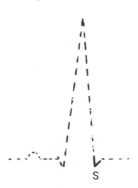

Now, the complete picture looks like this.

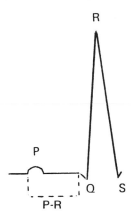

The P waves tells us the atria have depolarized. The P-R interval represents the time it takes for atrial depolarization and for the SA impulse to travel from the SA node through the atria and through the AV junction. And voila! When the traveling impulse reaches the Purkinje fibers, ventricular depolarization occurs—shown on the monitor as the QRS. Ventricular muscle contraction normally follows electrical depolarization.

Depending upon which EKG lead one is examining, one may not observe an actual Q wave. In other words, the QRS may look like this. There is no observable Q wave (initial negative deflection). Technically speaking, this is an "RS" wave . . .

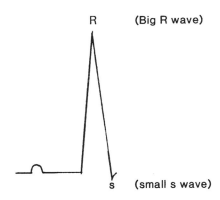

. . . but it is referenced as a QRS complex.

Likewise, in predominantly negatively deflected leads—V_1, V_2, and V_3—the QRS will appear different owing to the placement of the electrode, the proximity to the heart muscle and the direction of the depolarization wave. (Refer back to p. 8.)

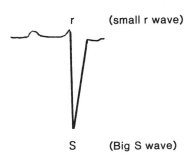

Though the above complex is also referred to as a QRS complex, technically there is only a small R and a large S wave! An R wave is the first upward deflection, and an S wave is a negative-downward deflection that follows, regardless of wave size.

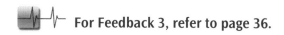

Practice Exercise 3

A. Draw and label the waves representing ventricular activation or depolarization.

B. Ventricular depolarization begins when the SA initiated impulse reaches _____

_____ .

For Feedback 3, refer to page 36.

For Feedback 3, refer to page 36.

input section   **1.4   The ST Segment, the T Wave and U wave . . . (followed by a word about the QT interval and QRS interval and QRS-ST segment)**

Only a few more *minor* details. Following ventricular activation (depolarization), there must be a period of rest or recovery (repolarization).

Simple physiology—cells work—they get tired—they rest! So, the remaining portions of a normal EKG cycle appear as illustrated below.

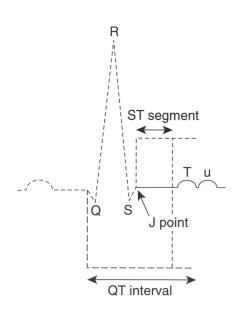

The ST segment (straight line between the S wave and T wave) represents an early phase of ventricular muscle recovery. During this time, the ventricular cells are in a state of "inaction" (refractory state), unresponsive to any further electrical stimulation. The ST segment begins at the J point (junction of the end of the QRS with the beginning of the ST segment) and ends at the beginning of the T wave.

The T wave is the recovery phase (repolarization) following ventricular activation (depolarization). The top (apex) of the T wave is the earliest time the ventricles can respond to another electrical stimulus.

Various pathologies and conditions producing changes in the ST segment and T wave will be studied in later Sections. Whew!!

Occasionally, a U wave may be visible following the T wave. If visible, the U wave is smaller than the T wave, though oriented in the same direction. The U wave is thought to represent repolarization of the Purkinje fibers.

The QT interval represents the total time for ventricular depolarization and repolarization. It further represents the absolute refractory period. The QT interval is measured from the intiation point of the QRS to the termination point of the T wave. The QT interval should measure no greater than ½ of the R-R interval (the distance between two R waves). The QT interval is also discussed on pages 124, 264, and 305.

Let's do the whole thing—an entire EKG cycle! When I see this complex on the monitor, I can now intellectually describe the whole physiologic process.

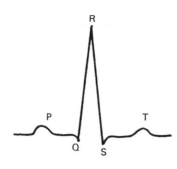

Ready? Okay . . . . "My good man/woman, EKG monitor interpretation is based on simple application of a basic physiologic principle. Ion shift at the myocardial cell membrane level allows one to record electrical potential via specially designed electrodes. Atrial excitation begins at the SA node and spreads down the conduction system. The initially recorded wave, the P wave, represents depolarization of the atria. The straight line following the P wave represents time for atrial repolarization and impulse conduction to the ventricles. The QRS complex represents ventricular depolarization. Following ventricular depolarization is the repolarization phase evidenced by the ST segment and T wave!"

> **REMEMBER**, the EKG is simply a representation of the electrical events occurring within the myocardium!

Sounds fairly intellectual, right?!

Practice Exercise 4

A. Label each wave.

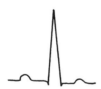

P.S. If you are unsure, look at the top of the page!

B. Atrial excitation begins in the _____.

C. The P wave represents _____.

D. The P-R interval represents _____

_____

_____.

E. The QRS represents _____.

The Q wave is the first _____ deflection.

The R wave is the first _____ deflection.

The S wave is the _____ deflection following the R wave.

F. The ST segment represents _____.

G. The T wave represents _____.

H. The PQRST complex ⎍ represents one _____.

⎍ **For Feedback 4, refer to page 36.**

input section 1.5 Paper Time

Now that the PQRST cycle has been more or less exhausted, we need to think about EKG paper—henceforth, this will be referred to as "paper time." In order for this whole process to make good sense, some convention of measure must be applied. EKG recording paper is run at a standard speed of 25 mm. per second to standardize the measurement of the various electrical events. EKG paper is subdivided both horizontally and vertically with 1 mm. and 5 mm. (dark lines) spaced lines. The vertical lines represent time intervals, much like a clock! 🕐

So, moving horizontally across the EKG paper denotes *time*. One must understand the concept of paper time in order to calculate heart rate from the EKG paper.

In the following illustration, notice the three second marker intervals at the top of the EKG paper. Every three seconds this mark will appear. The distance between three of these markers is 6 seconds.

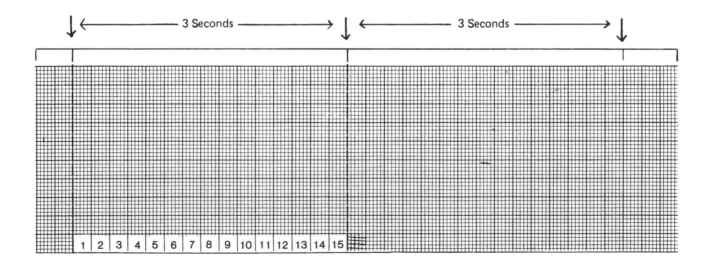

Each larger square represents *0.20 seconds*. That makes sense if one counts the number of large squares between each three second marker. (See bottom illustration page 24.)

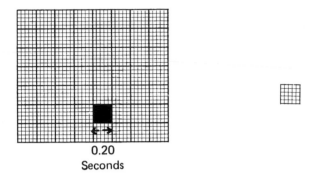

0.20
Seconds

There are 15 large squares between each three second marker (15 × 0.2 seconds each = 3.0 seconds).

Now look at one of the smallest squares. Each small square represents 0.04 seconds.

Again, that makes sense if one counts the number of small squares moving across one big square. There are five small squares (5 × 0.04 seconds = 0.2 seconds or one large square).

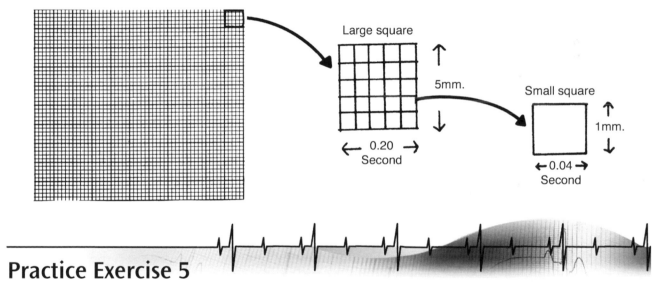

Practice Exercise 5

Paper time is actually quite easy . . . if you practice!
    Before looking back, complete the following statements.

A. Moving horizontally across EKG paper denotes _____.

B. Every _____ seconds I will see a time marker on the EKG paper.

C. The amount of time between three of these time markers is _____ seconds.

D. Each large square represents _____ seconds.

E. I understand that there are 15 large squares between two _____ second markers.

    Therefore, _____ seconds lapse between those markers (15 × 0.20 seconds =   ).

F. The smallest square on the EKG paper represents _____ seconds.

G. There are _____ small squares (in one row) within a large square.

H. There are _____ large squares in a six second time interval.

I. Three small squares represent _____ seconds.

J. Four small squares represents _____ seconds.

K. Five small squares represent _____ seconds, which is the same as _____ large square(s).

L. How much time is represented by five big squares?_____.

M. How much time is represented by 13 big squares?_____.

   . . . If you can answer question N without looking back, you have a sound understanding of paper time.

N. How much time has elapsed when there are five big squares and three small squares?

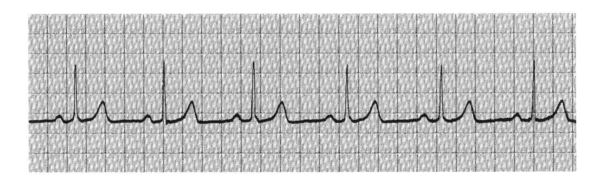

_____

For Feedback 5, refer to page 37.

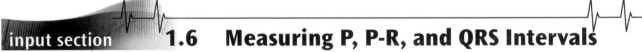

input section   **1.6   Measuring P, P-R, and QRS Intervals**

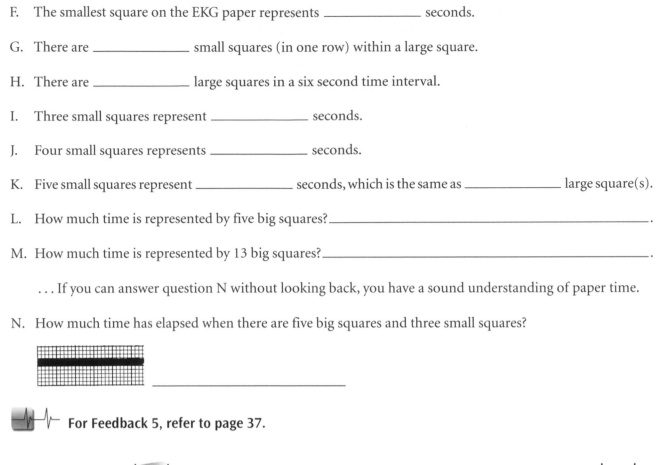

Although we will not go into great detail, it is important to think about *atrial activation*. You will remember that the P wave represents atrial depolarization (depolarization of both the left and right atria).

   The *normal* P wave does not exceed 0.12 seconds in duration (no more than three small squares) or more than 2.5 mm. in height. Any increase in duration or amplitude suggests *atrial hypertrophy*. Though it is not always possible to distinguish right from left atrial hypertrophy on an EKG, one can make several generalizations. Basically, atrial hypertrophy represents an enlargement of one or both of the atrial chambers due to excessive strain or workload.

With left atrial hypertrophy (often seen in mitral stenosis), one may observe a wide, notched P wave called *P mitrale,* best seen in leads I and II. Following is an example of left atrial hypertrophy.

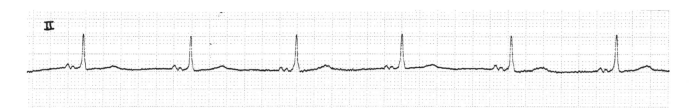

Right atrial hypertrophy is most commonly associated with chronic pulmonary disease. P waves associated with right atrial hypertrophy are usually tall (greater than 2.5 mm. in height) and *peaked* in leads II, III, and AVF.

Though the duration and amplitude of P waves is interesting, I do not expect you to commit this to memory . . . however, you should be aware that abnormalities may occur in the P wave itself! *Whew!*

Remember the P-R interval? The P-R interval represents the time required for atrial activation, atrial recovery and impulse transmission through the AV node and across the bundle of His.

In a healthy adult heart, the impulse will travel from the sinus node to the Purkinje system in 0.12 to 0.20 seconds.

To be within normal limits then, the P-R interval must measure 3–5 small squares in width or between 0.12 and 0.20 seconds in duration.

Look at the following EKG strip. The P-R interval is almost 4 small squares wide. The P-R interval is measured from the beginning of the P wave to the beginning of the Q wave . . . or if there is no Q wave, to the beginning of the upward R wave. (For assistance with measurement, see the diagrams at the top of page 28.)

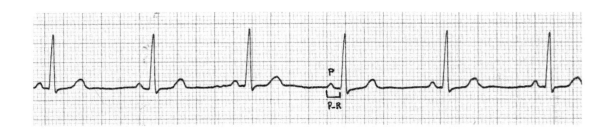

The P-R interval in the above strip is *almost* 0.16 seconds in duration (.04 × 4 = 0.16 seconds).

That means the P-R interval is within normal limits. In other words, the impulse is traveling through the conduction system at a healthy speed.

As a contrast, examine this next strip. Here the P-R interval measures 0.24 seconds (6 × .04 = 0.24) indicating a *delay* in impulse conduction or a *conduction defect.*

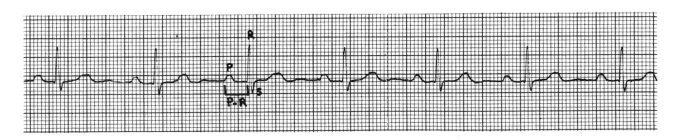

And, as you might guess, an abnormally short P-R interval represents accelerated impulse conduction. For now, we are only concerned with the accurate measurement of the P-R interval. Pathology will be discussed later in the text.

Correctly Measuring the P-R Interval and QRS Interval

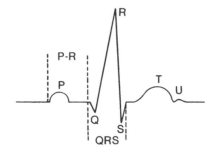

The P-R interval is measured from the beginning of the P wave to the beginning of the QRS . . . in this instance, to the beginning of the Q wave.

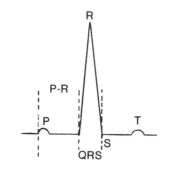

In this example, the P-R interval measurement is taken from the beginning of the P wave to the beginning of the R wave (the beginning of the R wave upstroke).

Remember, *to be within normal limits the P-R interval must measure 3–5 small squares in width, or 0.12 to 0.20 seconds in duration.*

We will be concerned with one other major paper time measurement. The QRS, you will recall, represents ventricular depolarization. Unless a conduction defect is present (abnormal, slow conduction), the QRS will measure *less* than 3 small squares wide, or less than 0.12 seconds in duration. The QRS is measured from the beginning of the Q wave to the end of the S wave. If a Q wave is not present, measure the distance between the R and S waves. Please refer to the above diagrams.

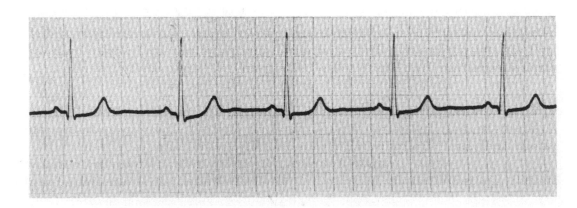

In the above rhythm strip, the QRS measures *approximately 0.10 seconds* or 2½ small squares. Therefore, ventricular depolarization occurs within the expected period of time (*less than 0.12 seconds or less than 3 small squares*).

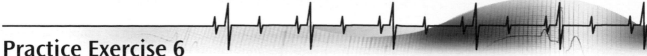

Practice Exercise 6

A. To be within normal limits, the P-R interval must measure _____ to _____ small

squares in width or _____ to _____ seconds in duration.

B. P-R interval less than _____ small squares in width or greater than _____ small
squares in width represents an abnormality in the impulse conduction.

C. Evaluate the boxed cardiac cycle below. The P-R measures _____ small squares or

_____ seconds.

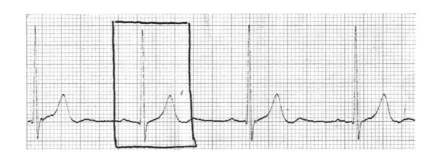

D. The QRS waveform represents _____ _____.

E. To be within normal limits, the QRS must measure _____ _____ small squares less

than _____ seconds in duration.

F. The QRS in the above boxed cardiac cycle measures _____ small squares which

is _____ seconds.

For Feedback 6, refer to page 38.

input section 1.7 Calculating Heart Rate

Now, let's try some fun things with heart rate!

There are several methods for calculating heart rate from a cardiac monitor strip.

> **NOTE:** When in doubt about any heart rate, take the patient's pulse . . . and remember, an apical
> pulse is usually the most accurate.

When we are dealing with a *regular* rhythm, the process of calculating heart rate can be simplified. Every three seconds a marker appears on the top of the EKG paper. *Count the number of QRS complexes or cardiac cycles in a six second time interval. Multiply that number by 10* to find the number of complexes in one minute. That number is the approximate heart rate.

Figure the heart rate in the following EKG strip. Note the circled three second markers.

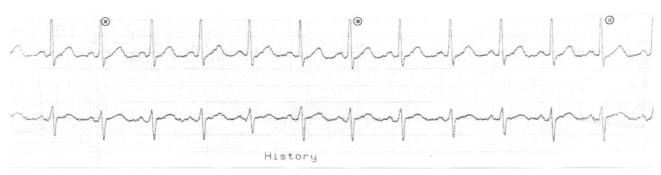

History

In the previous strip there are 7 complexes within a six second time interval.

Therefore, 7 × 10 equals 70.

This patient's heart rate is approximately 70 beats/minute.

Another way to calculate heart rate is the "rule of 1500." To use this rule, identify two consecutive QRS complexes. Count the number of small boxes between the two QRS complexes. Divide the number of boxes into 1500 to determine heart rate.

Now using the strip above, the same one you used to determine an approximate rate of 70, count the number of boxes between the third and fourth QRSs. I count 22 boxes. Divide 22 into 1500 and you will determine a heart rate of 68.

As you can see, both methods yield similar rates. These are estimated rates because you are not looking at a full minute of rhythm.

> **REMEMBER:** This method should *only* be used when the rhythm is **REGULAR** and it is an estimate of heart rate.

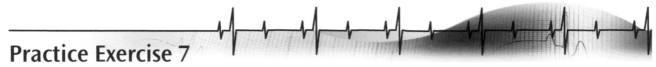

Practice Exercise 7

Now try some practice! Figure the heart rate on each of the following EKG strips. Do not look back until you have completed the exercise.

A. Reference the strip below then decide if the rhythm is regular. Imagine all the tall upright waves (R waves) are sticks lying in a row.

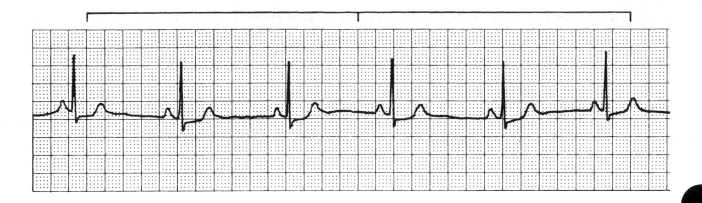

Each marker at the top of the EKG paper represents _____ seconds.

There are _____ complexes in the six second time interval displayed. Therefore, _____ × 10

equals _____. The approximate heart rate is _____ beats/minute.

Using the rule of 1500, the heart rate is approximately _____ beats/minute.

B. Using the same methods, calculate the heart rate in the following strip. First count the number of small boxes between the fourth and fifth QRSs.

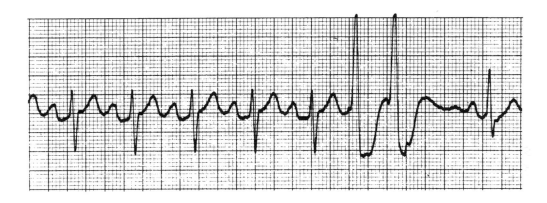

The heart rate is _____

Now count the number of small boxes between the sixth and seventh funny looking QRSs. These beats are PVCs and will be discussed in Section 4.

The heart rate of the two PVCs is _____

 For Feedback 7, refer to page 39.

A Brief Review

I forgot to tell you . . . if you get tired, you can interrupt your study at any point. That's why the material is organized in this fashion. You can stop and go as you please. You're almost an expert now anyway!

Following is a brief review summarizing what we have covered thus far!

1. The sinus node is the pacemaker in the normal heart. Thus, the term sinus rhythm implies that the electrical impulse originates in the sinus node.
2. The P wave is the first wave formation in the normal EKG complex. The P wave represents depolarization of the atria. The P waves seen on an EKG strip should all appear identical, and should be equidistant to the attached QRS complexes.
3. The P-R interval of each EKG complex represents the time necessary for the sinoatrial impulse to travel from the sinus node and through the AV junction. In normal conduction, that time should be *0.12–0.20 seconds.* Now, how many small EKG squares is that? Remember, each small square represents 0.04 seconds . . . so, 0.12 seconds equals three small squares, and 0.20 seconds equals five small squares. Thus, a normal P-R interval will measure between *3–5 small squares* in width or 0.12–0.20 seconds in duration.
4. The QRS represents depolarization of the ventricles. Every normal rhythm should have a QRS preceded by a P wave and followed by a T wave . . . all occurring in a regular fashion. The normal QRS should measure *less* than *0.12 seconds,* or less than 3 small EKG squares. (If the QRS is 3 or more small squares in width or duration, it indicates a delay in the conduction system.)
5. The T wave represents the recovery state after ventricular depolarization. The T waves should all be upright and appear identical. The ST segment will be flat, neither elevated nor depressed.
6. A normal heart rate is 60–100 beats per minute. Typically, the sinus node will initiate an impulse 60–100 times per minute, and each time, the impulse will be conducted down through the AV junction, through the bundle of His, down the bundle branches to the Purkinje fibers to initiate ventricular depolarization.

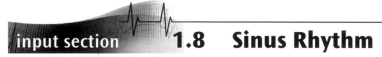

input section   1.8   Sinus Rhythm

Now, let's think about a sinus rhythm or a normal rhythm. This next strip illustrates a sinus rhythm.

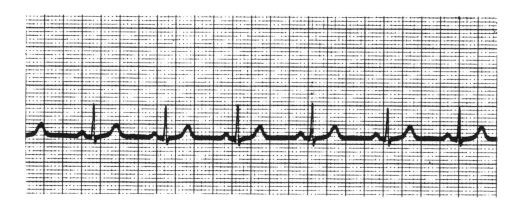

A sinus rhythm will have all of the following identifying features.

Rate:	60 to 100 beats per minute
Rhythm:	Regular
P Waves:	A P wave will precede each QRS complex. All P waves will be uniform in appearance.
QRS:	All QRS complexes will appear uniform in configuration.
Conduction:	Each P wave will be followed by a normal QRS complex.

Sinus rhythm is given its name because it originates in the sinoatrial node. The SA node is the normal pacemaker of the heart because it has the highest inherent rate of discharge or automaticity (60 to 100 times per minute). Though other tissues have pacemaking capability, their inherent rates of impulse-formation are significantly less than the sinus rate. ***Thus, the fastest pacemaker always assumes control of the rhythm!***

Here is another example of sinus rhythm.

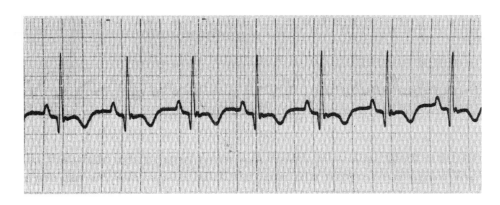

In the above strip, the heart rate is between 75 and 100, but closer to 100 beats per minute. Various pathologies (which will be discussed later in the text) occur even when the rhythm is normal! Notice that the T waves of this strip are inverted as compared to the sinus rhythm example at the top of the page.

Practice Exercise 8

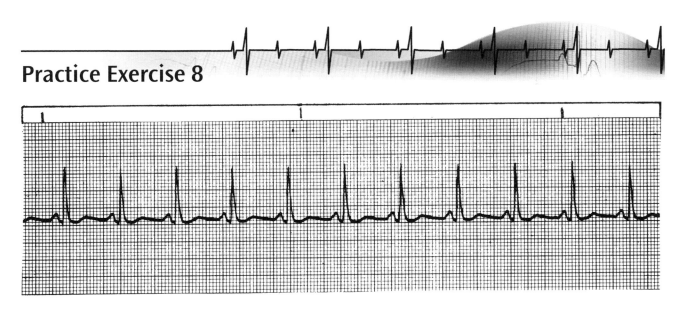

Reference the above rhythm strip when answering these questions.

A. The heart rate in this strip is _____ beats per minute.

B. The rhythm is regular/irregular (circle one).

C. Each QRS complex is *preceded* by a _____ wave.

    Do all the P waves look uniform or alike? _____ yes _____ no (check ✔ one)

D. Is each P wave followed by a normal QRS complex? _____ yes _____ no (check ✔ one)

E. Do all QRS complexes appear uniform? _____ yes _____ no (check ✔ one)

F. VOILA! This is a _____ rhythm!

For Feedback 8, refer to page 40.

Following is some introductory information for Section 2!

In order to accurately interpret dysrhythmias, there are *five* basic steps one must follow. As you become more proficient in EKG interpretation, you may combine, reorder . . . or even think of new steps. However, for now, it will assist you to follow these five steps when analyzing any rhythm!

1. ***First,*** *determine whether the rhythm is regular or irregular.* If the rhythm is irregular, try to determine what makes it irregular. Are there early (premature) beats? Are there pauses? Are abnormal beats present? The simplest method for determining rhythm regularity is to measure the distance between two consecutive R waves (R-R interval) and compare that distance with other R-R intervals in the strip (see below). In a regular rhythm, the R-R intervals will all measure the same.

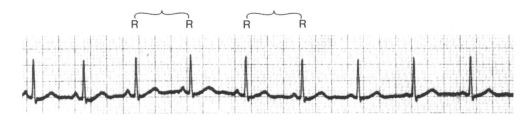

2. ***Second,*** *determine the heart rate.* Remember . . . if the rhythm is irregular, it is necessary to count the rate for one full minute. (In the previous strip, the rate is 90.)
3. ***Third,*** *one must evaluate atrial activity. What atrial activity is evident?* Are there P waves that occur uniformly across the monitor tracing? Are the P waves alike in appearance? If no distinct P waves are present, is there any evidence of atrial activity, or is the baseline preceding the QRS flat? If atrial impulses are present, are they regular or irregular? Is the atrial activity occurring so rapidly that there are more atrial impulses than QRS complexes? If actual atrial wave forms are difficult to identify, does the baseline appear wavy, sawtooth or static-y?
4. ***Fourth,*** *determine ventricular activity. What ventricular activity is evident?* Are the QRSs of normal duration (less than 0.12 seconds)? Do the QRSs occur uniformly across the monitor tracing? Does a QRS follow every P wave or atrial wave deflection? Are all of the QRSs pointing in the same direction?
5. ***Finally,*** it is important to *determine the relationship between atrial and ventricular activity.* Is each P wave producing a QRS, or are there P waves that are not followed by QRS complexes? Is each QRS preceded by a P wave, or is there evidence of independent ventricular activity? Is the P-R interval of all conducted beats constant, does it vary, or is there no established relationship?

The above five steps will be repeatedly followed as various rhythm abnormalities are explored.
The above five steps will be repeatedly followed as various rhythm abnormalities are explored.
The above five steps will be repeatedly followed as various rhythm abnormalities are explored.
The above five steps will be repeatedly followed as various rhythm abnormalities are explored.
The above five steps will be repeatedly followed as various rhythm abnormalities are explored.
The above five steps will be repeatedly followed as various rhythm abnormalities are explored.

REMEMBER: One need not apply a sophisticated name to any rhythm. A simple descriptive analysis (answering the questions in the above five steps) conveys the most accurate information!

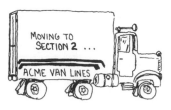

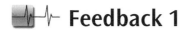 **Feedback 1**

Very good!

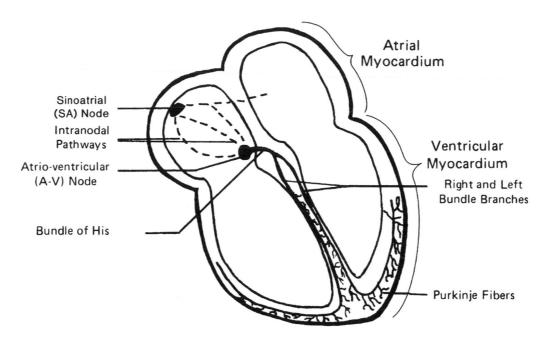

The impulse originates in the sinoatrial (SA) node and travels down the intranodal pathways, activating the atria. The impulse then travels through the AV node, slowing slightly. Impulse conduction speeds up as it leaves the AV node, passing to the bundle of His. From the bundle of His, the impulse travels rapidly down the right and left bundle branches to the Purkinje fibers.

Each cardiac cycle consists of two phases—activation or *depolarization,* and recovery or *repolarization.*

Normally, the SA node fires **60** to **100** times per minute.

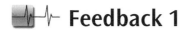 **Feedback 2**

If your answers look like this, you're doing a super job!

A. Atrial excitation (in the healthy heart) begins in the <u>sinoatrial or SA node</u>.

B. As the impulse spreads across the atria, it causes atrial muscle contraction following <u>depolarization</u>.

C. The monitor picture associated with atrial depolarization is the <u>P wave</u>.

D. ⌒ (a "P" wave.)

E. In the healthy heart, the <u>P wave</u> will note the beginning of each new cardiac cycle.

F. (a P-R interval)

G. The P-R interval represents the time it takes for the impulse to depolarize the atria and travel from the atria, through the <u>AV node</u> to the ventricles.

P.S. If your answers varied from these, review the material one more time!

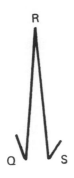 Feedback 3

A. If you have drawn a QRS complex, good for you!

= **Ventricular Depolarization**

B. Ventricular depolarization begins when the SA initiated impulse reaches the ventricles (after traveling through the atria, through the AV junction, through the bundle of His, down the bundle branches to the Purkinje fibers). Ventricular muscle contraction follows electrical depolarization.

Feedback 4

Excellent work! Your answers should be similar to mine.

A.

B. Atrial excitation begins in the SA (sinoatrial) node.

C. The P wave represents atrial depolarization.

D. The P-R interval represents the time for atrial recovery and the time necessary for the impulse to pass from the SA node to the AV node.

E. The QRS represents ventricular depolarization.
The Q wave is the first downward deflection.
The R wave is the first upward deflection.
The S wave is the negative or downward deflection following the R wave.

F. The ST segment represents the early phase of ventricular muscle recovery (repolarization).

G. The T wave represents the recovery phase following ventricular activation (repolarization).

H. The PQRST complex represents one cardiac cycle.

The following summary is included to tie together any loose ends.

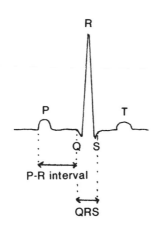

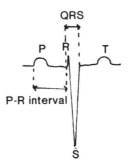

Remember, wave forms may be either positive or negative depending upon which lead one is viewing.

P-Wave—Artial excitation starts at the SA node and spreads through both atria. The P wave represents depolarization of the atria. If P waves are present, and of normal size and shape, it can be assumed that the stimulus began in the SA node.

P-R Interval—The period of atrial repolarization is represented by the P-R interval. It also represents the time for the impulse to pass from the SA node, through the AV junction, through the bundle of His, down the bundle branches to the Purkinje fibers. The normal P-R interval is usually between 0.12–0.20 seconds.

QRS Complex—These waves represent depolarization of the ventricular muscle. The initial *downward* deflection is the Q wave. The R wave is the first positive or *upward* deflection. The S wave is the *downward* wave following the R wave. The normal QRS duration is less than 0.12 seconds.

ST Segement—This segment represents the early phase of repolarization (recovery of the ventricular muscle).

T wave—The recovery phase following ventricular activation.

Note: Electrical depolarization occurs before cardiac muscle contraction . . . and, electrical repolarization follows cardiac muscle contractions.

⎍⎍ Feedback 5

How did you do? Probably excellent, as usual! I hope your answers match mine.

A. <u>time</u>

B. <u>3 seconds</u>

C. <u>6 seconds</u>. That may be confusing, but | 3 | 3 | there are only two 3 second intervals between three markers!

D. <u>0.20 seconds</u>

E. 15 large squares between two <u>3</u> second markers. Therefore, <u>3</u> seconds lapse between these markers (15 squares × 0.20 seconds [per square] = 3.0).

F. 0.04 seconds

G. 5 small squares

H. 30 large squares in a 6 second time interval

I. 0.12 [0.04 seconds (one small square) × 3 small squares = 0.12 seconds]

J. 0.16 [0.04 seconds (one small square) × 4 small squares = 0.16 seconds]

K. 0.20 seconds which is the same as one large square

L. 1.0 second [0.20 seconds (per big square) × 5 big squares = 1.0 second]

M. 2.6 seconds [0.20 seconds (per big square) × 13 big squares = 2.6 seconds]

N. 1.12 seconds. There are two ways to figure this.

   1. You could figure the 5 big squares first
       0.20 seconds per big square × 5 big squares   = 1.0 second

       Then figure the small squares:
       0.04 seconds per small square × 3 small squares   = 0.12 seconds

                                            Total   = 1.12 seconds

                                     or

   2. You could simply say there are a total of 28 small squares.
       So, 0.04 seconds per small square × 28 small squares = 1.12 seconds

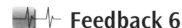 Feedback 6

If your answers match mine, you're doing a great job! If they don't, a little more practice is in order!

A. To be within normal limits, the P-R interval must measure 3 to 5 small squares in width or 0.12 to 0.20 seconds in duration.

B. A P-R interval less than 3 small squares in width or greater than 5 small squares in width represents an abnormality in the impulse conduction.

C. The P-R interval of the EKG cycle measures 5 small squares or 0.20 seconds (the upper limit of normal).

D. The QRS wave form represents ventricular depolarization.

E. To be within normal limits, the QRS must measure LESS than 3 small squares or less than 0.12 seconds in duration.

F. The QRS of the boxed cardiac cycle measures slightly less than three small squares which is slightly less than 0.12 seconds.

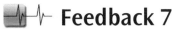 # Feedback 7

Keep up the good work! 🙂

A. Each marker at the top of the EKG paper represents <u>three</u> seconds. There are <u>5</u> complexes in the six second time interval displayed. Therefore, 5 × 10 equal <u>50</u>. The approximate heart rate is <u>50</u> beats/minute, using both methods.

B. The heart rate between the fourth and fifth QRS is 100. The rate of the PVCs is 150.

P.S. Here is a little "cheat sheet." Count the number of small squares (small boxes) between two R waves of a regular rhythm, then read across the chart to determine heart rate.

P.P.S. A copy of this guide is located at the back of the book. Cut it out and hang it near your monitor.

A Trusty Guide for Determining Heart Rate

No. of Boxes	Heart Rate	No. of Boxes	Heart Rate
5	300	25	60
6	250	26	57
7	214	27	55
8	187	28	53
9	166	29	52
10	150	30	50
11	136	31	48
12	125	32	47
13	115	33	45
14	107	34	44
15	100	35	42
16	94	36	41
17	88	37	40
→ 18	83	38	39
19	79	40	37
20	75	44	34
21	71	46	32
22	68	48	31
23	65	50	30
24	62		

Count the number of *small* EKG squares between two R waves on the following strip.

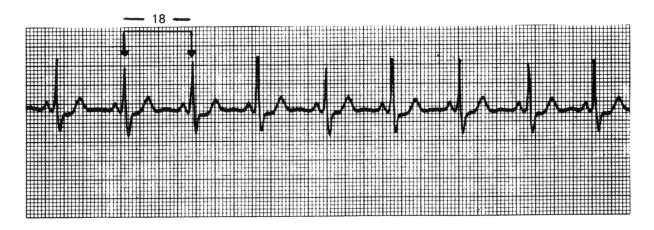

In this strip there are <u>18</u> small squares between R waves. Looking back to the Trusty Guide, one can quickly see that the heart rate is <u>83</u>.

REMEMBER, this method of determining heart rate applies *only* when the rhythm is *regular!*

Remember, there are 1500 small EKG squares in one minute. So, if one counts the number of small squares between two R waves (i.e., 18 in the previous example) and divides that number into 1500, one arrives at the heart rate. Remember this method works *only* when the rhythm is regular.

$$18\overline{)1500}^{\,82}$$

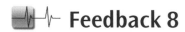 ## Feedback 8

Excellent work!

A. The heart rate in this strip is *approximately 90* beats per minute.

B. The rhythm is **regular**.

C. Each QRS complex is preceded by a <u>P</u> wave. All the P waves look uniform.

D. Each P wave is followed by a normal QRS complex.

E. All the QRS complexes appear uniform.

F. This is a **sinus rhythm**!

Notes

_____

_____

_____

_____

_____

_____

_____

_____

_____

_____

_____

_____

_____

_____

_____

_____

_____

_____

_____

_____

Notes

_____

_____

_____

_____

_____

_____

_____

_____

_____

_____

_____

_____

_____

_____

_____

_____

_____

_____

_____

Sinus and Atrial Dysrhythmias

Objectives

When you have completed Section 2, you will be able to describe or identify

1. a method for interpreting dysrhythmias
2. sinus arrhythmia
3. sinus bradycardia
4. sinus tachycardia
5. wandering atrial pacemaker (W.A.P.)
6. premature atrial contractions (P.A.C.s)
7. atrial tachycardia and re-entry mechanisms 🎓
8. atrial flutter
9. atrial fibrillation
10. atrial flutter-fibrillation
11. sick sinus syndrome (brady-tachy syndrome)
12. Wolff-Parkinson-White Syndrome (bypass re-entry mechanisms)🎓

2.1 Steps for Interpreting Dysrhythmias

You're back! From this point forward, the content will build upon principles learned in the first section. All abnormal rhythm patterns explored will be compared to sinus rhythm.

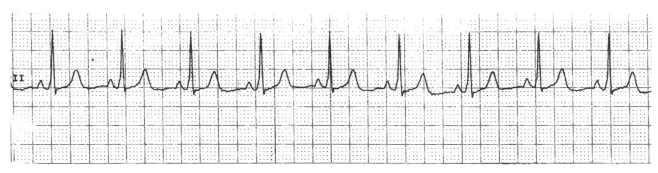

Sinus rhythm

You will remember, sinus rhythm is a *regular* rhythm with a rate of 60–100 beats per minute. Each QRS complex is preceded by a P wave. All P waves are uniform in appearance. All QRS complexes are uniform in appearance and each P wave is followed by a QRS.

As we begin to interpret the various abnormal rhythm patterns, *five* steps will be followed.

1. *Determining rhythm regularity.* If the rhythm is irregular, one must determine what makes it irregular. Are there early (premature) beats? Are there unexpected pauses? Are abnormal beats occurring? The simplest method for determining rhythm regularity is to measure the distance between two consecutive R waves (R-R interval) and compare that distance with other R-R intervals. In a regular rhythm, the R-R interval measurement will remain constant (as illustrated in the bottom diagram on page 46).

2. *Determining heart rate.* Remember . . . if the rhythm is irregular, it is necessary to count the rate for one full minute.

3. *Determining atrial activity.* Are P waves occurring uniformly across the tracing? Are the P waves alike in appearance? If no distinct P waves are present, is there evidence of atrial activity, or is the baseline preceding the QRS flat? If atrial impulses are present, are they regular or irregular? Is the atrial activity occurring so rapidly that there are more atrial deflections than QRS complexes? If actual atrial wave forms are difficult to identify, does the baseline appear zig-zag, jagged, or bumpy?

4. *Determining ventricular activity.* Are the QRS complexes of normal duration (less than 0.12 seconds)? Do the QRSs occur uniformly across the tracing? Does a QRS follow every P wave?

5. *Determining the relationship between atrial and ventricular activity.* Is each P wave producing a QRS, or are there P waves that are not followed by QRS complexes? Is each QRS preceded by a P wave, or is there evidence of independent ventricular activity? Is the P-R interval of all conducted beats constant, does it vary, or is there no established relationship?

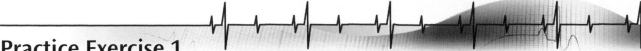

Practice Exercise 1

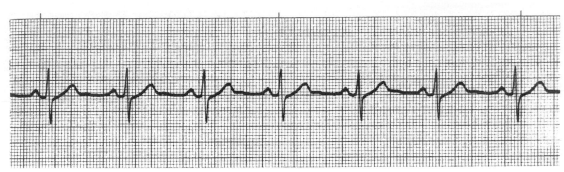

Study the above strip and then answer the following questions.

A. The heart rate is _____ beats per minute.

B. The rhythm is regular / irregular (circle one).

C. Each QRS complex is preceded by a _____ .

D. All P waves are _____ in appearance.

E. Each P wave is followed by a _____ .

F. All QRS complexes are _____ in appearance.

G. The P-R interval is _____ and measures _____ seconds.

H. Therefore, this is a _____ rhythm!

To interpret any rhythm, I use the same five principles.

1. First, I determine if the rhythm is _____ .

2. Second, I must determine the heart _____ .

3. I next determine _____ activity.

4. Then I look to determine _____ activity.

5. The final step involves determining if a relationship exists between _____ and _____ activity.

 For Feedback 1, refer to page 78.

For Feedback 1, refer to page 78.

input section **2.2** **Sinus Arrhythmia**

The first dysrhythmia to be explored is ***sinus arrhythmia.***

A sinus arrhythmia is a *slightly* irregular rhythm that is initiated by the SA node. Usually the slight variation in rhythm is related to **respiration**. The heart rate will increase slightly with inspiration, and decrease slightly with expiration. When you inspire a greater volume of blood enters the atria and heart rate increases to deal with the increased volume. When you expire the volume entering the atria returns to normal, as does heart rate. A sinus arrhythmia is a normal finding in children and young adults. A *slight* sinus arrhythmia may be found throughout adulthood. Any factor which *increases* vagal tone will exaggerate a sinus arrhythmia.

Looking closely at this rhythm strip, you will note the following:

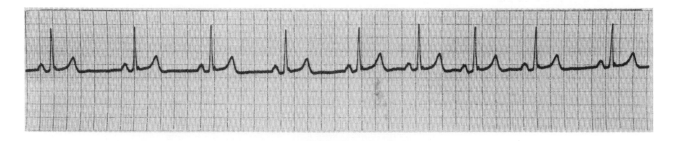

1. The heart rate falls somewhere between 60 and 100 beats per minute.
2. **The rhythm is irregular.**
3. The P waves are all uniform in appearance.
4. The QRS complexes are all of normal configuration and duration.
5. Each P wave produces a QRS. The P-R interval measures approximately 0.16 seconds and is consistent across the strip (so, atrial activity is related to ventricular activity!).

> The only abnormal finding is that the rhythm is *slightly* irregular, showing irregular spacing of the normal P waves.

The easiest method for determining rhythm irregularity is to measure the distance between two P waves (P-P interval) and then compare that distance to the distance between two other P waves (other P-P intervals).

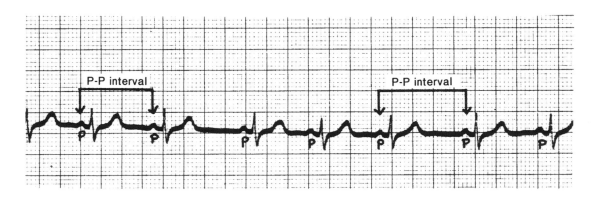

OR

Measure the distance between two R waves (R-R interval) and then compare that distance to the distance between two other R waves (other R-R intervals).

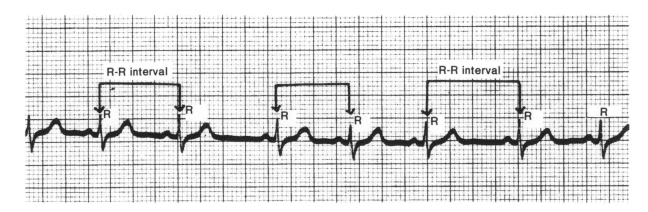

Easy, huh?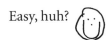

The following strip demonstrates the time measurement between each R-R interval. One can easily see the slight irregularity, though everything else appears normal.

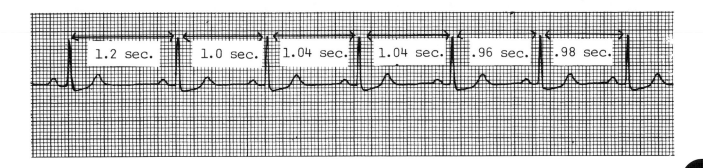

| 1.2 sec. | 1.0 sec. | 1.04 sec. | 1.04 sec. | .96 sec. | .98 sec. |

Remember, each small square on the EKG paper represents 0.04 seconds.

To review then, a sinus arrhythmia is simply a sinus rhythm that is slightly irregular! Since it is usually associated with respiration, *no treatment is required.*

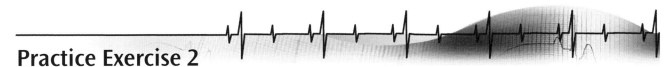

Practice Exercise 2

Okay, now it's your turn! Review the next two rhythm strips, then answer the questions following each strip.

1.

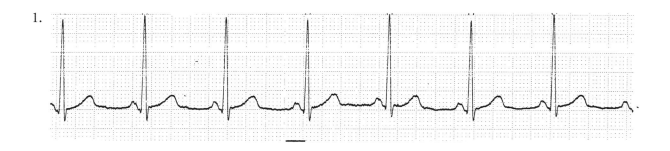

A. The heart rate in this strip is *approximately* _____ beats per minute.

B. The P waves are all _____ in appearance.

C. A _____ wave precedes each QRS complex.

D. The QRS complexes are _____ in appearance.

E. A _____ follows every P wave.

F. The rhythm is regular/irregular (circle one).

G. This is a _____ rhythm.

2.

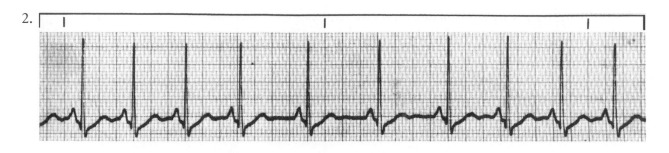

A. The heart rate in this strip is *approximately* _____ beats per minute.

B. The P waves are all _____ in appearance.

C. A _____ wave precedes each QRS complex.

D. The QRS complexes are _____ in appearance.

E. A _____ follows every P wave.

F. The rhythm is regular/irregular (circle one).

G. This is a _____ rhythm.

3. Usually the irregularity found in sinus arrhythmia is related to _____.

For Feedback 2, refer to page 78.

input section   2.3   Sinus Bradycardia

Bradycardia is a term used to describe a heart rate less than 60 beats per minute. *Sinus bradycardia* is a normal rhythm with the exception that the heart rate falls below 60. The impulse originates in the sinus (SA) node, but the impulses are fired at a slower rate due to vagal stimulation.

Sinus bradycardia is common in athletes and other persons accustomed to regular physical exercise. Vagal stimulation can be induced by pressing on the carotid artery or bearing down with the abdominal muscles. Vagal stimulation, resulting in bradycardia, can occur due to pain or fear, a bowel movement or during coughing. Cardiac drugs such as digitalis, beta-blockers and calcium-channel blockers can also have bradycardia as a desired effect or undesired side effect.

Here is a rhythm strip demonstrating a *sinus bradycardia.*

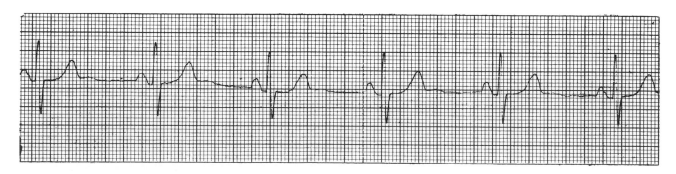

1. The rate is approximately 48 beats per minute (I referenced the chart on page 39).
2. The rhythm is regular.
3. The P waves are all uniform in appearance and precede each QRS complex.

4. The QRS complexes are uniform in appearance (and measure 0.10 seconds).
5. Each P wave produces a QRS. The P-R interval measures approximately 0.18 seconds and is consistent across the strip. Thus, atrial activity is assumed to be related to ventricular activity.

> The only abnormality is that the heart rate is approximately 48, which falls below the lower limits of normal, 60 beats per minute. So, we have a sinus bradycardia.

Using the five principles for dysrhythmia interpretation, one could say:

- The rate is approximately 48 per minute.

- The rhythm is slow and regular.

- The atria are activated regularly. P waves precede each QRS complex and they are uniform in appearance.

- There is a QRS complex following each P wave. The QRS complexes are occurring regularly at a rate of 48 per minute. All QRS complexes appear uniform and measure 0.08 seconds.

- There is a definite relationship between atrial and ventricular activity because each P-R interval is 0.18 seconds. In other words, the impulse originating in the sinus node moves down the conduction system to activate ventricular tissue in the same amount of time during each cardiac cycle.

Usually sinus bradycardia is observed and not treated. Treatment will be initiated only if the patient becomes symptomatic (decreased blood pressure, mental confusion or disorientation, lethargy, loss of consciousness, and so forth). Should the patient become symptomatic, a physician should be notified immediately.

In most instances, intravenous (IV) atropine is the drug treatment of choice to increase the heart rate when symptoms are acute. (One must closely monitor ability to void following the administration of atropine, as atropine is a smooth muscle relaxant.) If unresponsive to atropine, transcutaneous pacing is typically initiated.

> **REMEMBER**, sinus bradycardia can be a desired effect in some patients. Always speak to the physician before holding a cardiac medication for a heart rate of less than 60. Beyond a heart rate of less than 60, the physician will want to know if the patients blood pressure is low, if fatigue is present or if the patient is confused.

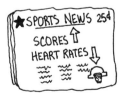

Practice Exercise 3

A. The term bradycardia implies that the heart rate is less than _____ beats per minute. Here are two strips for you to inspect.

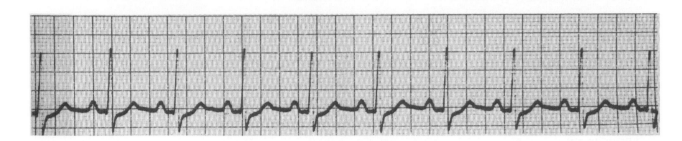

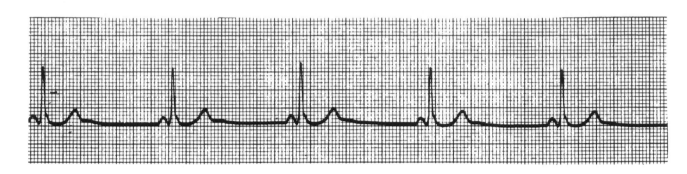

B. The first strip demonstrates a sinus rhythm. Explain how the second strip is both similar to and different from the first. (Use the steps previously discussed!)

_____

_____

_____

_____

_____

_____

_____

_____

_____

_____

The second strip demonstrates a _____ (rhythm).

For Feedback 3, refer to page 79.

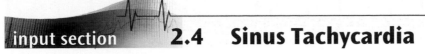

2.4   Sinus Tachycardia

Tachycardia is a term used to describe a heart rate *greater than* 100 beats per minute. *Sinus tachycardia* is a regular sinus rhythm with a rate greater than 100 beats per minute. *Usually a sinus tachycardia will not exceed the rate of 160 per minute.*

Some of the more common causes of sinus tachycardia are exercise, excitement, anemia, fear, heart failure, pain, fever, shock, infection, and foods—such as coffee or tea, and tobacco! For each Fahrenheit degree the body temperature rises, the heart rate will increase approximately eight to ten beats per minute. I bet you didn't know that!

The following rhythm strip demonstrates a sinus tachycardia.

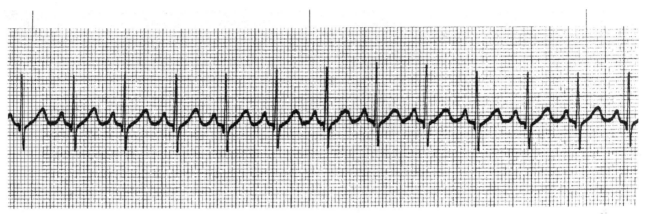

Using the five steps for dysrhythmia interpretation, one could say:

1. The rate is rapid, approximately 107 beats per minute.

2. The rhythm is regular.

3. The P waves are all uniform in appearance.

4. The QRS complexes are all uniform in appearance and duration.

5. Each P wave precedes the QRS by the same interval. In other words the P-R interval is constant, measuring approximately 0.14 seconds.

> The major abnormality is that the heart rate is 107, which falls above 100 beats per minute. Thus, we have a *sinus tachycardia.* (I have used the Trusty Guide on page 39 to determine the heart rate!)

If a heart rate of exactly 100 accompanies a sinus rhythm, it is usually called a *borderline sinus tachycardia.*

Should one find a patient's heart rate greater than 100 beats per minute, one must assume the role of *detective* to discover the underlying cause. The treatment for sinus tachycardia consists of *treating its cause* (i.e., lowering an elevated temperature or treating congestive heart failure, as examples).

If the patient has extreme anxiety, low blood pressure, labored breathing, or complains of chest pain, a physician should be notified immediately. The increased heart rate associated with a sinus tachycardia results in increased myocardial oxygen consumption.

Practice Exercise 4

A. Examine this rhythm strip closely, then describe *all* that you see! Looks normal to me, what do you think?

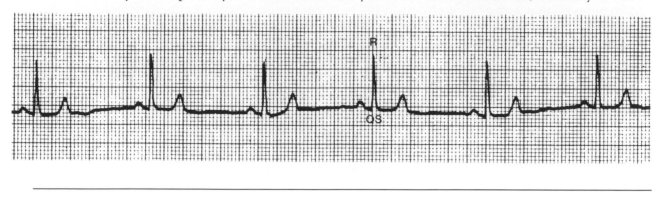

_____

_____

_____

_____

_____

_____

This rhythm is a _____.

B. Again, critically analyze the following strip and describe your findings.

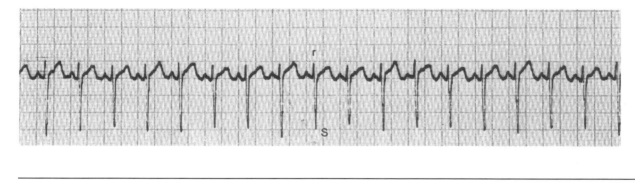

_____

_____

_____

_____

_____

This rhythm is a _____.

C. The treatment for sinus tachycardia consists of _____

_____

_____

_____

GOOD WORK!

 For Feedback 4, refer to page 80.

input section 2.5 Wandering Atrial Pacemaker (W.A.P.)

Before moving forward, we should look briefly at *wandering atrial pacemakers.* Basically, a *wandering atrial pacemaker* rhythm is a variation of a sinus rhythm that has no clinical significance. Rather than seeing uniform P waves across the EKG strip, the *P waves vary in appearance.* This P wave variation suggests that the pacemaker is wandering within the sinus mechanism and the surrounding atrial tissue. Notice that the first P wave of the strip, and the final three P waves are alike. This P wave comes from the sinus node. Now note the second, third and fourth P waves. They are notched on top and clearly different from the first P wave on the strip. These two different P waves come from different pacemaker sites. You may see multiple different looking P waves, so two isn't the limit!

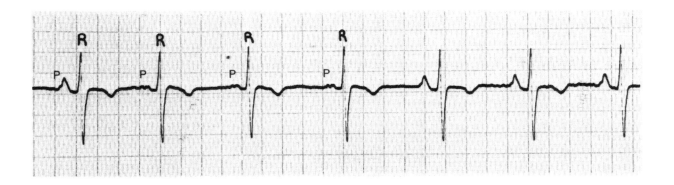

Commonly, a *wandering atrial pacemaker* is observed when the sinus rate slows. You will remember that other tissues within the atria have pacemaking capabilities . . . , *but* it is always the pacemaker with the *fastest* rate of discharge that controls the rhythm. In a wandering atrial pacemaker rhythm, various pacemakers (located within the atria) are discharging at similar rates. Thus, no single pacemaker site is dominant.

As you look at the above strip, you will notice that the rhythm is slightly irregular. (If you are unsure, measure the P-P or R-R intervals.) Looking further, the P waves tend to vary in shape or contour. Because of this variation, we assume that no single pacemaker within the atria is dominant. *How do I know that the various pacemakers are located within the atria?* . . . because each cardiac complex begins with a P wave . . . and P waves represent atrial depolarization!

The other fact one should be aware of is that the P-R interval may vary throughout a wandering atrial pacemaker rhythm. Since the P-R interval represents the time for impulse conduction from the pacemaker site through the system to the AV node, it makes sense that if the pacemaker site changes, so will the time for impulse conduction!

Since ventricular activation is usually unaltered, the QRS complexes are of normal duration (less than 0.12 seconds). Owing to the fact that a wandering atrial pacemaker is a variation of normal, no treatment or intervention is required. Whew! Typically, a wandering atrial pacemaker is associated with pronounced pulmonary disease.

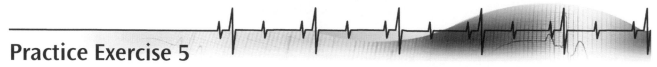

Practice Exercise 5

Without looking back, draw a rhythm strip demonstrating wandering atrial pacemaker. Sounds like fun . . . right?

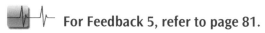 **For Feedback 5, refer to page 81.**

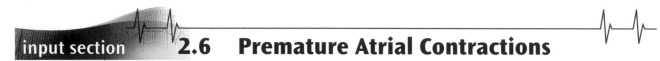

input section   2.6   Premature Atrial Contractions

We are now going to continue exploring *ectopic* activity. . . . electrical stimuli originating outside the normal conduction system.

A *premature atrial contraction,* henceforth to be known as a P.A.C., is an atrial impulse arising from an ectopic or abnormal atrial focus. As the name implies, the P.A.C. is *premature* in its relationship to the underlying sinus rhythm. In addition to occurring early or prematurely, the P.A.C. has an *abnormal appearing P wave.* In other words the P wave looks distinctly different from the P wave of the sinus rhythm since the route of atrial depolarization is different for the abnormal beat. That may sound confusing, so inspect the following rhythm strip.

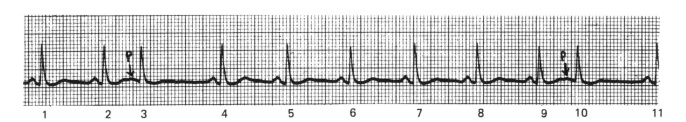

The first thing one notices is that the rhythm is *irregular.* Beat 3 and beat 10 occur early or prematurely. This is a technical interpretation based solely on quick "eyeball inspection"! You will notice the premature beats (3 and 10) have P waves . . . but, they look distinctly different from the other P waves in the strip. P.A.C.s may have P waves that are inverted, slurred, taller or wider than the normal P wave. On this strip, the P wave of the P.A.C. appears flat.

Premature atrial contraction is one of the few logical names used in EKG interpretation! Because the P.A.C. occurs early interrupting the underlying rhythm, it is called *premature.* And because there is a P wave we know the atria have depolarized.

A premature atrial impulse is *usually* conducted normally through the AV junction on to the ventricles. Do you know how I know that? *Voila!* because the P-R interval of the P.A.C. is usually between 3–5 small EKG squares (0.12–0.20 seconds) and because its QRS is usually narrow (*less than* 3 small squares). However, be advised that multiple rhythm abnormalities often occur together. It is not uncommon that the QRS associated with a P.A.C. will be widened, 0.12 seconds or greater. This is referred to as a P.A.C. that is *aberrantly* conducted, meaning that conduction moves down an abnormal pathway and thus takes longer than normal. Because width of a complex is measured in time, when conduction takes a longer time, the QRS will be widened!

In the following strip, every other beat is a P.A.C. (bigeminy P.A.C.s). Notice that the P waves of the premature beats tend to be less pronounced than the P waves of the sinus beats. For future reference, *bigeminy* is a term describing ectopic events occurring regularly in an every other beat pattern.

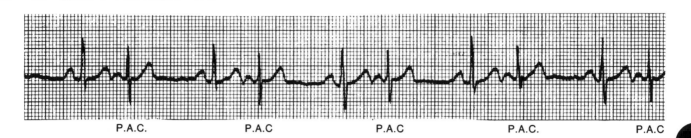

Premature atrial contractions may arise from a single focus (location) or several foci within the atria. All P.A.C.s arising from a single focus will have similarly appearing P waves. Conversely, if P.A.C.s arise from different sites, the appearance of their premature P waves will vary. When P.A.C.s arise from a single focus, there is a *tendency for a constant coupling interval.* So what is a *coupling interval?* Well, it's simply the interval or distance between the P.A.C. and the previous sinus beat. (This business about coupling intervals is for your trivia file ☺.)

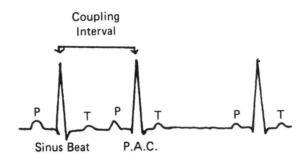

Examine the following rhythm strip. Notice that the *coupling interval* is constant and the P waves of the P.A.C.s appear similar. We therefore assume that the P.A.C.s are arising from the same ectopic atrial site.

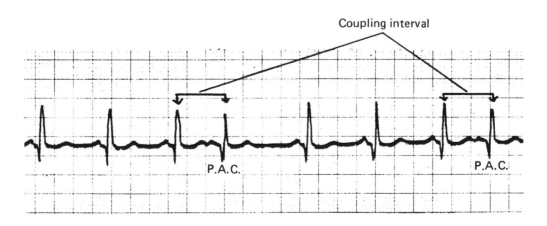

The other obvious finding associated with P.A.C.s is the slight pause or delay occurring before the next sinus beat.

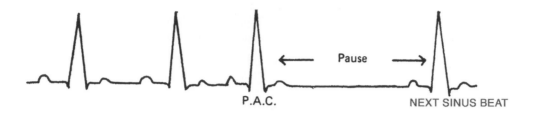

This pause tends to partly compensate for the prematurity. In other words, the P.A.C. firing prematurely disrupts the regular sinus cycle; the pause allows time for the sinus mechanism to reset the rhythm.

Premature atrial contractions may be observed in healthy individuals or may be associated with heart disease. P.A.C.s associated with rheumatic heart disease may be a forerunner to atrial fibrillation. P.A.C.s may also be noted in patients with pulmonary disease, right heart disease, and myocardial infarction. Drugs such as epinephrine and digitalis, stimulants such as coffee, tea, alcohol, tobacco, or emotional distress or fatigue may likewise precipitate P.A.C.s. To be on the safe side, always notify a physician when a patient begins having P.A.C.s and when they begin increasing in frequency! However, P.A.C.s. may precipitate rapid atrial dysrhythmias which will be covered later in this Section! Treatment, if indicated, typically involves the administration of cardiac drugs.

Examine this next strip.

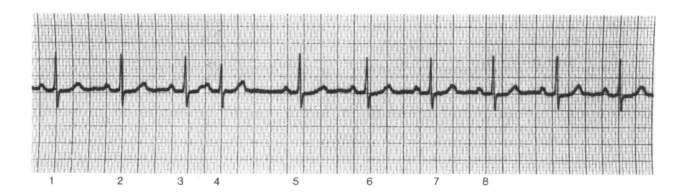

The P waves are *not* uniform in appearance. The P wave of beat 4 is premature in its relationship to the underlying rhythm and appears different from the other P waves. If you look closely, you will notice that the premature P wave falls on the T wave of the preceding beat. A P wave precedes every QRS complex. The QRS complexes are uniform in appearance, but do not occur regularly. There is a pause following the complex initiated by the premature P wave. The underlying rhythm is a sinus rhythm interrupted by a lone P.A.C.

Detecting P.A.C.s is usually not difficult. However, confusion may arise if, for some reason, a premature atrial impulse fails to be conducted. That sounds like a mouthful, so inspect this next strip closely.

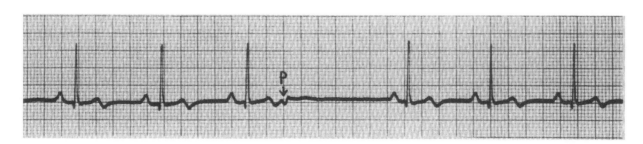

First, examine atrial activity. Refer back to the previous strip and locate all of the P waves. You will note that a premature P wave (appearing distinctly different from the other P waves) follows after beat 3. What is this? Well, it's a P wave—and P waves represent atrial depolarization. It occurs prematurely. So it's a premature atrial contraction that *fails to conduct* to the ventricles. In other words, since a QRS does not follow the premature atrial impulse, one concludes that the impulse was blocked or interrupted enroute to the ventricles. So this is an example of a *blocked P.A.C.* Like conducted P.A.C.s, there is a pause following the blocked P.A.C.

P.S. If this is confusing to you, it may help to remember that you will never find two T waves occurring together!

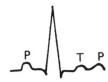

> **NOTE:** If a well-defined "bump" follows the T wave—most likely, it is a P wave!

Look closely at this second strip. Notice the blocked P.A.C. This strip is a tough one! By looking closely, however, you will notice that the T wave of the fourth complex is distorted . . . it has an extra "bump." This extra "bump" is assumed to be a P wave! In other words, the premature P wave is sitting on the downslope of the T wave. Thus, we again have a blocked P.A.C.!

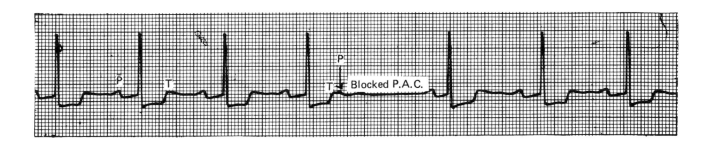

In this example, the premature atrial impulse does not conduct to the ventricles because the cardiac tissue has not fully recovered or repolarized. In other words, if the myocardial cells do not have sufficient time to repolarize, they may be refractory to (unable to receive) the next stimulation. (The patient belonging to this rhythm strip had a digitalis level of 4.7ng/ml.!!) **Ugh!** It is important to note that digitalis toxicity may be the culprit in either instance! A serum digitalis level is required to determine precise concentrations and to rule out digitalis toxicity. When digitalis toxicity is suspected, further doses of the drug are usually discontinued or held.

Enough on the subject of blocked P.A.C.s Let's try some practice.

Practice Exercise 6

A. Now, try your hand at interpretation! Describe all that you see.

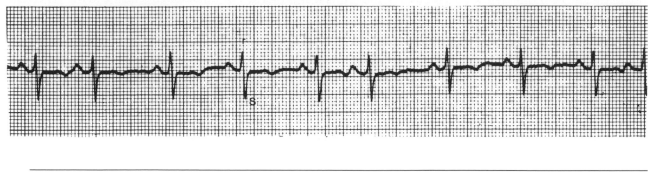

_____

_____

_____

_____

_____

_____

_____

_____

B. Circle the blocked P.A.C.s and indicate any suspicions you may have.

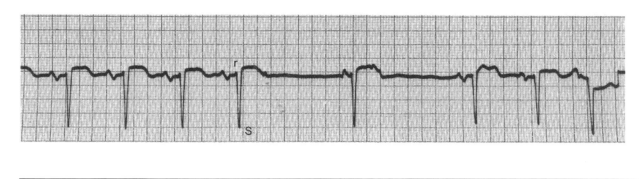

_____

_____

_____

_____

It sometimes helps to sing a few bars of "**keep on smiling....**" ☺

 For Feedback 6, refer to page 81.

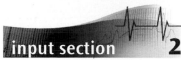

2.7 Atrial Tachycardia and Re-entry Mechanisms

You now have a basic understanding of ectopic atrial activity, the P.A.C. When the atria are repeatedly and rapidly stimulated by an ectopic pacemaker, an atrial tachycardia results. Atrial tachycardia can be initiated by: a single ectopic atrial pacemaker (P.A.C.) firing rapidly and repeatedly; multiple ectopic atrial pacemakers firing rapidly and repeatedly; or, a circus-like stimulation (re-entry phenomenon) of the atria.

Although the SA node is the heart's natural pacemaker, it rarely fires faster than 160 beats per minute. A regular, rapid (faster than 160 beats per minute) rhythm with clear P waves is assumed to be initiated by an ectopic atrial pacemaker.

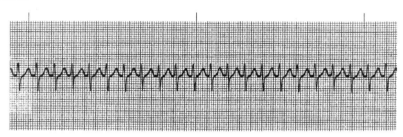

Atrial tachycardia rate 166.

From *ECG Workout: Exercises in Arrhythmia Interpretation,* 3rd edition by Jane Huff, RN, CCRN. Copyright © 1997 by Lippincott-Raven Publishers. Copyright © 1993, 1985 by J. B. Lippincott Company. All rights reserved. Reprinted with permission.

Atrial tachycardia is basically a rapid and regular *sustained* rhythm with a rate between *160 and 220* per minute. In addition to occurring in a sustained fashion, atrial tachycardia may both begin and end abruptly. When this occurs, the short runs of atrial tachycardia are said to be occurring in *paroxysms.* Hence, short bursts or runs of atrial tachycardia are referred to as P.A.T. (*paroxysmal atrial tachycardia*).

Atrial tachycardia may be associated with coronary artery disease, valvular disease (e.g., rheumatic mitral disease) . . . or may be found in otherwise healthy individuals! In fact, any of the following factors may precipitate atrial tachycardia: emotional stress, drug actions, coffee, tea, tobacco, alcohol, and so forth.

Most patients with a sustained atrial tachycardia experience a fluttering sensation in the chest along with light-headedness due to the rapid ventricular rate. The rapid heart rate reduces cardiac output because the volume of blood ejected with each contraction (*stroke volume*) is decreased as a result of the shortened ventricular filling time. That sounds a bit complicated! Actually it's a great deal like your average household toilet. If you stand there flushing your toilet 180 times per minute, you can imagine what happens . . . not much! You must allow time (between flushes) for the reservoir to refill; otherwise, there's not much action or "toilet output" at the bottom. . . . Right? . . . Just like cardiac output—there must be an appropriate ventricular filling time.

The rapid rate increases the oxygen demand and consumption of the cardiac muscle which, in turn, may cause ischemia of the myocardium and may precipitate an anginal attack (chest pain). Ultimately, the ventricle can fail.

Examine the rhythm strip of atrial tachycardia below.

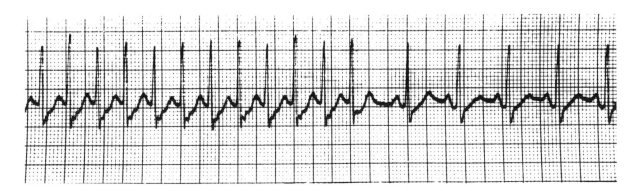

The first two-thirds of the above rhythm strip demonstrate atrial tachycardia at a rate of approximately 200 per minute. The rapid rhythm breaks spontaneously into a sinus tachycardia (approximate rate of 115 per minute). You will recall that characteristically, atrial tachycardia has a heart rate that falls between 160 and 220 per minute. Whenever one finds a rapid rhythm with *clearly distinguishable upright P waves* occurring before the QRSs, the rhythm is assumed to be of atrial origin! You will notice that the QRS complexes in both the atrial tachycardia and the sinus tachycardia are of normal duration (narrow), since ventricular activation occurs normally. A word of caution: Because underlying pathology may complicate electrical activity, one may find an atrial tachycardia with a widened QRS known as atrial tachycardia with *aberrant conduction*.

Atrial tachycardia may terminate abruptly without treatment. If it persists, a physician should be notified immediately. If the patient is alert, he or she may be asked to perform the *Valsalva maneuver*. This maneuver requires that the patient hold his breath and bear down—it's basically like having a bowel movement. This maneuver increases vagal tone which may terminate the rapid rhythm. Another technique for increasing vagal tone (a vagal maneuver) is to place a *cold* or *ice* compress on the patient's face. By stimulating a vagal response, the AV junction may slow its rate of impulse conduction, thereby slowing the heart rate. This application of cold or ice water to the face stimulates the *mammalian diving reflex*, a primitive reflex that stimulates the trigeminal nerve (cranial nerve V) which activates the vagues nerve (cranial nerve X) which may result in slowed conduction! If these techniques are unsuccessful, synchronized cardioversion or, alternatively, beta blockers, calcium channel blockers, amiodarone, sotalol or digoxin may be administered. When the patient's condition is rapidly deteriorating, synchronized cardioversion is the treatment of choice, though amiodarone or diltiazem represent treatment options.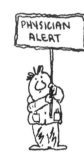

Always alert the *managing* physician to even brief periods of atrial tachycardia.

Multifocal Atrial Tachycardia (MAT)

Rather than a single ectopic site (P.A.C.) firing repeatedly, atrial tachycardia may also be precipitated by multiple ectopic sites or foci firing repeatedly. Multifocal atrial tachycardia is the terminology used when a rapid, irregular rhythm (greater than 100 beats per minute) presents with **at least 3 morphologically different (different in appearance) P waves**, signifying at least three different ectopic atrial sites or pacemakers. Typically, the QRS complexes are within normal limits, though they will widen with aberrant conduction.

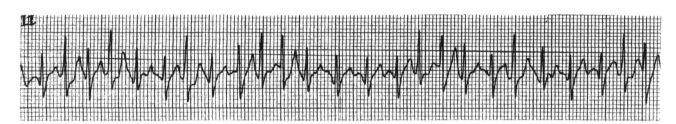

Multifocal atrial tachycardia. Notice the rapid rate and variation in P wave morphology.

As with all dysrhythmias, a name is less important than an accurate description of the rhythm!

Multifocal atrial tachycardia is most often observed in the elderly with coronary artery disease in conjunction with chronic lung disease. It may also be associated with hypokalemia, pulmonary embolism, pneumonia and congestive heart failure. Treatment, if indicated, is based on the symptoms. Beta-blockers, calcium channel blockers or amiodarone are drug options when CHF is absent and cardiac output is not significantly compromised. Treatment options for patients with CHF or compromised cardiac output (ejection fraction <40%) include amiodarone or diltiazem (a calcium channel blocker). Owing to the multiple atrial foci, cardioversion is rarely successful.

Adding to both diagnostic and treatment complexity, atrial tachycardia and upcoming atrial dysrhythmias (atrial flutter and atrial fibrillation) may be precipitated or caused by a *re-entry mechanism.* A re-entry mechanism results from an abnormal (accessory) connection between normal conducting fibers in the atria, creating a circular conducting pathway. *Under certain conditions,* a stimulus will travel rapidly and repeatedly around the circular pathway (circuit), like a race car around a race track, rather than down the normal conduction pathway. A stimulus traveling this rapid, circular pathway can precipitate atrial tachycardia. When atrial tachycardia is caused by this circular activation of atrial tissues, treatment involves disrupting the abnormal circuit, as discussed on page 64.

A re-entry dysrhythmia caused by an accessory circuit is a *DIFFICULT* concept (even for the experts!). The following example of **re-entry mechanics** attempts to demystify cardiac physiology and is included as optional, higher level reading. You may **skip** down to **TREATMENT OF RECURRENT ATRIAL OR SUPRAVENTRICULLAR TECHYCARDIA** . . . or take two deep breaths and read on !

Atrial Re-Entry Mechanisms

(Advanced Study)

Re-entry type dysrhythmias arise from one of two types of conduction system anomalies, both formed during embryonic development:

1. accessory circuitry (an abnormal connection between conducting fibers which creates a localized abnormal conduction path or circuit) located anywhere within the conduction system
2. actual bypass tracts (around the normal conduction system) that connect the atria directly to the ventricles.

The second type of anomaly will be discussed near the end of this Section. Here, we will focus on accessory circuitry in the atria.

The presence of an accessory conducting circuit (an abnormal connection between two conducting fibers) predisposes *the owner* to various rapid atrial or supraventricular dysrhythmias. In effect, this extra circuitry, under specific conditions, can precipitate a rapid, *circus-like* stimulation of the atria which, in turn, produces a rapid ventricular rate. A *right-timed* P.A.C. coupled with an ability to conduct in a portion of the circuit, are the usual conditions necessary to initiate a circus movement atrial tachycardia. **Circus movement tachycardias** are often abbreviated as CMTs.

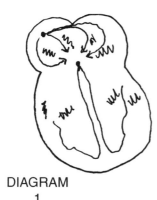

DIAGRAM
1

In normal healthy conduction, a sinus impulse travels through the atria along specialized conducting fibers or tracts, producing atrial depolarization (〜) , then travels across the AV node (slowing slightly) and the bundle of His, down the right and left bundle branches, out to the Purkinje fibers to initiate ventricular depolarization (〜) . See Diagram 1.

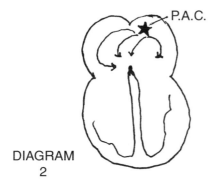

DIAGRAM
2

When a P.A.C. arises from an excitable focus (somewhere in either atria), the stimulus progresses (propagates) across the atria, traveling along the specialized fibers or tracts (atrial excitation pathway) from the point of ectopic origin to the AV node. From there, the remainder of the conduction sequence is normal. See Diagram 2.

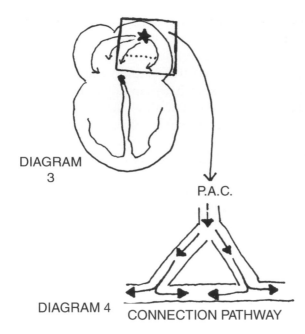

DIAGRAM 3

Suppose, however, an anomalous connection exists between two specialized conducting fibers or tracts of the P.A.C. conduction route. Refer to the dotted line (. . . . . .) in Diagram 3. Even though this abnormal connection exists, conduction is uninterrupted (progressing around and out of the circuit) when the tissues are in a uniform state of recovery (repolarization or receptivity). Refer to Diagrams 3 and 4.

P.A.C.

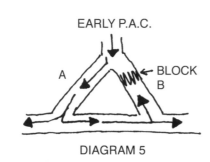

DIAGRAM 4   CONNECTION PATHWAY

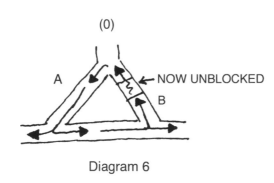

EARLY P.A.C.

A ← BLOCK B

DIAGRAM 5

Certain conditions, however, will cause the anomalous connection to behave as a *true* electrical circuit. In this instance, an early timed P.A.C. finds one "leg" or conducting fiber of the circuit in a *not-yet-recovered* or not fully re-polarized state. That portion of the circuit is refractory or unable to receive a stimulus until fully recovered. In other words, a forward moving (antegrade) stimulus attempting to activate that "leg" or fiber (labeled **B**) would be blocked temporarily (unidirectional block). It is this temporary blockage that creates *electrical circuit behavior.* Refer to Diagram 5.

(O)

A ← NOW UNBLOCKED B

Diagram 6

In this situation (a blockage secondary to refractory tissue), the wave of excitation travels normally across the fully repolarized (unblocked) leg (labeled **A**) of the circuit causing depolarization of atrial cells as it moves forward toward the AV nodal pathway. However, because of the abnormal circuitry, the wave of excitation also flows backward (retrograde) toward the blocked area (labeled B). If, by this time, the tissue in the blocked area is fully recovered, the moving stimulus activates the once blocked area, causing depolarization. The wave of excitation slows slightly during depolarization, then continues on to the point of (O)rigin (See Diagram 6).

So, now back at the point of origin (**O**), the whole cycle can begin again. Ugh!! If the atrial tissues in "leg" A of the circuit are fully recovered from the previous stimulation, the progressing wave of excitation (pre-excitation) will assume control of the rhythm, continuing a counter-clockwise loop around the circuit, producing a rapid atrial tachycardia. The rapid rate is a result of the accelerated pace of atrial activation created by the anomalous circuit. Whew!

If, however, the atrial tissues in "leg" A are not fully recovered (partial state of repolarization) when the stimulus comes around the circuit, the circus-like activation will cease! In other words, the abnormal stimulation is interrupted and the normal underlying pacemaker resumes control of the rhythm.

You *may* want to ponder this *demystified cardiac physiology* again over coffee (or other stimulants)! **The important points to remember are covered below.**

- Anomalous circuitry (a re-entry mechanism) within the atrial conduction system may be responsible for rapid, atrial dysrhythmias, often described as *circus-like* atrial activation.
- Timing is everything!! In the presence of abnormal circuitry, refractory tissue can both start (see "leg" B, diagram 5) or terminate (see "leg" A, diagram 6) circus like atrial activation.
- A re-entry mechanism is also referred to as a *pre-excitation* syndrome.
- A re-entry mechanism (anomalous conducting circuit) is diagnosed by electrophysiology (EP) studies.

IF YOU FEEL SUSCEPTIBLE TO UNIDIRECTIONAL BLOCK,

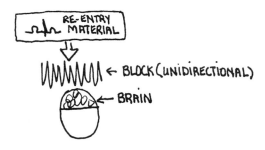

PLEASE UNDERSTAND YOU ARE PROGRESSING IN A NORMAL, ANTEGRADE (FORWARD) FASHION!!

Finally, examine this strip.

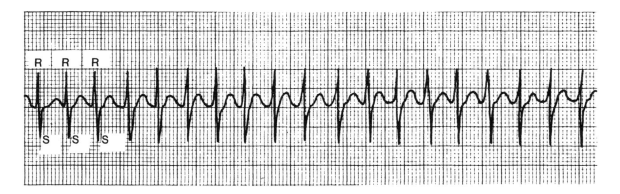

The heart rate in the above strip is approximately 187 beats per minute which makes me think of atrial tachycardia. But, where are the P waves? P waves may or may not be there! If *definite* P waves are not observable, one cannot call the rhythm *atrial* tachycardia. So what will we call it? How about just describing what we see?

This is a rapid, regular rhythm with a heart rate of 187 beats per minute. The QRS complexes are borderline, measuring slightly less than 0.12 seconds. Oftentimes, rapid regular rhythms with normal duration QRSs are referred to as *supraventricular* (SVT) rhythms. The term *supraventricular* implies that the rhythm originates above the level of the ventricles.

Treatment of Recurrent Atrial or Supraventricular Tachycardia

Patients with recurrent tachydysrhythmias or those unresponsive to drug therapy are often studied in the electrophysiology lab. These studies are called electrophysiology studies and abbreviated EP studies. The EP lab is much like a cardiac catheterization lab. The patient is placed on an x-ray table with fluoroscopic capability (ability to shoot a moving, real time x-ray). However, the EP lab also has sophisticated electrocardiography equipment that allows for the precise anatomic location of dysrhythmias.

A venous cutdown, usually femoral, is performed allowing for the insertion of special catheters into the femoral vein. A catheter is threaded into the vein and venous flow helps to advance the catheter up through the abdominal vena cava up to the superior vena cava into the right atrium, and eventually into the right ventricle. This special catheter is capable of reading endocardial (from within the heart chambers) electrical activity. These "inside" EKGs identify the abnormal depolarizations or bypass pathways causing the tachydysrhythmia.

Once the site of pathology is confirmed, *radiofrequency ablation* (RFA) is employed. RFA delivers high frequency energy via a catheter inserted into the heart. RFA destroys the tissue causing the dysrhythmia. In particular, RFA is incredibly effective in terminating dysrhythmias caused by a re-entry phenomenon. Ablation destroys the tissue that allowed reentry to occur. Following ablation of the tissue, the cardiologist again attempts to induce the rhythm. If the abnormal rhythm cannot be induced, the treatment is considered successful.

Ablation is considered curative for most SVTs. However, in some patients, continued drug therapy (anti-arrhythmics) is necessary.

In Summary of Atrial Tachycardia

If this is your first foray into EKG interpretation, the lengthy discussion of atrial tachycardia may have drained your battery! *Not to worry.* Since re-entry phenomena and multifocal ectopic activity reappear throughout the text, it seemed fitting to sensititize you early on! The following brief (and simple) summary captures the highlights of atrial tachycardia.

Atrial tachycardia originates in one of three ways:

1. A single ectopic atrial focus fires rapidly and repeatedly (rapid fire P.A.C.s), assuming control of the rhythm by virtue of its accelerated rate (faster than the sinus pacemaker). You will recall that the fastest pacemaker controls the rhythm. The monitor picture shows a rapid (characteristically, 160–220 beats per minute), regular rhythm with uniform P waves.
2. A rapid, regular atrial rhythm can be precipitated by an initiating P.A.C. when an abnormal conduction circuit is present. The abnormal circuit allows the wave of excitation (initiated by the P.A.C.) to rapidly and repeatedly activate the atria in a circus-like fashion (requires a *right-timed* P.A.C. and the presence of anomalous circuitry). The monitor picture shows a rapid (characteristically, 160–220 beats per minute), regular rhythm with uniform P waves.

The monitor cannot distinguish single focus versus re-entry atrial tachycardia since the electrical activity appears the same!

3. A rapid, slightly irregular atrial tachycardia can be precipitated by multiple ectopic sites firing rapidly (characteristically, 160–220 beats per minute). Rather than appearing uniform, at least three different P wave presentations will be visible.

QRS Morphology

In the normal healthy heart, the QRS is narrow, measuring less than 0.12 seconds. Typically, the QRS associated with atrial (or supraventricular) tachycardia occurs within normal limits (WNL). However, rapid atrial (or supraventricular) stimuli may encounter the conduction pathway only partially recovered (partially repolarized) between repeat stimulations. When conducting tissues are partially refractory, impulse conduction occurs more slowly, requiring more time. Thus, one may find a widened QRS associated with rapid atrial and supraventricular dysrhythmias. This widening of the QRS secondary to conduction pathway refractoriness is known as **aberrancy** (atrial tachycardia with aberrancy.)

These concepts will be revisited throughout the text! Now, on other rapid atrial dysrhythmias!

Practice Exercise 7

Just relax. Okay, now study the strip below. Describe everything that you see using the questions that follow as a guide.

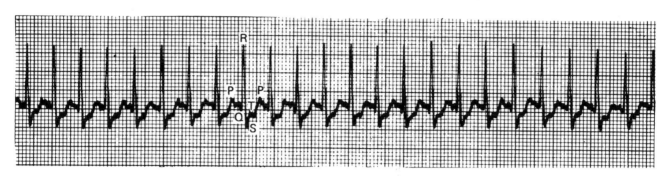

A. Describe the rhythm pattern and cardiac complexes _____

_____

_____

B. What is the heart rate? _____

C. What can you say about atrial activity? _____

_____

_____

_____

D. What can you say about ventricular activity? _____

_____

_____

_____

E. This rhythm is _____.

F. Treatment is aimed at slowing down the heart rate. A method that might be used is the Valsalva maneuver.

Describe this maneuver. _____

_____

_____

_____

G. Atrial tachycardia may be precipitated by which of the following events or conditions? (Check all that apply.)

☐ A P.A.C. firing rapidly and repeatedly

☐ A P.A.C. entering a re-entry circuit

☐ Emotional stress

☐ Stimulants

☐ EKG practice exercises

H. Explain the difference between atrial tachycardia and multifocal atrial tachcardia. _____

_____

_____

_____

I. Describe RFA and its therapeutic use. _____

_____

_____

_____

_____

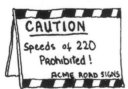 **For Feedback 7, refer to page 82.**

input section 2.8   Atrial Flutter

Remember the normal conduction system?

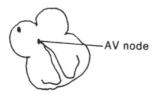

AV node

Before we go any further, you must commit the following to memory.

The AV node *is physiologically unable* to conduct greater than approximately 220 impulses per minute. (This is a *general* rule.) If the heart rate exceeds 220 impulses per minute, some of the impulses will not be conducted through to the ventricles. This is called a normal *physiologic block*. Physiologic block is a protective mechanism that *guards* the ventricles from the effects of rapid stimulation!

CAUTION
Speeds of 220
Prohibited!
ACME ROAD SIGNS

Atrial flutter is a rapid *regular* atrial rhythm that arises from an excitable ectopic site (focus) in the atria or results from a *re-entry circuit* around the tricuspid valve of the right atrium.

It is important to remember that the fastest pacemaker will control the heart rate. The *atrial rate* in atrial flutter is usually between *220–350* impulses per minute.

Following what we said above, all of these impulses will not be conducted to the ventricles because the AV node is incapable of conducting more than 220 impulses per minute.

The rapid *atrial* impulses of atrial flutter appear *saw-toothed* in shape and are labeled "F" waves. ("F" waves stand for flutter waves.) Flutter waves are continuous—they never stop. Consequently, they may even distort the QRSs! Flutter waves are more pronounced in leads II, III, and aVF . . . in other leads, the "saw-toothed" appearance is less visible.

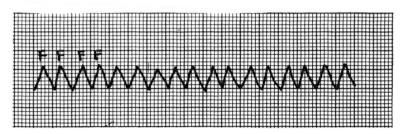

Saw-toothed atrial flutter waves

Since the AV node is unable to conduct greater than 220 impulses per minute, certain flutter impulses will not be conducted, or will be blocked from reaching the ventricles. *Usually,* only ½, ⅓, or ¼ of the atrial impulses will be conducted through the AV node to the ventricles.

To make this easy to understand, *let's say that the atrial flutter rate is 300* (300 F waves per minute).

If ½ of those atrial impulses are conducted (2:1 conduction), the ventricular rate will be 150.

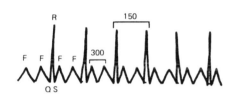

In other words, for every two flutter waves, there is one QRS. This is called 2:1 conduction. The first flutter wave is blocked; the second flutter wave conducts to the ventricles producing ventricular depolarization (a QRS).

> A 2:1 conduction with 300 'F' waves and a ventricular rate of 150 is the most common finding in atrial flutter.

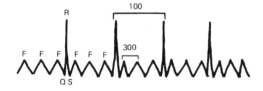

If ⅓ of those impulses are conducted, the ventricular rate will be 100.

For every three flutter waves, there will be one QRS. The first two flutter waves are blocked; the third one conducts to the ventricles producing ventricular depolarization. In other words, there will be 3 flutter waves for every 1 QRS, or a 3:1 conduction.

Or, if ¼ of those atrial impulses are conducted (4:1 conduction), the ventricular rate will be 75.

For every four flutter waves, there will be one QRS. The first three flutter waves are blocked; the fourth flutter wave conducts to the ventricles producing ventricular depolarization. This is a 4:1 conduction.

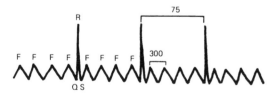

So, the atrial activity appears saw-toothed in leads II, III, and aVF. There are flutter waves *rather than* P waves! The QRS complexes are normally *narrow* (less than 0.12 seconds), and the ventricular rhythm is *usually regular.* If, however, the degree of *physiologic block* in the AV node varies, the ventricular rhythm may be somewhat irregular. In other words, the AV node may arbitrarily allow flutter impulses to be conducted to the ventricles.

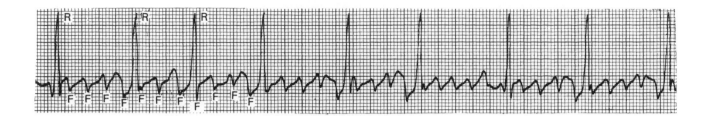

The above monitor tracing indicates atrial flutter with variable physiologic block in the AV node (atrial flutter with varying degrees of block). As you can see, with variable block the ventricular response is irregular. You know what this means . . . to determine an accurate heart rate one would need to count for one full minute!

Regardless whether the QRS complexes occur regularly or irregularly, the rhythm is atrial flutter. *The diagnosis of atrial flutter is based on the rapid, regular, continuous atrial impulses occurring at a rate of 220–350 per minute.*

When describing atrial flutter, it is important to specify the rate at which the atrial flutter waves are occurring and indicate both the *rate* and *regularity* of the ventricular response.

Atrial flutter can be acute or chronic. It commonly occurs in acute myocardiac infarction (AMI), after pneumonectomy post cardiac surgery, mitral valve disease, COPD and hyperthyroidism.

Following is a strip demonstrating atrial flutter with a regular ventricular response (4:1 atrial flutter—four flutter waves for every QRS).

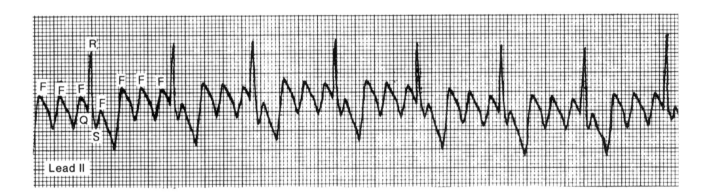

Let's describe what is happening!

Oh! I forgot to tell you something. This is going to sound *truly* illogical, but . . . if I turn an atrial flutter tracing upside down, it's easier for me to see the flutter waves. When no one is watching, try it!

Okay. Lets analyze the atrial activity.

Well, there are no P waves. Instead, there are rapid, saw-toothed continous flutter waves. To calculate the atrial flutter rate, use the "rule of 1500" method. Count the number of small boxes between two consecutive 'F' waves and divide into 1500.

F F F F F
ΛΛΛΛΛ

So, the atrial flutter rate in the above strip is 300! Because physiologic block limits the AV node capacity of conducting greater than 220 impulses per minute, some of those 300 impulses will be blocked or will not conduct. If you look closely, there are four flutter waves for every QRS (4:1 conduction).

What about ventricular activity? The ventricular rate is regular at a rate of 75 per minute. The QRS complexes are within normal limits (less than 0.12 seconds). In atrial flutter, the *ventricular rate is usually between 60–150 per minute*. Atrial and ventricular activity are related because the interval between the conducted flutter wave and its QRS is always constant.

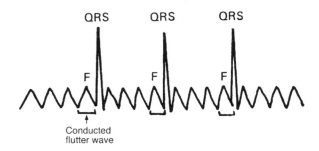

The distance between the atrial flutter wave preceding each QRS and the QRS measures the same indicating that atrial activity is related to ventricular activity. In other words, the atrial impulse (flutter wave) prior to the QRS, conducts down through the AV node to the ventricles producing ventricular depolarization (QRS).

Vagal maneuvers, such as carotid pressure or the Valsalva maneuver, may interrupt atrial flutter . . . or may assist in the diagnosis of atrial flutter.

Look at this next strip!

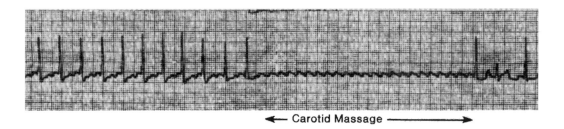

Note the prominent flutter waves during carotid massage. Carotid message is a *rarely* employed "physician-only" procedure owing to the risk of embolism.

Atrial flutter may be treated in a variety of ways, but the *object* of initial treatment is to slow conduction of the 'F' into the ventricles. Similar to the discussion of atrial tachycardia, a rapid heart rate may predispose the patient to a diminished cardiac output, LV failure, ischemia, and angina. If the patient is acutely symptomatic, the best method of treatment is synchronized cardioversion. The DC (direct current) cardioversion interrupts the chaotic firing of the ectopic atrial focus, allowing the sinus pacemaker to resume control.

In a more stable clinical presentation, drugs such as verapamil, diltiazem, digitalis and beta-blockers may be administered to slow the ventricular response. These drugs produce further block in the AV node, reducing the number of conducted atrial impulses. In other words, the drug effect might change a 2:1 conduction to a 3:1 or 4:1 conduction pattern. (For example, an atrial flutter rate of 300 in a 2:1 conduction pattern would produce a ventricular rate of 150. If the increased block resulted in a 3:1 conduction pattern, three flutter waves per QRS, the ventricular rate would be 100. In a 4:1 conduction pattern, the ventricular rate would be 75.)

$$2\overline{)300} = 150; \ 3\overline{)300} = 100; \ 4\overline{)300} = 75$$

If the ventricular rate is well tolerated, initial drug therapy may be focused on converting the rhythm. Drugs such as procainamide, disopyramide, propafenone, sotalol, amiodarone, flecainide, ibutilide, and quinidine may be given in attempt to convert the rhythm.

> **NOTE:** Prior to drug therapy, it is important to determine whether the patient is currently taking digoxin. Though rare, digoxin toxicity can cause atrial flutter!

If atrial flutter is recurrent and found (through electrophysiologic studies) to be associated with a re-entry mechanism, the treatment of choice is ablation (discussed on page 64) which destroys the anomalous conducting pathway.

Only one other major point to make about atrial flutter. This is really a secret . . . a method to impress your friends!

> **BONUS:** Any time you observe a regular rhythm with a heart rate between 150–190, *always* think about atrial flutter! (See the rhythm strip below)

Flutter waves may be hiding . . . see for yourself!

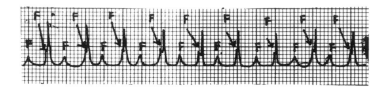

Finally, note the atrial flutter waves occurring at a rate of 250 per minute in the next strip. The two leads (lead II and V_1) are presented to make the point that atrial activity is best viewed from leads II, III and aVF. You will notice that the flutter waves are indistinguishable in lead V_1.

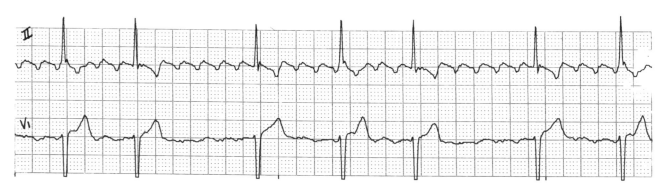

Practice Exercise 8

Atrial flutter is a fun rhythm 🙂 to detect.

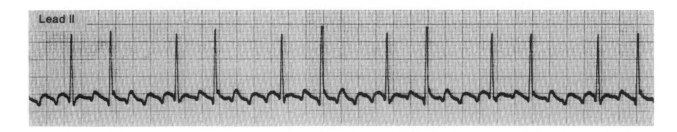

A. Use your skills to describe this strip in detail! _____

_____

_____

_____

_____

_____

B. The atrial rate in atrial flutter varies between _____ and _____ impulses per minute. The AV node is unable to conduct greater than _____ impulses per minute. Beyond this rate, a _____ block occurs.

For Feedback 8, refer to page 83.

2

input section   2.9   **Atrial Fibrillation**

By now, you may be feeling a bit overwhelmed! That, however, is a natural reaction. Knowing that you are nearing the end of Section 2 may improve your outlook! Atrial fibrillation is an easily identified dysrhythmia.

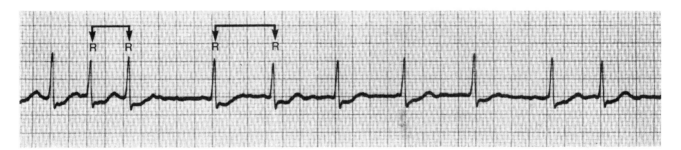

Atrial fibrillation

The above strip demonstrates *atrial fibrillation* (sometimes abbreviated as "A fib"). There are no P waves; instead there are *bizarre* and *irregular* atrial deflections referred to as fibrillation. Fibrillation has no rhythmic pattern; thus *atrial activation is chaotic.* The atria appears to quiver due to chaotic impulses—up to 400–600 impulses/minute. In atrial fibrillation, the baseline appears fuzzy, or like static.

We must refer back to the discussion concerning physiologic block. Owing to physiologic block, the AV node is incapable of conducting more than *220* impulses to the ventricles per minute. Thus, the 400–600 atrial impulses per minute cannot all be conducted. Most usually, this physiologic block will permit 120–160 impulses through to the ventricles each minute. However, if associated with a re-entry mechanism (an anomalous conduction circuit), the ventricular rate may be faster. The ventricular response (QRSs) associated with atrial fibrillation will occur irregularly. This is due to the refractory state of the AV node when the impulse arrives at the AV node. Thus, the R-R interval will *always* vary, as depicted in the above tracing. Because fibrillation occurs *continuously,* it may deform the QRS complexes, the ST segments, and the T waves!

In atrial fibrillation, there is no coordinated activation process in the atria. The tissue within the atria is electrically fragmented into various stages of excitation, refractoriness (resting state), or responsiveness. In other words, the tissues are "out of phase" with each other. Normally, all the fibers within a heart chamber will be in essentially the same electrophysiologic state—they will all be in a state of excitation, all in a state of refractoriness, or all in a partial state of responsiveness.

In many instances, the ventricular response rate will be rapid (120–160 beats per minute). Like previously discussed rapid rhythms a rapid ventricular response may decrease cardiac output and precipitate LV failure, ischemia, and chest pain. Remember the toilet analogy . . . page 59.

With uncontrolled atrial fibrillation, cardiac output is compromised because of both the rapid ventricular rate and the loss of synchronized atrial activation (atrial kick). It is common to find a *pulse deficit* associated with atrial fibrillation. A pulse deficit exists when the apical pulse is faster than the radial pulse, when the two pulses are counted simultaneously. When the cardiac output is compromised, not all cardiac contractions will be felt radially.

Let's try describing what we see, using the five steps for dysrhythmia interpretation.

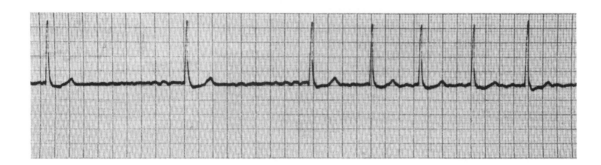

One can visually determine that the rhythm is irregular. As a matter of fact, atrial fibrillation is described as being *irregularly irregular!* In order to accurately determine heart rate, one would need to count the ventricular complexes (QRSs) over the course of one full minute. Preferably, the heart rate should be determined by simultaneously counting the patient's apical and radial pulses for one minute.

Next, evaluate atrial activity. There are no P waves, and thus, no P-R intervals. The baseline appears to *undulate.* There are rapid, small irregular atrial waves with no common pattern. An evaluation of ventricular activity reveals that the QRS complexes are normal in shape and duration (measuring less than 0.12 seconds), though they occur irregularly. The interval between the R waves (R-R interval) varies.

Evaluation of the relationship between atrial and ventricular activity reveals a *bizarre* conduction pattern. Most of the atrial impulses (fibrillation waves) that reach the AV node are blocked from further progression (owing to the fact that the AV node in unable to conduct greater than 220 impulses per minute). The atrial impulses that pass through the AV node are normally conducted, as demonstrated by QRS complexes of normal duration.

Atrial fibrillation is one of the most commonly observed dysrhythmias and its occurrence increases with advancing age. Symptoms associated with atrial fibrillation vary and may include palpitations, fatigue, dizziness, and congestive heart failure (CHF). Though an easily recognized dysrhythmia, the etiology of atrial fibrillation is more complex. It may occur in otherwise healthy individuals, may be associated with drug and alcohol toxicities, may result from electrolyte imbalances, or be associated with significant pathologies such as coronary artery disease, pulmonary disease, hypertensive heart disease or rheumatic heart disease. Whew!

Owing both to the underlying pathology and the duration of the pathology, the treatments for atrial fibrillation vary. **In all instances, the aim of treatment is the reduction of the rapid ventricular response and the restoring of hemodynamic equilibrium.** In emergent situations (hemodynamic collapse or evidence of ischemia), synchronized cardioversion will usually be the first line of treatment. In a stable clinical situation, efforts will be made to determine the duration of atrial fibrillation. If the dysrhythmia is of recent onset (usually less than 48 hours), synchronized cardioversion is the treatment of choice. Caution is required if the patient is not anti-coagulated, due to the risk of thrombo-embolism.

When the duration is unknown, diagnostic procedures are commonly conducted. Those procedures include a transesophageal echocardiogram (TEE) to rule out blood clot formation in the left atrium caused by the out-of phase atrial depolarization and the compromised atrial muscle contraction. When there is no evidence of thrombus formation, synchronized cardioversion, drug therapy, or procedures such as radio-frequency ablation (RFA, discussed on page 64) or cryotherapy (creates electrical barriers in the atria using laser cold probes) may be employed to abolish the site causing the dysrhythmia. As an alternative to diagnostic studies, a patient may be placed on an anticoagulant prior to cardioversion or chemical conversion. Drugs commonly employed for chemical conversion include flecainide, propafenone, procainamide, sotalol, amiodarone, ibutilide and others.

Importantly, recent randomized controlled studies have demonstrated that restoring atrial fibrillation to a sinus rhythm does not improve the long term survival rate not reduce the incidence of stroke. Those study finding have shifted the treatment for long standing atrial fibrillation away from conversion to a **rate control strategy**. In other words, treatment is aimed at controlling the ventricular response rate to atrial fibrillation; the atrial fibrillation continues, but fewer atrial impulses are conducted through the AV junction to the ventricles resulting in a slower heart rate. Rate control drug therapy involves beta-blockers and calcium channel blockers.

☆ **The following are the important points remember.**

- Atrial fibrillation is an easily recognized, irregularly irregular rhythm.
- Atrial fibrillation has many causes.
- Long-standing atrial fibrillation predisposes the patient to risk of stroke.
- Generally, therapy is aimed at reducing the rapid ventricular response and restoring hemodynamic stability.
- Specific therapy depends on the underlying cause and the duration of the dysrhythmia.

Find one more example of atrial fibrillation below. Notice how the baseline *undulates* or appears to quiver!

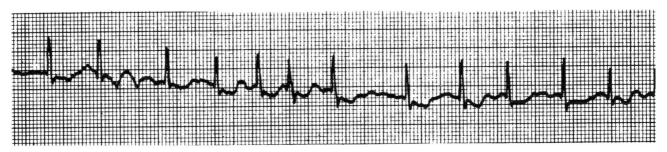

Notice the undulating baseline.

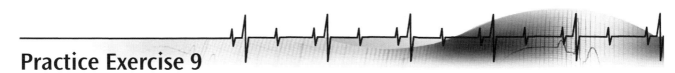

Practice Exercise 9

A. Atrial fibrillation impulses occur _____ to _____ times per minute. The AV node is unable to conduct greater than _____ impulses per minute owing to a normal _____ block.

B. If on a monitor tracing one sees *no clear P waves, an undulating baseline and a varying R-R interval,* one can suspect _____.

C.   Examine this rhythm strip closely. Then, describe what you see.

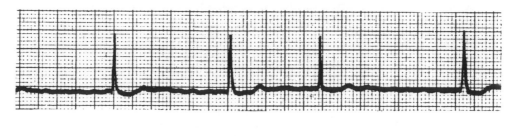

_____

_____

_____

_____

_____

_____

_____

For Feedback 9, refer to page 83.

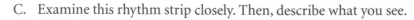

2.10 Atrial Flutter-Fibrillation ("flutter-fib")

Occasionally, a rhythm strip will be encountered that looks suspiciously like atrial flutter (F waves observed across the strip). Yet, when one attempts to measure the rate and *regularity* of the F waves, they *do not* measure out! In other words, the F waves do not occur regularly. Oftentimes, this rhythm is referred to as *impure flutter,* or more commonly, *atrial flutter-fibrillation.* It is unclear whether such a phenomenon truly exists, or whether the classification has been created for convenience sake! In all probability, the underlying disorder is that of a coarse atrial fibrillation. Fortunately, treatment is similar for the two atrial dysrhythmias.

See what you think! Try measuring the regularity of the *flutter* waves on the next strip.

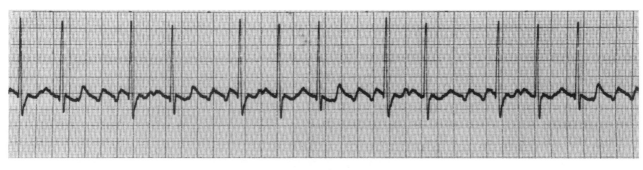

P.S.   There is no practice exercise associated with input 10. Whew!

2.11 Sick Sinus Syndrome (Brady-Tachy Syndrome)

Sick sinus syndrome is more a classification category rather than a specific diagnosis. Sick sinus syndrome is thought to be related to degeneration of the SA node cells, and is therefore usually found in patients with coronary artery disease. The rhythm of a patient with sick sinus syndrome may display sinus bradycardia, sinus tachycardia, sinus pause, atrial or supraventricular tachycardia, escape beats, etc. In other words, the monitor tracing is a "*mixed bag*" of slow and rapid rhythms arising *above* the level of the ventricles (this means that the QRS duration is within normal limits indicating normal ventricular depolarization).

Let's look at a sample strip.

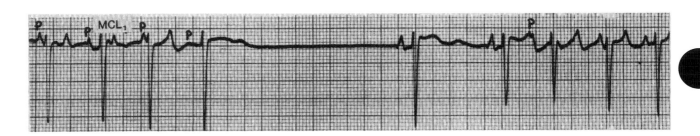

Notice the inconsistent and erratic nature of the sinus pacemaker. If you think this is a difficult rhythm strip, you are absolutely right!

Many times the patient exhibiting a sick sinus syndrome presents with a history of syncope or fainting and periods of fluttering sensations in the chest. In many cases, diagnosis is made from the analysis of continuous Holter monitor tracings (the patient wears a portable monitor while he or she goes about normal activities). Once sick sinus syndrome is identified, the object of treatment is to maintain a stable heart rate. Drugs such as atropine have little long term success in speeding up a slow sinus pacemaker discharge rate. Suppressive drugs utilized to slow rapid rhythms would further suppress the slow phases of the rhythm. Gets complicated, right?

Because of the varying nature of sick sinus syndrome, the treatment of choice involves the combination of a ventricular pacemaker (to augment heart rate during slow rhythms) and suppressant drugs (to control the rapid periods of the rhythm).

Since sick sinus syndrome is a collection of other dysrhythmias, there is no practice exercise! Such a deal!

2.12: Bypass Re-Entry Mechanisms (Wolff-Parkinson-White Syndrome) Advanced Study

Earlier in this Section, atrial re-entry mechanisms were considered as possible causes for atrial tachycardia, atrial fibrillation and atrial flutter. Here, we will consider an *example* large scale (global) re-entry mechanism caused by an accessory connection (**bypass**) between the atria and the ventricles. A bypass route connecting the atria and ventricles (bypassing the AV node) can be responsible for rapid supraventricular tachycardias (originating in either the atria of the AV junction). Wolff-Parkinson-White (WPW) Syndrome is one such re-entry dysrhythmia caused by an anomalous bypass between the atrial and ventricles.

Wolff-Parkinson-White (WPW) Syndrome is another one of those *somewhat complicated* re-entry or pre-excitation phenomena and is included here as **information, only**! An anomalous congenital connection (known as the Kent bundle) connects the atria and ventricles, bypassing the AV node. You will recall that impulses passing normally through the AV node are slowed before progressing down the conduction system. The presence of a bypass pathway can expedite conduction. A WPW supraventricular tachycardia is often precipitated by a premature impulse, often arising in the atria. Conduction of that impulse follows both the normal and bypass conduction pathways, though traveling in different directions and at different times!

The majority of WPW tachycardias demonstrate a forward (antegrade) conduction over the AV node and bundle of His pathway and a backward (retrograde) conduction over the accessory path (Kent bundle) as demonstrated in the diagram below. The sequence begins with a premature beat. The impulse (wave of excitation) conducts from the point of origin through the AV junction, across the bundle of His and down the bundle branches to the Purkinje system. Somewhere in the ventricles, the wave of excitation also encounters the bypass connection and spreads rapidly backward along the bypass path to the atria where it again initiates atrial activation and the cycle begins again! This repeated cycle of rapid retrograde conduction (circus movement stimulation) increases the rate of atrial and ventricular conduction. Other than the rapid rate, EKG findings associated with retrograde conduction across the anomalous pathway are subtle. Inverted P waves may be observed in leads II, III and a VF and the lateral leads.

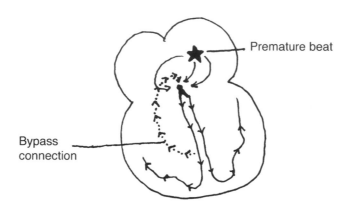

In other cases of WPW, an early-timed premature beat may find the normal conduction system refractory (not fully recovered). Because refractory tissues are immune to stimulation, the advancing premature stimulus is temporarily blocked. In this instance, the premature impulse travels rapidly forward (around the AV node) down the bypass pathway to initiate ventricular depolarization. The wave of excitation then enters the normal conduction system (Purkinje system) backwards or retrograde which causes depolarization of the remaining ventricular tissue. Examine the diagram below. Essentially, this sequence of stimulation produces a dual or double stimulation (one stimulus occurring earlier, traveling forward and faster; one stimulus traveling backward, later and slower) of the ventricles. The retrograde stimulus then continues propagating backward through the normal conduction pathway, back to re-excite the atria. The counter-clockwise rapid sequence then repeats, repeats, repeats, etc.

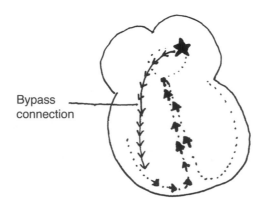

As you might suspect, this abnormal conduction and dual stimulation of ventricles produces characteristic EKG changes. In this conduction sequence, one finds a short P-R interval (less than 0.12 seconds), and a slurred beginning of the QRS known as a *delta wave*. The slurring of the initial portion of the QRS contributes to the widened QRS (a characteristic finding).

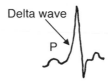

Perhaps an *imperfect* analogy may aid understanding of this type of abnormal conduction. Think of a hotel or airport with a large continuous (timed) revolving door (large enough to accommodate several folks with luggage). Typically, even though the speed of the revolving door is timed or pre-set, one can make the revolving door move faster by pushing on the door. Next to revolving doors, a regular door exists (for bellmen to re-enter the lobby or terminal). For the purpose of this analogy, assume the bellman's door cannot be opened from inside the hotel or terminal.

OK. Father and rambunctious five year old exit the hotel, entering the revolving doors together. While the father walks at the pre-set pace of door revolution, the five year old slips past the rubber revolving door guard, exists first, runs back (retrograde) into the hotel through the bellman's door, re-enters the revolving door, pushing on the door to accelerate the pace of door revolution. (Thus the revolving the door has been both powered by the normal mechanism and by a bypass mechanism.) This is so much fun, the five year old continues to repeat the process, causing the door to revolve at a faster pace than intended. This rapid circus movement will likely continue until intervention occurs. Hope the analogy helped!

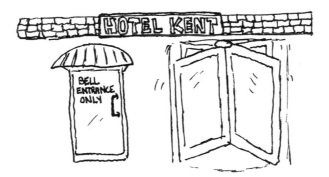

Other accessory pathways (other than the Kent bundle) can exist between the atria and ventricles, also creating rapid rhythm anomalies. As was noted earlier, one can only identify the presence of a re-entry mechanism (localized or bypass tract) through invasive diagnostic procedures. Often, it is the recurrence of a rapid supraventricular rhythm (or the inability to disrupt or control the rhythm with drug intervention) that prompts diagnostic and interventional studies and procedures.

There are three main therapeutic interventions for treating rapid WPW and related bypass re-entry dsyrhythmias. The most effective interventions are surgical ablation or radiofrequency ablation (RFA) which destroy or disrupt the anomalous bypass pathway, thereby disabling the abnormal atrial–ventricular conduction route. Drug therapy (a less effective alternative) intended to disrupt or slow rapid supraventricular dysrhythmias requires forethought. Drugs which act by slowing conduction across the AV node can exacerbate rapid conduction along the bypass tract. Thus, drug therapy often involves a combination of agents, those which block conduction in the accessory bypass path (class 1C or III drugs) combined with an AV nodal blocker.

The above discussion of accessory path anomalies is informational. You will be relieved to know, there is no accompanying practice exercise!

⌁ Feedback 1

If your answers are similar to mine, you have the basics down pat! If you are "shaky" on any of the points covered, review Section 1 one more time. (You'll be happy you did!) ☺

A.   The heart rate in this rhythm strip is approximately <u>70</u> beats per minute.

B.   The rhythm is regular.

C.   Each QRS complex is preceded by a <u>P wave</u>.

D.   All P waves are <u>uniform</u> in appearance.

E.   Each P wave is followed by a <u>QRS</u>.

F.   All QRS complexes are <u>uniform</u> in appearance.

G.   The P-R interval is <u>constant</u> and measures 0.12 seconds.

H.   Therefore, this is a **sinus** rhythm.

The five principles used in dysrhythmia interpretation are:

1.   First, determine if the rhythm is <u>regular</u>.

2.   Second, determine the heart <u>rate</u>.

3.   Next determine <u>atrial</u> activity.

4.   Then determine <u>ventricular</u> activity.

5.   The final step involves determining if a relationship exists between <u>atrial and ventricular</u> activity.

⌁ Feedback 2

You're doing great!

1. A.   The heart rate in this strip is **approximately** <u>70</u> beats per minute.

    B.   The P waves are all <u>uniform</u> in appearance.

    C.   A <u>P</u> wave precedes each QRS complex.

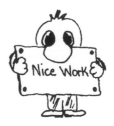

D. The QRS complexes are <u>uniform</u> in appearance.

E. A <u>QRS</u> follows every P wave.

F. The rhythm is (regular.)

G. This is a **sinus rhythm**.

2. A. The heart rate in this strip is **approximately** <u>90</u> beats per minute.

B. The <u>P</u> waves are all <u>uniform</u> in appearance.

C. A P wave precedes each QRS complex.

D. The QRS complexes are <u>uniform</u> in appearance.

E. A <u>QRS</u> follows every P wave.

F. The rhythm is (irregular)

G. This is a **sinus arrhythmia**.

3. Usually, the irregularity found in sinus arrhythmia is related to <u>respiration</u>.

Just for review, here are the EKG criteria for a sinus arrhythmia.

EKG Criteria for Sinus Arrhythmia

Rhythm: Slightly irregular. The P-P interval or R-R interval varies in duration.
Rate: 60–100.
P waves: Normal configuration.
QRS: Normal configuration and duration.
Conduction: Each P wave is followed by a QRS; the P-R interval is constant.

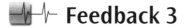 **Feedback 3**

Nice work!

A. The term *bradycardia* implies that the heart rate is less than <u>60 beats</u> per minute.

B. Rhythm strip 2 is similar to strip 1 in the following ways:

1. In each strip, the P waves appear uniform.

2. A P wave precedes each QRS.

3. In each strip, the QRS complexes appear uniform.

4. A QRS complex follows each P wave.

5. The rhythm is regular in each strip.

Rhythm strip 2 differs from rhythm strip 1 in this way:

In rhythm strip 1 (sinus rhythm), the heart rate falls between 60 and 100 beats per minute.

In rhythm strip 2, the heart rate is 41 beats per minute, falling below the normal range of 60–100 beats per minute. (I have used the Trusty Guide on page 39 to determine the heart rate!!)

The second strip demonstrates a sinus bradycardia.

Just for review, following are the EKG criteria for a sinus bradycardia.

EKG Criteria for Sinus Bradycardia

Rhythm:	Regular.
Rate:	Less than 60.
P waves:	Normal configuration.
QRS:	Normal configuration and duration.
Conduction:	Each P wave is followed by a QRS; the P-R interval is constant.

 ## Feedback 4

What a pro!

A. The P waves are all uniform in appearance.

   A P wave precedes each QRS complex.

   A QRS complex follows every P wave.

   QRS complexes measure approximately 0.08 seconds in duration.

   The P-R interval is constant and measures 0.16 seconds.

   The rhythm is regular.

   The heart rate is 50 beats per minute.

   This is a sinus bradycardia!

   Did I fool you? Hope Not!!!

B. The P waves are all uniform in appearance.

   A P wave precedes each QRS complex.

   A QRS complex follows every P wave.

   The rhythm is regular.

   The heart rate is 150 beats per minute.

   QRS complexes (rS complexes) are approximately 0.08 seconds in duration.

   The P-R interval is constant and measures approximately 0.12 seconds.

   This is a **sinus tachycardia**.

C. The treatment for sinus tachycardia consists of <u>finding and treating its underlying cause</u> (i.e., fever, heart failure, anxiety, etc.).

Just for review, following are the EKG criteria associated with a sinus tachycardia.

EKG Criteria for Sinus Tachycardia

Rhythm:	Regular.
Rate:	100–160.
P waves:	Normal configuration.
QRS:	Normal configuration and duration.
Conduction:	Each P wave is followed by a QRS; the P-R interval is constant.

Feedback 5

How did you do? Remember, in wandering atrial pacemaker (W.A.P.), all QRS complexes will be preceded by a P wave. . . . It's just that the P waves may look different! The rhythm will be slightly irregular owing to the varying atrial pacemaker. See my art below!

This is what my *freestyle* W.A.P looks like

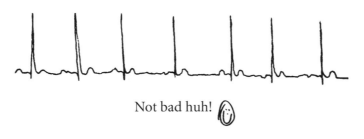

Not bad huh!

Feedback 6

Nice work! If you are becoming frustrated, remember . . . **All great minds are frustrated!**

A. Beat 2, beat 6, and beat 10 are premature. The contour of the P waves in the premature beats is slightly different from the normal P waves. The underlying rhythm is a sinus rhythm. A QRS complex follows every P wave. All the QRS complexes are uniform in appearance, measuring approximately 2½ small squares or 0.10 seconds. The P-R interval of the underlying rhythm measures approximately 0.20 seconds, the upper limits of normal. The P-R interval of the premature beats is slightly longer. A slight pause follows each P.A.C.

B. In this example, the premature atrial impulses occur during the repolarization phase of the preceding beats. Thus, the ventricular tissue is unable to respond to the stimulation. Therefore, the P.A.C.s are blocked or not conducted. The P-R interval of all conducted beats measures 0.24 seconds, indicating delayed conduction.

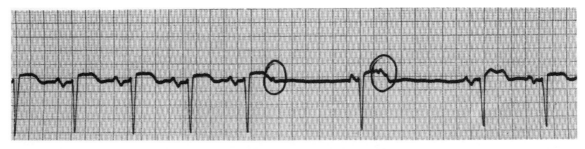

Non-conducted or blocked P.A.C.s interrupt a sinus rhythm.

Just for review purposes, here are the EKG criteria for P.A.C.s.

EKG Criteria for Premature Atrial Contractions

Rhythm:	Irregular owing to the disruption caused by premature beats.
Rate:	Usually normal (60–100 beats per minute).
P waves:	The P waves appear prematurely and differ in contour from the normal P waves.
QRS:	Usually normal configuration and duration.
Conduction:	A normal QRS usually follows the abnormal P wave. There is a slight pause or delay before the next normal beat. (Of course, if the P.A.C. is blocked, it is not followed by a QRS!)

Feedback 7

How did you do? Sometimes this material is difficult. If you feel a bit insecure, try reading the section one more time.

A. The rhythm is regular. There is a PQRST cycle in each cardiac complex.

B. The heart rate is approximately 200 beats per minute.

C. Each QRS is preceded by a P wave. All P waves look uniform.

D. Each P wave is followed by a QRS. All QRS complexes appear uniform. The QRS measures 0.12 seconds.

E. This rhythm is *probably* an atrial tachycardia, though if you answered supraventricular tachycardia, you are *absolutely* correct!

F. The Valsalva maneuver consists of having the patient hold his or her breath and bear down.

Just for review, here are the EKG criteria for atrial tachycardia.

EKG Criteria for Atrial Tachycardia

Rhythm:	Regular.
Rate:	160–220 beats per minute.
P waves:	May be buried in the QRS complexes or T waves and not visible; or may be similar to the contour of sinus P waves.
QRS:	Usually normal, but may be widened.
Conduction:	A ventricular complex follows each P wave by the same interval.

G. Atrial tachycardia may be precipitated by any of the following events or conditions.

☒ A P.A.C. firing rapidly and repeatedly   ☒ Stimulants

☒ A P.A.C. entering a re-entry circuit   ☒ EKG practice exercises

☒ Emotional stress

H. Atrial tachycardia is a regular, rapid rhythm (rate 160–220) with visible, uniform P waves. The dysrhythmia is a result of: a single ectopic site within the atria firing repeatedly; or, a P.A.C. entering an anomalous circuit, creating a re-entry phenomenon. The QRS is usually within normal limits. Multifocal atrial tachycardia is a rapid, irregular rhythm (rate >100 beats per minute) produced by multiple (at least 3) ectopic sites within the atria firing repeatedly. Distinctly different P waves are visible.

I. RFA, radio frequency ablation, is a treatment for supraventricular tachyarrhythmias. RFA involves delivering high frequency energy via catheter into tissue causing the dysrhythmia. RFA destroys the tissue causing the dysrhythmia. It is particularly effective in destroying anomalous conducting circuits responsible for re-entry tachycardias.

Feedback 8

Excellent work!

A. There are no P waves. Rather, there are saw-toothed atrial waves ("F" waves) occurring regularly at a rate of 300 per minute. The QRS complexes occur irregularly owing to variable physiologic block. The QRS complexes appear uniform and measure approximately 0.08 seconds. One would need to count the heart rate for one full minute!

B. The atrial rate in atrial flutter varies between <u>220</u> and <u>350</u> impulses per minute.

The AV node is unable to conduct greater than <u>220</u> impulses per minute. Beyond this rate, a <u>physiologic</u> block occurs.

Just for review, here are the EKG criteria for atrial flutter.

EKG Criteria for Atrial Flutter

Rhythm:	Atrial activity occurs in a regular pattern. The ventricular rhythm may be regular or irregular, depending on the degree of physiologic block.
Rate:	The atrial rate ("F" waves) occurs between 220–350 per minute. The ventricular rate (QRSs) may vary from 60–150 depending on the number of impulses passing through the AV junction.
P waves:	There are characteristic atrial oscillations—"saw-toothed" waves ("F" waves) ranging between 220–350 per minute. *No isoelectric line is visible.*
QRS:	The QRS complexes appear uniform and usually measure less than 0.12 seconds.
Conduction:	Usually ½, ⅓, or ¼ of the flutter (atrial) impulses will be conducted to the ventricles.

Feedback 9

What a Pro you are !

A. Atrial impulses occur <u>400 to 600</u> times per minute. The AV node is unable to conduct greater than <u>220</u> impulses per minute, owing to a normal <u>physiologic</u> block.

B. If on a monitor tracing one sees no clear P waves, an undulating baseline and a varying R-R interval, one can suspect <u>atrial fibrillation</u>.

INTERPRETATION

C. This rhythm is irregularly irregular. There are no clear P waves or P-R intervals. Atrial activity appears rapid and chaotic. The baseline appears to undulate. The QRS complexes are normal in shape and are less than 0.12 seconds in duration. The QRS complexes occur irregularly—the R-R interval varies. One would need a full minute strip to accurately determine heart rate. Most of the atrial impulses reaching the AV node are blocked. Those impulses passing through the AV node are conducted normally.

Just for review, here are the EKG criteria for atrial fibrillation.

EKG Criteria for Atrial Fibrillation

Rhythm:	The ventricular rhythm is totally irregular.
Rate:	The heart rate varies according to the number of atrial impulses conducted through the AV node to the ventricles.
P waves:	No P waves or P-R intervals; instead, there are rapid, small, irregular waves.
QRS:	The QRS's are normal in shape and duration, but occur irregularly. The R-R interval varies.
Conduction:	The conduction is bizarre. Most of the atrial impulses which reach the AV node are blocked. Those impulses that pass through the AV node are normally conducted.

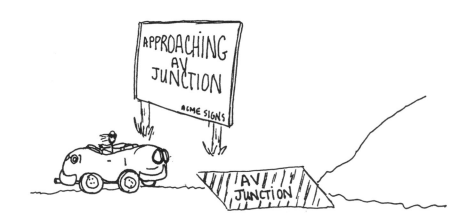

Notes

Notes

_____

_____

_____

_____

_____

_____

_____

_____

_____

_____

_____

_____

_____

_____

_____

_____

_____

_____

_____

Junctional Escape and Ectopic Rhythms

Objectives

When you have completed Section 3, you will be able to describe or identify

1. junctional escape rhythms and junctional escape beats
2. premature junctional beats
3. junctional tachycardia

3.1   Junctional Escape Rhythm

You're back again! Persistent creature, aren't you! Though there are several other abnormal atrial rhythms, those will be reserved for more advanced lessons! Whew!

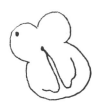The heart has many potential pacemaker centers—the SA node, the atria, the AV junctional tissues, and the ventricles. Only the *dominant* or the *fastest pacemaker* (highest automaticity) will normally control the heart. If the sinus node fails to discharge an impulse *or* if the sinus impulse fails to be conducted *or* if the sinus rate of discharge is inadequate, a lower and slower (more distal) pacemaker may assume the role of pacemaker. (Persistent or intermittent failure of the sinus mechanism may occur secondary to myocardial infarction, ischemia, hypoxia, vagal stimulation or degeneration of the SA node cells, as is often associated with sick-sinus syndrome.)

A lower or more distal pacemaker initiated rhythm is known as an *escape rhythm*—a safety mechanism of the heart. In some respects, a lower (escape) pacemaker resembles an emergency power generator that "kicks in" when the normal current fails. And, like a generator, the escape pacemaker is not necessary when normal electrical activity resumes.

 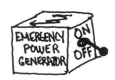   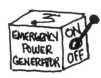

When an escape rhythm is initiated in the AV junctional tissue, it is known as a *junctional rhythm* or a *junctional escape rhythm*. The junctional pacemaker *usually* discharges an impulse 40–60 times per minute (though it may discharge slower or faster).

You are no doubt thinking that the term *escape* is a peculiar name for a rhythm. Basically, the term implies that a lower, more distal pacemaker has *escaped* from the control of the sinus node. In other words, although lower tissues have the ability to serve as pacemakers, their inherent rates of impulse discharge are slower than the sinus node. Therefore, the faster sinus impulse controls heart rate. In effect, the faster sinus impulse causes depolarization before lower, more distal pacemakers have the opportunity to generate pacemaking impulses! Only when the sinus pacemaker fails, slows or is interrupted will a lower pacemaker assume control of the rhythm.

An escape rhythm *always occurs* as a *secondary phenomenon*, never as a primary disorder. In other words, an escape rhythm serves as a safety mechanism when higher order pacemakers are disrupted or fail.

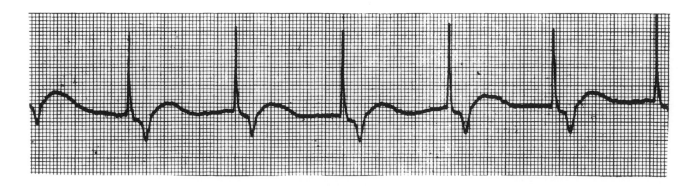

The previous rhythm strip demonstrates a junctional or junctional escape rhythm with a rate of 50 beats per minute. You will note that the rhythm is regular, there are no visible P waves and the QRS is of normal duration. One can expect to see a junctional escape rhythm *when the sinus pacemaker fails or is depressed.* If the patient has a sinus bradycardia (less than 60 beats per minute), his heart rate may be *slower* than the AV junctional pacemaker, which has the ability to initiate a rhythm at a rate of 40–60 beats per minute. In this case, the AV junctional pacemaker might become the dominant pacemaker because it has a faster rate. It is helpful to remember that the *AV node itself has no pacemaker fibers.* Only the lower portion of intranodal pathways and the bundle of His have pacemaker properties.

Before going further, let's explore a junctional escape rhythm in detail.

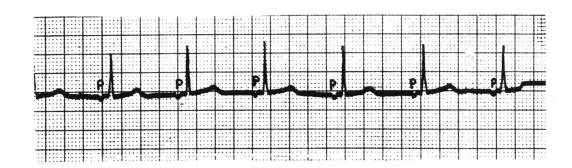

The first thing one notices is that the rhythm is *regular.* The customary junctional heart rate is between *40 and 60 beats* per minute. What about atrial activity? You will recall that P waves denote atrial depolarization.

In a true junctional rhythm, the P wave (if visible) is usually inverted 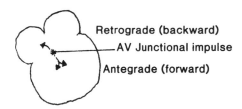 in leads II, III, and aVF. (Atrial activity is usually most clearly evident in leads II, III and aVF). In a junctional escape rhythm, P waves may occur *before, during,* or *after* the QRS. Because of its location, the AV junctional pacemaker impulse will be conducted both in an antegrade (forward) and a retrograde (backward) fashion.

Retrograde (backward)
AV Junctional impulse
Antegrade (forward)

In other words, when the impulse originates in the AV junction, the impulse must travel upward and backward to activate the atria, and downward to activate the ventricles. The impulse traveling to the ventricles will be conducted in a normal forward fashion following the normal conduction pathway. In other words, the QRS will be *"of normal duration"* (less than 0.12 seconds).

Atrial activation, however, is a bit more complicated. To fully understand atrial activation, one must recognize that the junctional impulse must travel in a backward or retrograde fashion to initiate atria depolarization.

The junctional pacemaking impulse travels in the *opposite* direction of a normal SA impulse. Retrograde or backward activation of the atria results in abnormal P waves, usually inverted in leads II, III and aVF.

Now, we must do a bit of abstract thinking! The junctional impulse must travel both to the atria and to the ventricles. If the junctional impulse reaches the (1) atria before the impulse traveling downward reaches the (2) ventricles, a P wave will appear just before the QRS complex. The P wave occurring before the QRS tells the observer that atrial activation occurred before ventricular activation. The inverted nature of the P wave suggests that atrial stimulation occurred in a backward fashion.

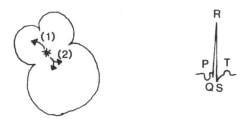

Additionally, the P-R interval of the junctional beat will be of *short* duration, *less than* three small squares, or *less than 0.12 seconds.* Some authorities believe the P-R interval will be 0.10 seconds or less! No doubt you are wondering why the P-R interval is short! Since the AV junctional pacemaker is in close proximity to the atria, the impulse "travel time" is short. Therefore, the P-R interval is short!

It should be pointed out that a P.A.C. may also have an inverted P wave occurring before the QRS if it is initiated low in the atria. When an ectopic impulse (P.A.C.) arises low in the atria, the time interval required for the impulse to travel through the conduction system would be normal (a PR of 0.12–0.20 or shorter)!

To review then, the above diagram demonstrates that the atria depolarize first (the P wave), followed by ventricular depolarization (the QRS). Notice that the P wave is inverted and the P-R interval is short.

The following rhythm strip demonstrates a junctional escape rhythm with a rate of 55 per minute. Notice the inverted P waves and the shortened P-R intervals occurring before each QRS. P waves occurring before the QRS indicate that atrial depolarization precedes ventricular depolarization.

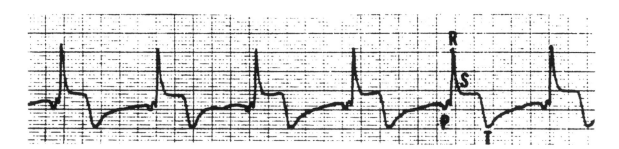

In contrast, let's suppose that the AV junctional pacemaker impulse reaches and activates the ventricles before it reaches and activates the atria.

The QRS represents ventricular depolarization. The P wave represents atrial depolarization. So when the ventricles depolarize before the atria, guess what we see?!

You're right. . . . the QRS coming before the P wave!

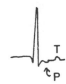

The rhythm strip below demonstrates a junctional escape rhythm, rate 88 per minute. Since the rate of this escape rhythm is faster than the inherent AV junctional rate (40–60), one might elect to call it an accelerated junctional escape rhythm or an accelerated junctional rhythm. *It is important to specify the rate of any rhythm!*

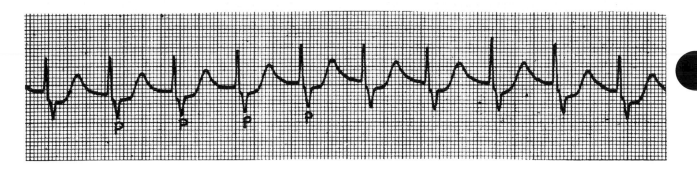

Looking at the above strip, one can now intellectually say this is a junctional escape rhythm with ventricular depolarization occurring before atrial depolarization (because the QRS comes before the P wave). If this is confusing to you, it simply means that you're in the same boat with everyone else! Usually escape rhythms are regular. You will notice that the rate is approximately 88 per minute, somewhat faster than a typical junctional rhythm. It is important to remember that even though a junctional pacemaker has a common or inherent rate (40–60 per minute), the pacemaker is not limited to those rate parameters!

Before progressing further, examine the above rhythm strip again. The rhythm is regular. The rate is 88 per minute. **This is a pop quiz!** Why isn't the above rhythm a sinus rhythm? The answer, of course, is that there is no upright P wave. You knew that, right?!

Finally, what would you expect to find if the junctional pacemaker impulse reached and activated the atria and ventricles at almost the same time?

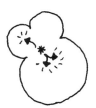

That's a tough one! Take time to think before reading on.

If the impulse traveling backward or retrograde reaches the atria at the same time that the impulse traveling forward or antegrade reaches the ventricles, the P wave will not be obvious. It is said to be "buried" or "hiding" in the QRS.

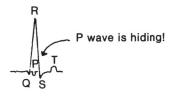

This "hiding" concept is a bit difficult to grasp, so let's move away from EKG's for a moment. Imagine that I'm in a shopping center, driving around in hopes of finding a parking space. I spy one, so I quickly drive toward it. However, I neglect to notice a big truck driving toward the empty space from the opposite direction!

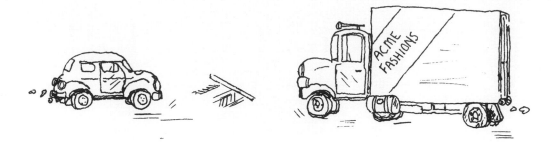

Later, when a rescue helicopter pilot is viewing the accident scene, he only sees the truck!

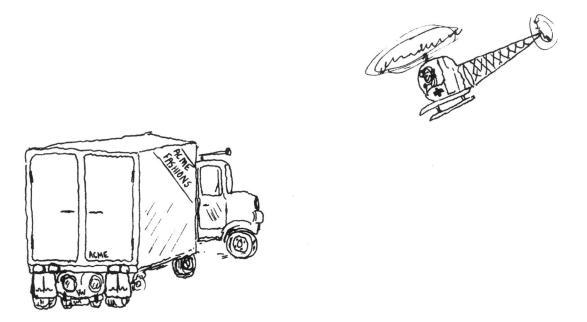

The VW is buried or hiding! But, we know it's there! It simply is not visible because the truck is so large.

The monitoring electrodes have a distant view of activity much like the helicopter pilot! External monitoring electrodes "sense" internal electrical events, but "sense" only one electrical event when two events occur simultaneously. Thus, when atrial and ventricular depolarization occur at the same time, the monitoring electrodes will sense one electrical event and the monitor will record the larger QRS.

Does that help? Hope so!

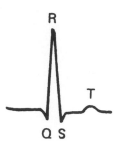

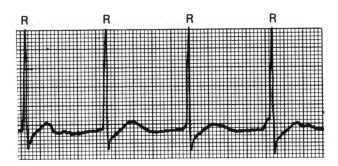

When I observe a monitor tracing like the one above, I know the rhythm *cannot* be of sinus origin because there are no upright ⌒ P waves occurring before the QRS complexes. In fact, there are no visible P waves!. Yet, the QRS is of normal duration (less than 0.12 seconds), so I know the ventricles were activated in a normal fashion. Therefore, this must be a junctional rhythm with P waves "hiding" in the QRS complexes. Thus, I conclude that atrial and ventricular depolarization have occurred during the same time frame. ☺

Some of the more frequently encountered causes of junctional escape rhythms are digitalis toxicity, hypoxia, acute infections, vagal influence, and myocardial infarction. A small artery nourishes the sinus node. In about 75% of the population, this small artery is supplied by the right coronary artery (RCA). It stands to reason that compromise of the RCA (disease or damage) may cause interruption of the sinus mechanism. This frequently results in a junctional escape rhythm (a lower, more distal pacemaker assumes control).

 If, for some reason, the SA node fails to discharge (sinus arrest) or if the impulse is blocked within the sinus mechanism (sino-atrial block), an AV junctional pacemaker may take over the rhythm, as evident in the following strip.

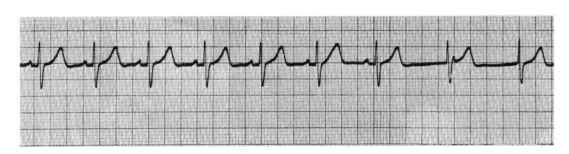

Notice that following complex 7, the sinus mechanism is disrupted, allowing an AV junctional pacemaker to escape or take control of the rhythm.

Here is another example.

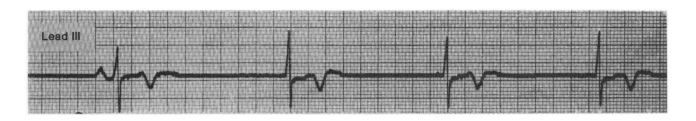

This rhythm strip demonstrates failure of the sinus pacemaker. Notice that the first complex is a normal sinus beat followed by a 2.0 second pause. A junctional escape pacemaker then emerges to assume control of the rhythm. Note that the rate of the junctional escape rhythm is approximately 37 beats per minute. (Though escape rhythms are generally regular, at *start up* one may observe some variation in rhythm regularity). There are no P waves visible either prior to or following the QRS. The QRS is of normal duration. Here, atrial and ventricular activation are occurring in concert (the P wave is hiding in the QRS).

To review then, any disruption or failure of the sinus pacemaker may result in an escape rhythm (a safety mechanism). In order to determine the origin of the escape rhythm, one must look closely at *all* of the wave forms. If the QRS is of normal duration (less than 0.12 seconds), we will soon learn that the rhythm cannot be initiated in the ventricles. The absence of normal, upright P waves in leads II, III, and aVF indicates that the rhythm is probably not of sinus or atrial origin. In other words, the rhythm is most likely of AV junctional origin. If a P wave is observed, it will occur prior to, or after the QRS, and will be inverted in leads II, III, and aVF. If the inverted P wave occurs before the QRS, the P-R interval *must measure less than* 0.12 seconds to qualify as a junctional rhythm.

Looking at this next strip, you can see that the QRS occurs before the P wave, so ventricular depolarization occurs before atrial depolarization. Easy, huh?

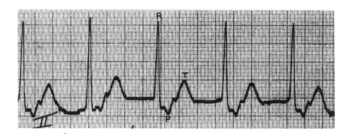

If you remember the discussion on premature atrial contractions (page 54), you will recall there is a pause following the P.A.C. which allows the sinus pacemaker to reset itself. When a premature beat is followed by a long pause, a junctional escape beat may occur before the sinus pacemaker can regain control. Do you know why that occurs?

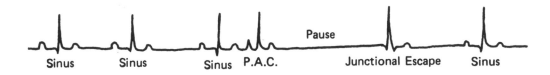

Well . . . the AV junction is behaving normally, conducting all impulses progressing down from the atria. Then unexpectedly, there is a pause—no impulse arrives at the AV junction. Since the AV junction can initiate pacemaker impulses 40–60 times per minute, it slips in a junctional beat (junctional escape beat) to ensure that the heart rate does not fall to an exceedingly unhealthy rate. Had the sinus pacemaker failed to resume control, the AV junctional pacemaker could have maintained the heart rate at 40–60 beats per minute!

The important point to remember is that escape beats or escape rhythms are *NEVER* primary phenomena. They always result *secondary* to another event or problem. Therefore, escape rhythms are never terminated. Abolishing an escape rhythm would be analgous to turning off the emergency generator when the power is out!! Rather, the aims of treatment are to support the escape pacemaker and to correct the primary disorder.

It is important to understand that a patient may experience hemodynamic instability owing to both a slow heart rate and the loss of atrial activity (atrial kick). Therefore, it may be necessary to augment the heart rate using either atropine or a transcutaneous pacemaker. Atropine may promote an increase in the rate of AV junctional discharge, thereby increasing heart rate! Dopamine may also be added to the drug regimen to augment low blood pressure.

Are you ready to try some practice? Hope so!

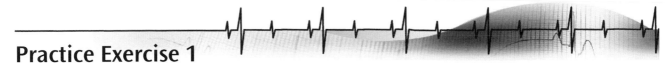

Practice Exercise 1

Examine this strip closely. I'll help!

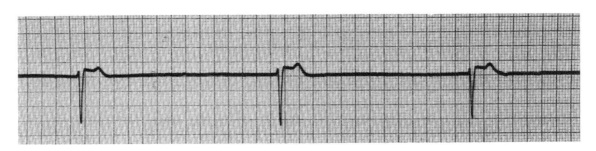

A. Is the rhythm regular? _____

The heart rate is approximately _____ beats per minute.

Determine atrial activity. Are there P waves? _____

_____

_____

Determine ventricular activity. _____

_____

_____

The QRS measures _____ seconds.

Because the QRSs are of normal duration, I know that the impulses are conducted normally

_____.

This rhythm strip must be a _____ rhythm.

Since there are no obvious P waves, I must conclude that atrial and ventricular depolarization are occurring

_____. Thus, the P waves are hidden in the QRS complexes.

Now, try this one on your own. Describe all that you see! (I added a label to assist.)

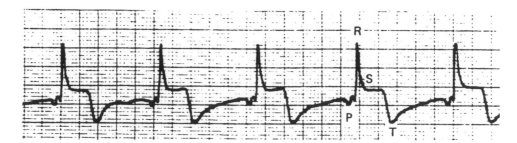

B. _____

_____

_____

_____

_____

For Feedback 1, refer to page 101.

input section   3.2   Premature Junctional Beats

Junctional beats can occur either early (premature) or late (escape). Escape junctional beats occur secondary to failure or disruption of a higher pacemaker. Premature beats, on the other hand, usually represent irritability of the involved tissue and interrupt the normal or underlying rhythm.

A *premature junctional beat* is an impulse that arises in an excitable or irritable site or focus in the AV junctional tissue. You will remember that the AV node itself has no pacemaking capability! Like junctional escape beats, a premature junctional beat must travel both retrograde and antegrade to activate the atria and ventricles, respectively. In other words, an inverted P wave may occur before, during, or after the QRS complex.

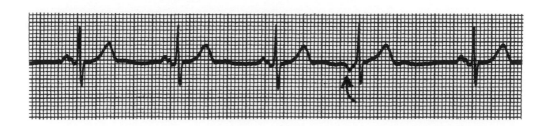

The location of the P wave indicates the sequence of atrial activation.

An occasional premature junctional beat may be found in the healthy individual. However, recurrent premature junctional beats are usually associated with rheumatic heart disease or coronary artery disease.

Examine this rhythm strip carefully.

The first thing that catches the eye is an early or premature beat occurring earlier than the next expected sinus beat (see arrow). Before diagnosing the premature beat, notice that the underlying rhythm is a borderline sinus bradycardia with a rate of approximately 58 beats per minute. It is always helpful to determine the basic or underlying rhythm and rate before analyzing abnormal beats.

So what about this abnormal beat? Is there a P wave? Yes, there is a P wave, but it's upside-down or inverted. Ah-ha! Maybe this is a premature junctional beat! 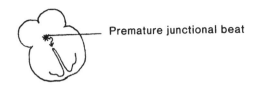 The P-R interval of the premature beat, measures a "hair" less than 3 small squares or 0.12 seconds. You will recall that to be qualified as a beat of junctional origin, *the P-R interval must be short*. The QRS of the premature beat appears similar to the QRS complexes in the normal underlying rhythm. This is to be expected since ventricular activation usually occurs in a normal fashion!

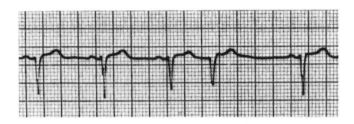

Premature junctional beat

Because the premature junctional impulse travels normally down the conduction pathway, ventricular depolarization is unaltered. Therefore, the QRS complexes are of normal duration.

Now, analyze the following rhythm strip.

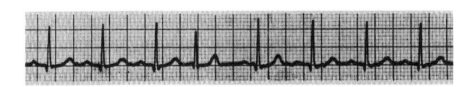

The underlying rhythm in the above strip is sinus rhythm, with a heart rate of approximately 75 beats per minute. If you have measured accurately, you will note that the QRS measures two small squares or 0.08 seconds. Beat 4 occurs prematurely. If you look closely at the premature beat, there is no obvious P wave, but the QRS is identical to the QRS complexes in the underlying rhythm. This must be a premature junctional beat! Because there is no obvious P wave in this premature junctional complex, we can assume that the atria and ventricles are depolarizing during the same period of time. In other words, the P wave is hiding in the QRS.

Next, examine this rhythm strip.

Here we see a premature junctional beat (the fourth complex) interrupting a borderline sinus tachycardia. You will notice that again, there is no evidence of a P wave occurring either before or after the premature beat. Thus, atrial and ventricular activation are occurring at the same time!

Usually premature junctional beats are merely observed and noted. If however, the patient becomes symptomatic, drug therapy may be initiated.

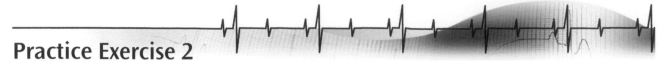

Practice Exercise 2

Now try some practice.

Describe everything that you see!

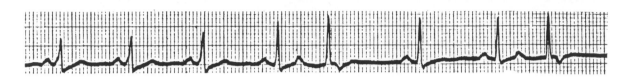

A. _____

_____

_____

_____

_____

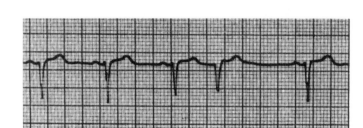

B. _____

_____

_____

_____

_____

For Feedback 2, refer to page 102.

input section 3.3 Junctional Tachycardia

When three or more rapid, ectopic junctional beats occur in succession, it is termed *AV junctional tachycardia*. It may be paroxysmal in nature, or it may persist. Usually the heart rate ranges between 120–200 beats per minute. If P waves are visible, they will occur before or after the QRS complexes. The QRS is *usually* of normal duration (less than 0.12 seconds) since the impulse is conducted normally through the ventricular conduction system. Junctional tachycardia may result from a single ectopic focus firing repeatedly. More commonly, however, junctional tachycardia occurs secondary to a re-entry circuit that allows a circus-like repeat stimulation.

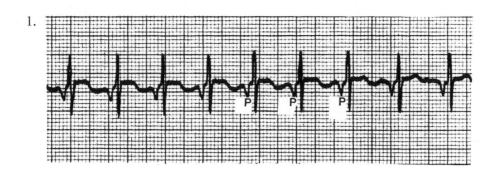

1.

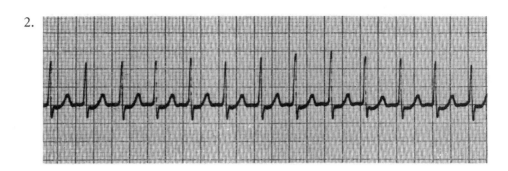

2.

Above are two rhythm strips demonstrating AV junctional tachycardia. Notice, the rhythms are *regular* and rapid.

Strip 1 demonstrates a heart rate of approximately 125 per minute. An inverted P wave precedes each QRS complex. The P-R interval is short, measuring less than 0.12 seconds. In this example, atrial depolarization occurs prior to ventricular depolarization.

Strip 2 shows a regular rhythm with a rate of 150 per minute. There are no P waves visible before or after the QRS complexes, and the QRS duration is within normal limits. In this instance, the atria and the ventricles are depolarizing at the same time (the P wave is hiding in a QRS).

We won't dwell on the subject of AV junctional tachycardia for one *good* reason! . . .

. . . When the heart rate is rapid, it is usually *impossible* to determine whether a P wave is related to the preceding QRS complex or whether it is occurring before the QRS. In fact, it is often difficult to discriminate the various wave forms when the heart rate is rapid!

Now, examine this strip.

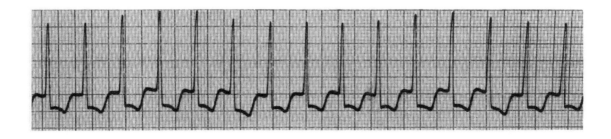

In the above rhythm strip, the various wave forms are difficult to discriminate! I am uncertain if P waves are present. Because the duration of the QRS is within normal limits, I know this is either an atrial or a junctional tachycardia. Therefore, I am simply going to call this rhythm a **supraventricular tachycardia** with a heart rate of approximately 136 per minute. (I used the heart rate guide on page 39!)

Often, it is impossible to discriminate atrial tachycardia from an AV junctional tachycardia. The terms *supraventricular tachycardia* simply means the heart rate is rapid, the QRS complexes are within normal limits (less than 0.12 seconds) and it is uncertain whether P waves are present. The term *supraventricular* indicates that the initiating pacemaker is above the ventricles, somewhere in the atria or AV junction (as evidenced by the narrow QRS, less than 0.12 seconds). Supraventricular tachycardia is one of the *few* terms worth remembering! You will also hear it called SVT!

In any event, the clinical significance of AV junctional tachycardia is similar to that of atrial tachycardia. The rapid heart rate reduces cardiac output because the volume of blood ejected with each contraction is decreased as a result of the shortened ventricular filling time . . . just like the flushing-toilet analogy page 59. However, it is important to note that the patient with junctional tachycardia will be compromised from two points of view: (1) the rapid ventricular rate, and (2) the loss of appropriately synchronized atrial activity (atrial kick).

A decrease in cardiac output can lead to left ventricular failure, and may precipitate chest pain due to the increased oxygen demand and consumption of the cardiac muscle. The treatment for any rapid supraventricular rhythm (atrial tachycardia, junctional tachycardia) is similar. The object of treatment is to reduce the rapid ventricular rate and restore sinus rhythm. Typically, a beta blocker, a calcium blocker or amiodarone will be administered. Amiodarone is the drug of choice in the presence of poor cardiac output or congestive heart failure. If unsuccessful, or if the patient is compromised, synchronized cardioversion may be employed.

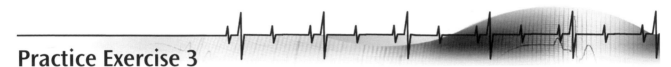

Practice Exercise 3

A   Describe this rhythm strip in detail!

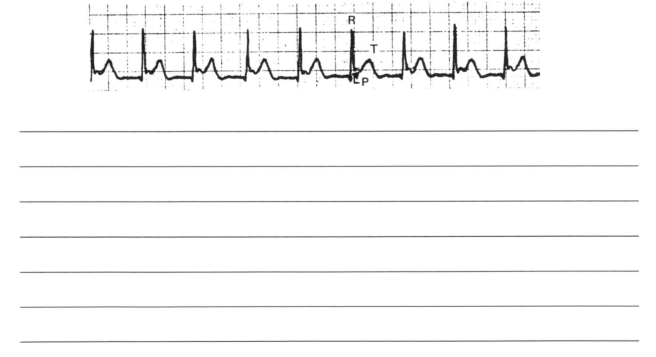

_____

_____

_____

_____

_____

_____

B.   If one observes a rapid rhythm with narrow QRS complexes and no distinguishable P waves, one can term

the dysrhythmia a _____.

 For Feedback 3, refer to page 103.

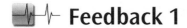 **Feedback 1**

Pass GO and collect $200.00. You're doing a great job! 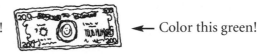 ← Color this green!
Strip 1

A. The rhythm is *slow* and regular.

The heart rate is approximately <u>21</u> beats per minute . . . $70\overline{)1500}$ with quotient 21

I don't see any P waves anywhere!

The ventricular complexes are occurring regularly and they all appear uniform.

The QRS measures <u>0.08</u> seconds.

Because the QRSs are within normal limits, I know that the impulses are conducted normally through <u>the ventricles</u>.

This rhythm is a <u>junctional escape</u> rhythm.

Since there are no obvious P waves, I must conclude that atrial and ventricular depolarization are occurring <u>in the same period of time</u>. Thus, the P wave is hidden in the QRS complex!

P.S. Treatment would consist of speeding up the heart rate!

Strip 2. . . . Hope your answers are <u>similar</u> to mine!

B. The rhythm is <u>regular</u>.

The heart rate is between <u>50–60</u> beats per minute.

An upside-down or <u>inverted</u> P wave precedes each QRS complex. All the inverted P waves appear uniform. The P-R interval is <u>short</u>, less than three small squares, or <u>less than 0.12 seconds</u>.

The QRS complexes are occurring <u>regularly</u>, and all are <u>uniform</u> in appearance.

The QRS measures slightly less than 3 small squares.

Because the QRSs are less than 3 small squares, I know that the impulses are conducted normally through the ventricles.

This is a <u>junctional escape rhythm</u>. The inverted P waves occurring <u>shortly</u> before each QRS complex indicate that the junctional pacemaker activates the atria before reaching and activating the ventricles.

Just for review, here are the EKG properties of a junctional escape rhythm.

Properties of a Junctional Escape Rhythm

- The rhythm is usually regular
- The pacemaker impulse formation is usually slower (40–60 beats per minute but may be slower) than that of the sinus pacemaker.
- It occurs secondary to failure or slowing of the sinus pacemaker.
- If visible, P waves are inverted or upside down in leads II, III, and aVF.
- P waves may occur before, during, or after the QRS.
- The QRS complexes occur regularly, are uniform in appearance, and normally measure less than 0.12 seconds.

Extra! Extra! Bonus on next page!

Bonus

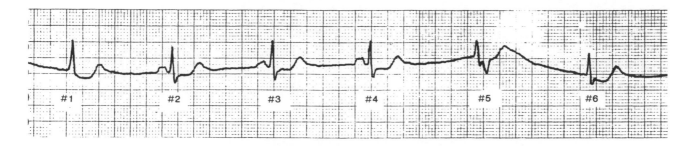

I saw this elderly patient today and she wasn't feeling well at all! I thought you might enjoy looking at her tracing with me.

Beats 2, 3, and 4 tell me that her underlying heart rhythm is a sinus bradycardia with a heart rate of less than 50 beats per minute. Apparently, her sinus node was feeling a bit "under the weather," so it periodically failed to fire an impulse. Consequently, the good ol' AV junction came through to save the day!

Beat 1 demonstrates a junctional escape beat that has no P wave. So, in this instance, the atria and ventricles were depolarizing in the same period of time. (The P wave is hiding in the QRS.) Beats 2, 3, and 4 demonstrate the underlying sinus bradycardia. Beat 5 shows a junctional escape beat with a retrograde P wave (the P wave follows the QRS). Thus, in this instance, the ventricles have depolarized before atrial depolarization occurs. The last beat (6) is similar to beat 1.

This patient has a pacemaker that wanders from the AV junction to the sinus node and back to the AV junction! More than likely, this patient has a sick sinus syndrome relating to degeneration of the sinus node.

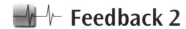 **Feedback 2**

Nice work!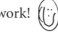

A. The underlying rhythm is a sinus rhythm, with a rate of approximately 80 per minute. Beats 5 and 8 are premature, interrupting the underlying regular rhythm. Inverted P waves occur after the premature beats. The QRSs of the premature beats are within normal limits. This must be premature junctional beats interrupting a sinus rhythm! Because the P waves of the premature beats occur following the QRS, I know that atrial depolarization occurred after ventricular depolarization, resulting in a loss of atrial kick.

B. The underlying rhythm is a sinus rhythm with a heart rate of approximately 75 beats per minute. The QRS complexes measure 0.08 seconds. Beat 4 is premature, interrupting the underlying regular rhythm. The premature beat does not have an obvious P wave. The QRS of the premature beat appears like the QRS complexes in the sinus rhythm. This is a premature junctional beat with atrial and ventricular depolarization occurring during the same period of time (the P wave is hiding in the QRS!).

Just for review, a premature junctional beat has the following properties:

Properties of a Premature Junctional Beat

- The premature beat interrupts the underlying rhythm; thus, the rhythm is irregular.
- An inverted P wave may occur before, during, or after the QRS complex of the premature beat.
- The QRS of the premature beat is usually similar to the QRS complexes of the underlying rhythm.

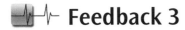

How are you doing? Fine, I hope!

A. This is a regular rhythm with a heart rate of approximately 115 beats per minute. The QRS complexes appear uniform and measure approximately 0.08 seconds. Inverted P waves follow each QRS complex, indicating that ventricular depolarization occurs prior to atrial depolarization. This is an AV junctional tachycardia!

B. If one observes a rapid rhythm with narrow QRS complexes (less than 0.12 seconds) and no distinguishable P waves, one can term the dysrhythmia a supraventricular tachycardia.

 To review then, an AV junctional tachycardia is a regular rhythm with a rapid rate. The P waves may occur prior to, during, or after the QRS complexes. The QRS complexes appear uniform and usually measure less than 0.12 seconds.

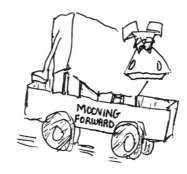

Notes

Ventricular Ectopic and Escape Rhythms

Objectives

When you have completed Section 4, you will be able to describe or identify

1. premature ventricular contractions (P.V.C.s)
2. fusion beats
3. ventricular tachycardia
4. ventricular re-entry mechanisms
5. torsades de pointes
6. ventricular flutter
7. ventricular fibrillation
8. pulseless electrical activity (PEA)
9. ventricular escape rhythm

4

4.1   Premature Ventricular Contractions

Now, back to the art of dysrhythmia interpretation!

This section addresses ventricular ectopic and ventricular escape rhythms. Sounds ominous, doesn't it? Actually, ventricular abnormalities are relatively easy, compared to what has been dealt with previously!

Probably everyone is familiar with ventricular extrasystoles or premature ventricular contractions (P.V.C.s). Ectopic ventricular excitation originates below the bifurcation of the bundle of His, outside the normal conduction system.

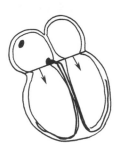

P.V.C.s represent abnormal electrical stimulation arising from an excitable focus or site, somewhere in either ventricle. There is no failure of the normal or underlying rhythm, merely additional premature beats arising from an irritable focus.

As the name *premature ventricular contraction* implies, P.V.C.s interrupt the normal rhythmic cycle. In addition, they may be coupled or related to the preceding sinus beats. You'll remember (from page 55) that a *coupling interval* is the distance between the premature beat and the preceding sinus beat. Remember?

Following is a rather dramatic illustration of P.V.C.s interrupting a normal rhythm. Notice that the coupling interval is constant. One can expect the coupling interval to be constant when the P.V.C.s are uniform in appearance, indicating that the ventricular stimulus arises from a single focus or location. P.V.C.'s arising from the same focus and having the same appearance are called *unifocal*.

Note the constant coupling interval illustrated below

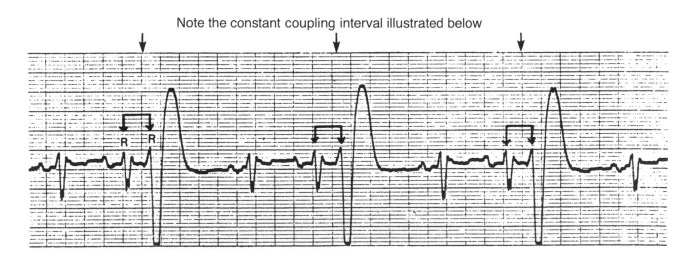

Most usually, P.V.C.s are extremely obvious owing to their *bizarre* appearance. One need know very little about interpreting EKGs to recognize the abnormality!

To confirm that these abnormal beats are indeed P.V.C.s, *they must prematurely interrupt the underlying rhythm, have a widened QRS (0.12 seconds or greater) and have no observable P wave prior to the wide QRS.*

Atrial depolarization is recorded on the monitor as a P wave ; ventricular depolarization is recorded as the QRS complex.

Since a premature ventricular impulse originates in the ventricles outside the normal conduction pathway, ventricular depolarization will occur from the point of origin, much like a rock thrown into a pool of water. This abnormal activation of the ventricles causes the QRS to be wide and bizarre. Further, since the P.V.C. originates in the ventricles, there will be no P wave prior to the QRS. So where are the P waves??? . . . or when do the atria depolarize? *One of two things may happen:*

1. A sinus impulse may fire while the ventricular ectopic impulse is moving across the ventricles. If this happens, the P wave may be "buried" in the QRS complex. In this case, the atria and the ventricles are stimulated by two separate impulses—the atria by the SA impulse, and the ventricles by the ectopic impulse (the P.V.C.). On the EKG strip, no P wave is obvious in the abnormal cardiac cycle.

   When myocardial activation occurs in this manner, there is very little disruption of rhythmicity. In other words, in a regular rhythm, the P.V.C. falls almost where one would expect the next sinus impulse to occur.

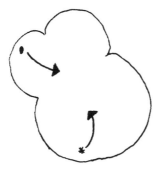 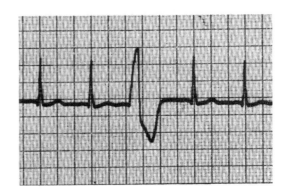

   In the above strip, note that no P wave occurs before or after the QRS. Rather, the P wave is buried in the QRS. When the P wave is "buried," there is no pause following the P.V.C and there is minimal disruption of the rhythm cadence.

2. The ectopic ventricular impulse may occur early in the cycle and be conducted backward (retrograde) through the AV junctional tissue across the atria before the sinus impulse fires. In this case, ventricular depolarization occurs prior to atrial depolarization. So, one would see a wide, bizarre QRS complex followed by a P wave, as demonstrated below.

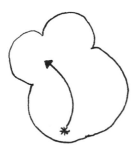 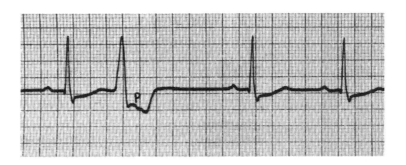

You will also notice, when retrograde conduction occurs, a long pause follows the premature beat. This pause is called a *compensatory pause,* and measures the distance of two normal R-R intervals. This pause allows the sinus pacemaker to reset the rhythm.

If this is difficult to understand, just remember that a P wave will never occur before the premature ventricular beat. A P wave may occur during or after the wide, bizarre QRS complex. You're probably wondering why I did not say that to begin with . . . right? **Right!**

The important point to remember is that all P.V.C.s indicate ventricular irritability. The visible presence or absence of a P wave merely indicates the sequence of atrial activation.

Now that you have an understanding of the P waves (atrial activation), we need to address the subject of the "widened" QRS. *All premature ventricular contractions will have a QRS measuring 0.12 seconds or greater.* A ventricular ectopic impulse (P.V.C.) initiates ventricular depolarization from the point of origin in either the right or left ventricle. The wave of excitation behaves much like a stone thrown into a pool of water, progressing outward. The wave of excitation thus travels outside the normal conducting pathway, requiring more time to achieve ventricular depolarization.

You will remember that moving horizontally across the EKG paper denotes time.

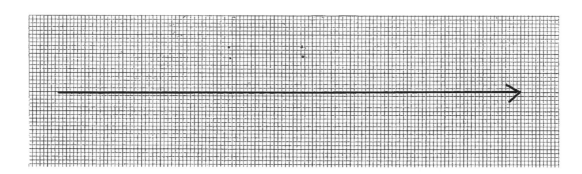

Thus, because the abnormal stimulus (P.V.C.) takes longer to achieve ventricular depolarization, the QRS will be widened—0.12 seconds or greater. (The speed of impulse movement through the myocardium varies from 0.5 to 1.0 meters per second, while the specialized conduction pathways conduct much faster, from 1.0 to 4.0 meters per second!) It should be noted that the wave of excitation produced by a P.V.C. originating in the right ventricle spreads generally from right to left. When viewed from a right precordial lead (V_1), the wave of depolarization moves away from the positive $\oplus$ electrode. The resulting QRS will be wide and negative in appearance. Conversely, when a P.V.C. arising from the left ventricle (spreading generally from left to right) is viewed from lead V_1, the QRS will be wide and positively directed, moving toward the positive $\oplus$ electrode.

To review then, a premature ventricular contraction (P.V.C.) presents as a wide, bizarre QRS that interrupts the underlying rhythm. A P wave will never occur before this abnormal QRS, but may occur during or following the QRS.

P.V.C.s can occur in normal hearts, especially during periods of fatigue or emotional distress. Likewise, persons who drink caffeine products or smoke may have P.V.C.s. (If you have ever experienced your heart "skip a beat," you may have experienced a P.V.C.!) When listening to a heart beat or feeling the pulse, you may hear or feel a pause following an early beat.

Persons taking such drugs as procainamide, digitalis, or drugs with known proarrhythmic effects, and persons with low serum potassium levels may experience P.V.C.s. Hypoxia may also result in ectopic ventricular activity. Manipulating the heart tissue itself (open heart surgery) or catheters situated within the heart chambers (pacemaker catheters, cardiac catheterizations, pulmonary artery catheters) may predispose to ectopic ventricular activity.

In healthy persons, P.V.C.s are relatively harmless. However, in patients with existing heart disease and especially myocardial infarction, *P.V.C.s may **warn of ventricular tachycardia or ventricular fibrillation**.* Ischemic tissue is thought to release a *substance* which is capable of increasing the automaticity of the Purkinje fibers. Thus, patients with ischemic disorders are prone to P.V.C.s.

Amiodarone administered intravenously is the current treatment of choice for ectopic ventricular activity. A bolus of amiodarone, usually 150 mg. I.V. is given over ten minutes to establish a blood level, followed by a continuous infusion. (Though amiodarone is preferred treatment, both lidocaine and procainamide remain acceptable alternatives.)

Usually, antiarrhythmic therapy is instituted when any of the following five scenarios are present:

1. P.V.C.s occurring with increasing frequency . . . (frequent P.V.C.s suggest increasing ventricular irritability and serve to decrease cardiac output.)
2. P.V.C.s occurring in rhythmic patterns, e.g., bigeminy P.V.C.s, where every other beat is a P.V.C.; trigeminy P.V.C.s, where every third beat is a P.V.C.; quadrigeminy P.V.C.s, where every fourth beat is a P.V.C., and so forth.

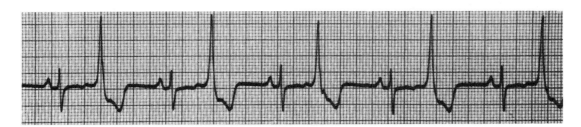

**Ventricular bigeminy . . . or bigeminy P.V.C.s. Notice that
all the P.V.C.s appear uniform or monomorphic or unifocal (identical).**

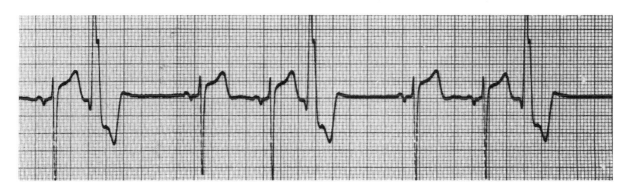

**Ventricular trigeminy . . . or trigeminy P.V.C.s.
(Another example of trigeminal P.V.C.s can be found at the bottom of page 107.)**

3. P.V.C.s falling close to the T wave of the preceding beat.

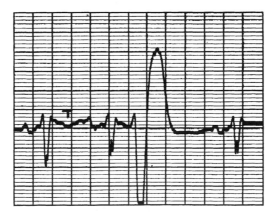

A P.V.C. falling on or near the T wave of the preceding beat is known as *the "R on T" phenomenon*. That is, the R wave of the QRS falls on or near the T wave. In the following strip you will notice that the T wave is inverted (upside down). That is significant too, as you will learn in a later section. The T wave is *vulnerable* to any electrical stimulation, particularly in the ischemic heart. A P.V.C. falling on a vulnerable T wave may precipitate ventricular tachycardia or ventricular fibrillation. (The apex of the T wave represents the earliest time the ventricles can respond to another stimulus.) Frequently, the ischemic heart is in various stages of repolarization. A P.V.C. occurring during this period can initiate depolarization resulting in ventricular fibrillation.

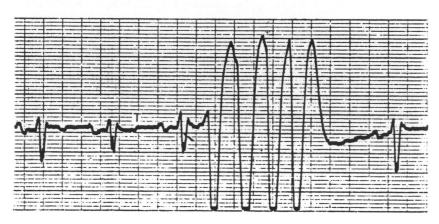

A P.V.C. falling on a vulnerable T wave produces a run of ventricular tachycardia!

(We'll discuss this later in more detail.)

4. P.V.C.s originating from *more* than one irritable site or focus.
   In other words, P.V.C.s are different in appearance. Commonly, this is referred to as ***multiformed, multifocal or multidirectional P.V.C.s.***

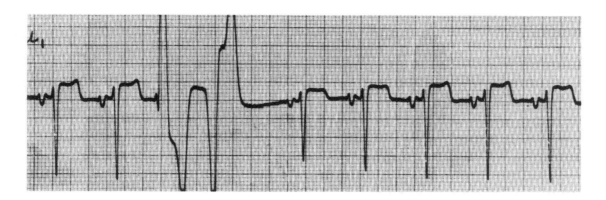

Sometimes this business of single and *multiformed* (or *multidirectional*) P.V.C.s is a bit confusing. So, to clarify the subject, I've borrowed an explanation from the Obstetrics Department! (If you can think of the ventricles as being a mama, you're all set!)

When twins develop from separately fertilized eggs, they appear uniquely different owing to their fraternal or ***multiformed*** relationship.

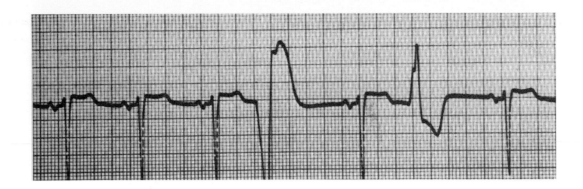

Multiformed (also known as multifocal) *P.V.C.s* originate from various irritable sites (or foci) within the ventricles, and appear uniquely different!

When, however, twins develop from a *single* fertilized egg, they appear identical.

Single origin P.V.C.s originate from the same irritable site (or focus) in either ventricle and are essentially identical in appearance.

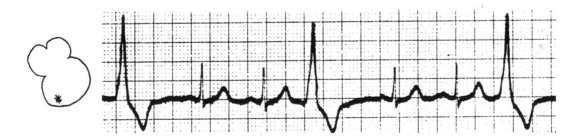

. . . Yes, I know, these analogies are a bit far-fetched . . . but, **I bet you remember them**!

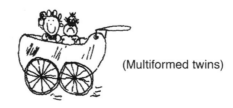

(Multiformed twins)

5. Two P.V.C.s occurring together, referred to as *paired P.V.C.s*, or a *couplet* of P.V.C.s. can also be an indication for antidysrhythmic therapy.

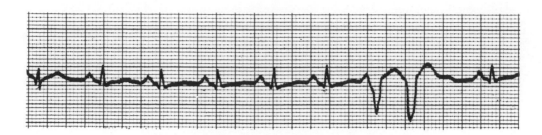

In the above example an ectopic focus in the ventricles has discharged two impulses in rapid succession. This clues us that the ventricular ectopic site is *extremely* irritable. (If it continues to initiate rapid impulses, the ectopic pacemaker will assume control of the heart rhythm!!)

To review then, the following situations or patterns are usual indications for antidysrhythmic therapy.

1. P.V.C.s increasing in frequency
2. P.V.C.s occurring in rhythmic patterns, e.g. bigeminy, trigeminy, etc.
3. P.V.C.s falling close to the vulnerable T wave
4. multiformed P.V.C.s
5. paired P.V.C.s

The reader should be aware that drug therapy and the indications for drug therapy continue to evolve, based on accumulated clinical data and new drug clinical trials. **For the most current recommended drug therapy, one should consult the American Heart Association's Advanced Life Support text.** As an example, past practice supported drug prophylaxis for dysrhythmias associated with acute myocardial infarction (AMI). Current practice does not favor the administration of prophylactic antiarrhythmic drugs in the presence of AMI.

> When P.V.C.s occur, they should be thought of as a **warning signal** until determined otherwise. They warn the observer that life threatening ventricular dysrhythmias may be imminent.

A physician should *always* be made aware when his or her patient begins experiencing P.V.C.s—the number per minute, their appearance (unifocal or multifocal), and their location in the cardiac cycle (i.e., falling near the vulnerable T wave). *Most importantly,* the care giver must directly evaluate the patient's clinical picture!

Before leaving the subject of premature ventricular contractions, the term "interpolated" ventricular extrasystoles or interpolated P.V.C.s. should be mentioned. When a P.V.C. occurs between two normally conducted sinus beats, and the rhythm of those sinus beats is not disrupted, the P.V.C. is said to be *interpolated*. In other words, the P.V.C. is *sandwiched* between two normal beats!

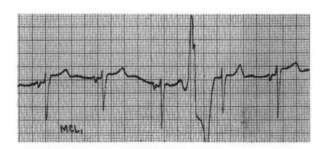

Interpolation results when the retrograde (backward) conduction of the P.V.C. is blocked from reaching and activating the atria by refractory tissue above the ventricles.

Commonly, the sinus beat following the interpolated P.V.C. will have a *prolonged* P-R interval owing to refractoriness of the AV node. The AV node has not fully recovered from the premature ventricular stimulation . . . thus, conduction takes longer! Interpolated P.V.C.s are only observed in slow rhythms.

Interpolated P.V.C.s have the same significance as other P.V.C.s. I thought you might find them interesting!

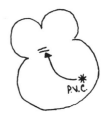

IMPORTANT NOTE: Higher than normal digitalis levels will frequently result in ectopic ventricular activity. In this instance, lidocaine and other antiarrhythmic drugs have little or no effect. Digitalis should be withheld when digitalis toxicity is suspected. Typical therapy involves correcting electrolyte imbalances and supporting the patient. Magnesium, in particular, may counter ventricular dysrhythmias associated with digitalis toxicity. In severe cases, dilantin or Digibind may be administered.

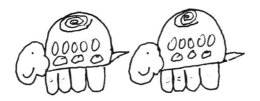

☒ Single formed (monomorphic)
☐ Multiformed (polymorphic)

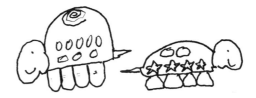

☐ Single formed (monomorphic)
☒ Multiformed (polymorphic)

Practice Exercise 1

How about some practice!

A. Describe this rhythm strip in detail.

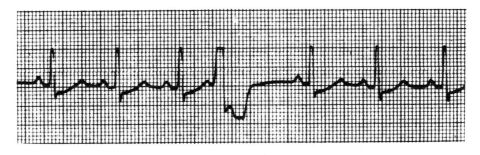

_____

_____

_____

B. Describe the abnormality in this rhythm strip.

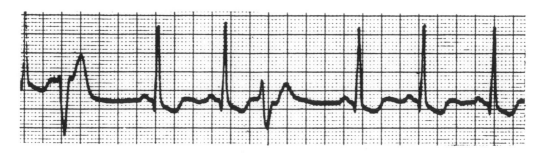

_____

_____

_____

_____

C. In the following rhythm strip, _____ is a premature ventricular contraction.

This is known as _____.

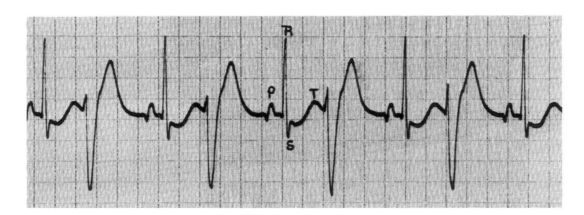

 For Feedback 1, refer to page 132.

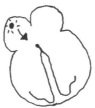

input section   **4.2   Fusion (Dressler) Beats**

To complicate life a bit further, we need to explore _fusion or Dressler beats_. So what's a fusion beat??

    In normal conduction, the ventricles are activated by a sinus impulse traveling down the conduction system.

When a premature ventricular contraction (P.V.C.) occurs, it initiates myocardial depolarization in a backward or retrograde fashion distorting the QRS complex.

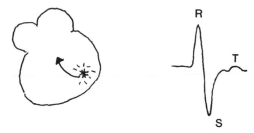

If a sinus impulse is initiated at the same time an ectopic focus in the ventricles initiates an impulse, ventricular depolarization (the QRS) will be produced by a double stimulation. That sounds confusing, so let's try an example. Let's say that the SA node initiates an impulse which activates the atria (producing a P wave), and that impulse travels ¼ of the way across the ventricles, beginning ventricular depolarization.

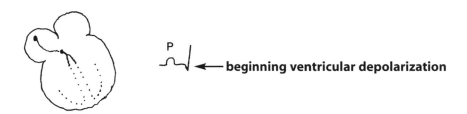

←—beginning ventricular depolarization

At the same time, a ventricular ectopic focus initiates an impulse (P.V.C.) causing retrograde or backward depolarization of the lower portion of the ventricles.

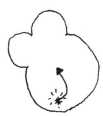

These two impulses, one traveling antegrade (forward) and one traveling retrograde (backward), collide somewhere in the ventricles.

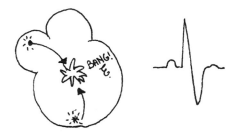

Thus, ventricular depolarization (the QRS) has been initiated by a double stimulation!

So what will the QRS look like? The QRS will resemble both the normal QRS and a wide, bizarre P.V.C. This "fused" QRS will be wider than the normal QRS, but less wide than a P.V.C.

Woops! I forgot something! What about a P wave? Will the fusion beat have a P wave? Of course! . . . because the SA impulse traveled through the atria (initiating atrial depolarization), through the AV junction into the ventricles before colliding with the premature ventricular impulse. So, the fusion beat will have a P wave, and that P wave will be equidistant from other P waves . . . in other words, the P-P interval will remain constant. Because of the double ventricular stimulation, the P-R interval, if visible, is abnormally short . . . the sinus impulse travels only part way down the conduction system! Examine this next rhythm strip.

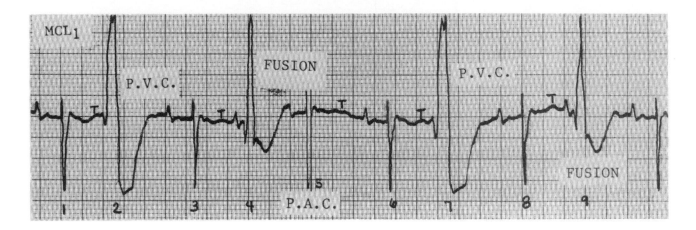

The above underlying rhythm is sinus rhythm, though it is difficult to tell! The rhythm is interrupted by frequent P.V.C.s and an occasional P.A.C. Beats 2 and 7 are P.V.C.s—they are wide and bizarre and have no preceding P waves. But what about beats 4 and 9? They resemble the P.V.C.s, except that they are not as wide. And, there are P waves preceding the QRSs! The P waves occur right on time! Beats 4 and 9 represent fusion beats (*collision beats*)! Notice that the P-R interval of the fusion beats is shorter than the P-R interval of the underlying rhythm. (⌣)

I almost forgot to tell you, fusion beats are also known as Dressler beats.
In review then, in order to identify a fusion beat, two phenomena must exist.

1. There must be a supraventricular pacemaker that conducts normally, producing normal QRS complexes.

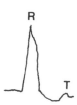

2. There must be an ectopic ventricular focus, producing wide, bizarre QRS complexes.

Then . . . if a beat with an abnormally short P-R interval and a QRS complex somewhere in between the shape and duration of the normal and the ventricular ectopic QRS is observed, it must be a fusion beat!
Amiodarone or lidocaine therapy will not only abolish the P.V.C.s, but will also abolish the fusion beats. Remember, a fusion beat is, in part, a P.V.C.!

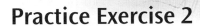

Practice Exercise 2

Step right up and try your luck!

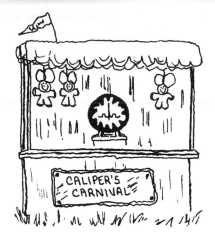

A. Study this rhythm strip. Then label all the beats.

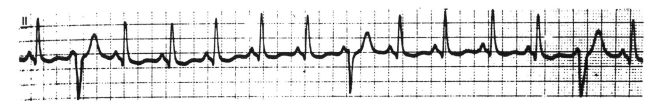

B. A fusion beat is _____

_____

_____

_____

_____

_____

 For Feedback 2, refer to page 133.

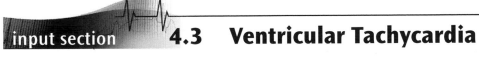

input section **4.3** **Ventricular Tachycardia**

Now, for some excitement . . . *Ventricular Tachycardia!*

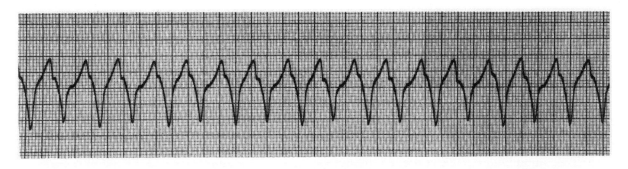

Ventricular tachycardia is most always associated with organic heart disease. It is probably one of the most difficult diagnoses to make, largely because one must make an instantaneous decision. The *important* fact is that ventricular tachycardia is a **life-threatening** dysrhythmia! Treatment *must* be initiated immediately when ventricular tachycardia is suspected.

The following criteria *help* to establish the diagnosis of ventricular tachycardia. (Refer to the rhythm strip at the bottom of the previous page).

1. The rate is usually rapid, between 140–200 beats per minute.
2. The P waves are usually buried in the QRS complexes making them obscure.
3. The QRS complexes are wide and bizarre.
4. The ventricular rhythm is *basically* regular.

> **IMPORTANT NOTICE:** Because virtually every criteria for ventricular tachycardia can be argued, **one must initiate treatment and *then* argue specific points.**

In ventricular tachycardia, the ventricles may be stimulated by an ectopic ventricular pacemaker firing repeatedly. Or, more likely, ventricular tachycardia is initiated by a single P.V.C. The repetitive ventricular stimulation is the result of a reentry mechanism within the ventricular myocardium.

To truly differentiate between ventricular and supraventricular activity, one must recognize atrial activity and its relationship to the QRS complexes. In ventricular tachycardia, the P waves (*if visible*) bear *no* relationship to the QRSs.

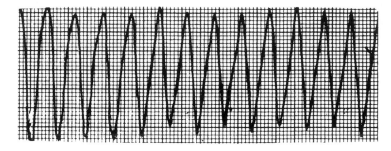

That's a difficult concept to grasp, so let's simplify it a bit! Let's say that the good ol' sinus pacemaker is firing along at a rate of 70. But, because an ectopic ventricular pacemaker is discharging an impulse at 180 times per minute, it takes control of the heart beat. (*The fastest pacemaker controls heart rate.*)

When the sinus impulses occur, they find the ventricular tissue refractory (or unable to respond) to further stimulation.

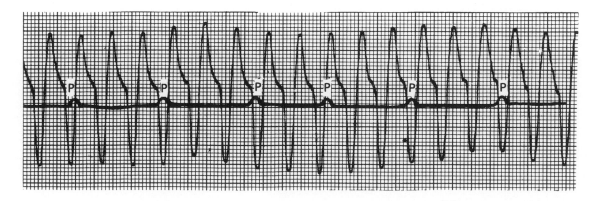

So, the P waves, *if visible,* bear no relationship to the QRSs. Usually, P waves are not visible—they're hiding within the QRS complexes! ☺

Long ago and far away, Schamroth (1971) suggested that the *best* evidence to support a ventricular tachycardia is the presence of a fusion beat during a tachycardia with bizarre QRS complexes. To refresh your memory, the third complex is a fusion beat.

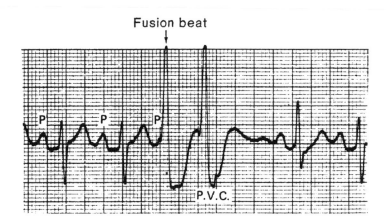

Fusion beat

P.V.C.

This above strip demonstrates two sinus beats followed by a fusion beat and a P.V.C. The P wave of the fusion beat occurs on time . . . it does not occur early or late. The QRS of the fusion beat is wider than the normal QRS, but less wide than the P.V.C. Remember, a fusion beat is the result of a normal beat and a P.V.C. colliding!

You'll remember that a fusion beat produces the QRS by double stimulation—one impulse originating in the atria, and one from an ectopic site or focus in the ventricles. A "run" of ventricular tachycardia may begin or end with a fusion beat, or a fusion beat may be seen in the tachycardia itself.

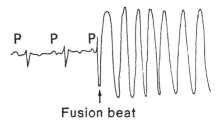

Fusion beat

Ventricular tachycardia beginning with a fusion beat.

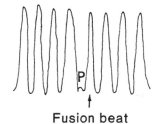

Fusion beat

Ventricular tachycardia evidence of a fusion beat.

Why does a fusion beat occur in the middle of ventricular tachycardia? Remember the P waves that are occurring at a slower rate, bearing no relationship to the QRSs? Well, a P wave happens to find the ventricular tissue polarized, so it initiates depolarization. But bang! Another ectopic impulse is fired. Thus, the two impulses collide, producing a fusion beat.

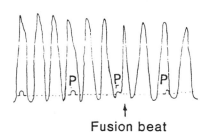

Fusion beat

A fusion beat is produced by a dual stimulation of the ventricles (sinus beat + P.V.C.). A P wave will be obvious, and the QRS of the fusion beat will not be as wide as the QRS of the ventricular beats. The P-R interval of the fusion beat will be abnormally short.

The presence of a capture beat is also evidence to support the identification ventricular tachycardia. So, what is a ***capture beat?***

A capture beat is a fusion beat's Big Brother!

In essence, a capture beat is a normally conducted beat (a sinus beat) that manages to slip through during a ventricular tachycardia. One of those P waves firing along at a slower rate, bearing no relationship to the QRSs, finds the tissue polarized. So *it initiates and completes* normal conduction before the next abnormal ectopic ventricular beat occurs!

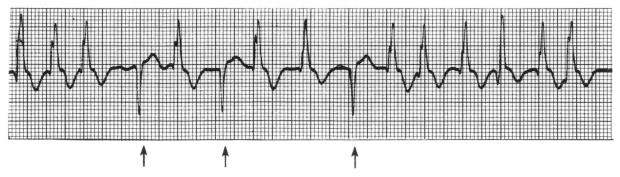

Capture Beats (three normally conducted beats occurring during ventricular tachycardia).

Because a capture beat conducts normally (in an antegrade fashion), the associated QRS has an entirely different contour than that of the PVC. The capture beat depolarizes the ventricles in an orderly, antegrade fashion. *A fusion beat is an incomplete capture beat!*

One must remember that ventricular tachycardia is a **life-threatening** dysrhythmia. It may rapidly progress to ventricular fibrillation; thus, treatment must be instituted *immediately*. If the patient is unstable (impaired cardiac function), amiodarone or lidocaine is administered intravenously followed by synchronized cardioversion. Synchronized cardioversion will be discussed in Section 7. Please reference Section 14 for antiarrhythmic drug details.

The patient with ventricular tachycardia may be asymptomatic and fully alert. They may also be anxious, short of breath, and have a low blood pressure—or, he may be essentially unresponsive with no attainable blood pressure. When the patient is unresponsive, direct defibrillation is applied. There is *no* time to waste! This is a cardiac arrest situation.

Ventricular tachycardia may be sustained or episodic in nature. It may suddenly appear and disappear without treatment.

Three or more P.V.C.s occurring together are considered ventricular tachycardia as evidenced in the following rhythm strip.

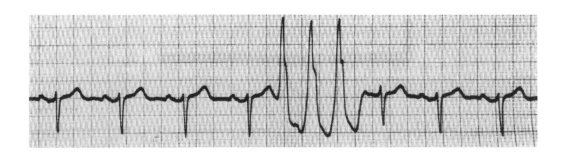

A P.V.C. falling on a vulnerable T wave (R on T phenomenon) may initiate a run of ventricular tachycardia as demonstrated in this next rhythm strip.

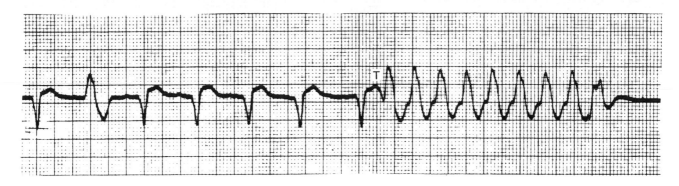

Though in the above examples, the ventricular tachycardia converted spontaneously, antiarrhythmic treatment is usually initiated.

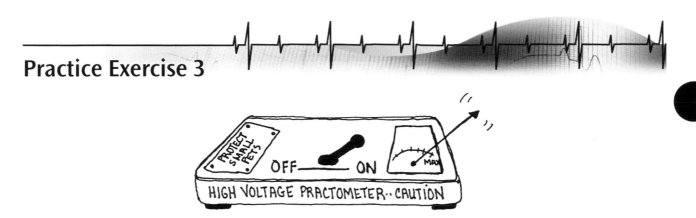

Practice Exercise 3

A. Describe this rhythm strip in detail (rate, rhythm, atrial activity and ventricular activity). Then, identity the probable treatment.

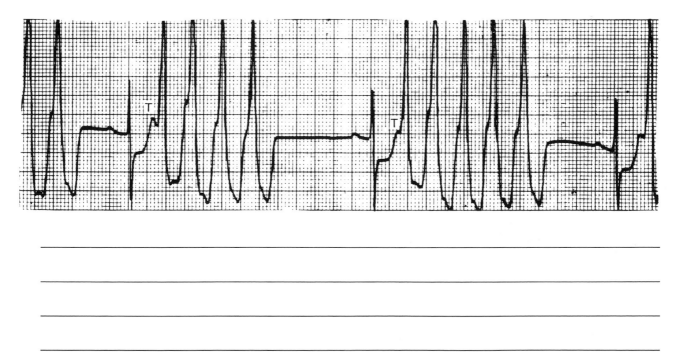

_____

_____

_____

_____

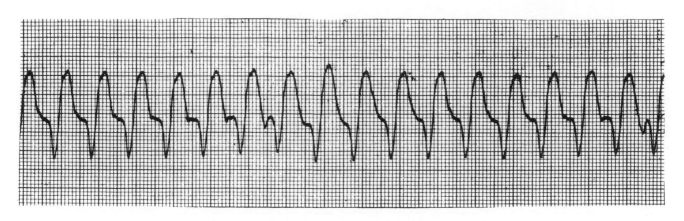

B.   This above strip demonstrates _____ with a heart rate of _____ beats per minute.

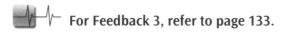   **For Feedback 3, refer to page 133.**

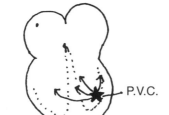

input section   4.4   **Ventricular Re-Entry Mechanisms (Advanced Study)**

At the beginning of this discussion (page 118), it was noted that ventricular tachycardia often occurs secondary to a re-entry mechanism (here we go again, here we go again, etc!) 🙂 A ventricular re-entry mechanism is a localized aberration and may be located anywhere within the ventricular myocardium. Briefly, a ventricular re-entry mechanism behaves in the following example way.

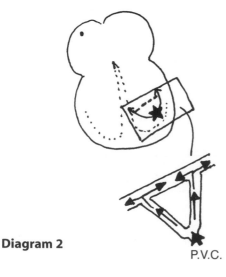

Remember, a P.V.C. arises outside the normal conduction pathway and therefore must travel in a backward or retrograde fashion to initiate ventricular depolarization, as depicted in Diagram 1.

Diagram 1

When an anomalous connection exists between two ventricular conducting fibers, a circuit (of sorts) or communicating loop is formed (see dotted line in Diagram 2). Under certain conditions, [(1) an initiating P.V.C. and (2) unequal refractoriness in portions of the circuitry], the anomalous communicating loop will *behave as an electrical circuit.*

Diagram 2

P.V.C.

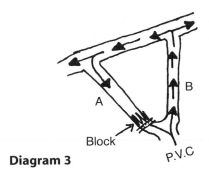

Diagram 3

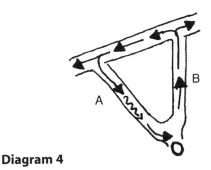

Diagram 4

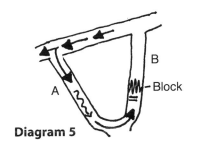

Diagram 5

If a well-timed P.V.C. occurs and begins conduction through the anomalous circuitry, it may find certain of the tissues partially refractory (not fully recovered). Tissues in a state of refractoriness are unable to receive a further stimulation until fully recovered.

In this example, the tissues in "leg A" of the circuit are in a state of partial refractoriness. Thus, the wave of excitation produced by the P.V.C. progresses normally across "leg B" of the circuit, but is *blocked* from entering "leg A" From "leg B", the wave of excitation begins a retrograde activation of ventricular tissues **and** loops around the abnormal circuit (moving antegrade) to "leg A". See Diagram 3.

If the tissues in "leg A" of the circuit are now fully recovered, the wave of excitation causes depolarization of the once blocked tissues. The speed of excitation slows during depolarization, then moves further forward to the point of (O)rigin, as depicted in Diagram 4.

If, "leg" B is now fully recovered, the wave of excitation loops around again, repeating (and repeating) the same sequence. This repeated circus-like ventricular stimulation produces a rapid ventricular tachycardia.

If, however, the wave of excitation finds "leg" B refractory, the stimulus is blocked and the rapid ventricular rhythm subsides as depicted in Diagram 5.

Radiofrequency ablation (RFA) is often the preferred therapeutic intervention. RFA destroys the anomalous tissue responsible for re-entry.

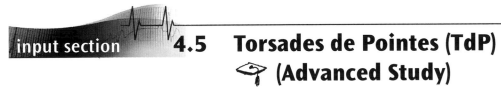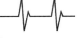

input section **4.5 Torsades de Pointes (TdP)** 🎓 **(Advanced Study)**

Torsades de pointes (TdP) is a rare polymorphic (multiformed) ventricular tachycardia associated with an underlying prolonged ventricular repolarization (a prolonged QT interval). The term *torsades de pointes* (twisting of points) aptly describe the appearance. The wide QRSs vary in appearance, moving from upright (positive) to negatively directed complexes and back again, described as twisting around the baseline.

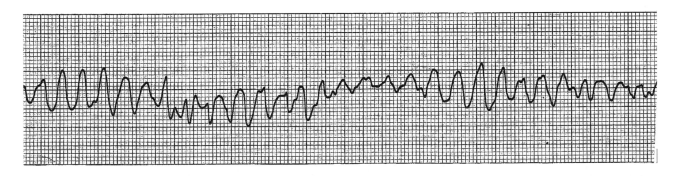

TdP commonly occurs in short bursts (5–15 seconds) and is therefore difficult to capture on 12 lead EKG. Characteristically, the rate ranges between 200 and 250 beats per minute. If the dysrhythmia persists, it may progress to ventricular fibrillation.

TdP can occur as an inherited disorder, a mutation in genes that control sodium and potassium channels. This type of disorder is termed an *inherited long QT syndrome,* discussed in Section 15. The dysrhythmia may also arise as a complication (**proarrhythmic** effect) of drugs that prolong the QT interval by blocking the potassium channel. This variation of TdP is termed an *acquired long QT syndrome.* (Drugs exhibiting a proarrhythmic effect are discussed on the next page).

You will recall from Section 1, the QT interval is a measurement that represents the total time of ventricular depolarization and complete repolarization. Measurement begins at the Q wave and ends at the conclusion of the T wave. (If no Q wave is present, the measurement begins at the R wave). The QT interval is *best* measured in leads V_2, and V_3.

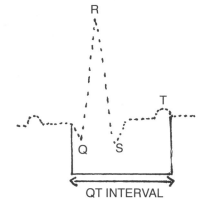

In a normal healthy rhythm, the QT interval measures less than one-half of the R-R interval (refer to page 20 for a quick review). However, the QT interval varies with age, gender, heart rate and a number of other subtle factors. In a healthy state, the normal male QT interval averages 0.39 seconds; it is considered prolonged at 0.45 seconds. The normal female QT interval averages 0.41 seconds; it is considered prolonged at 0.46 seconds. Because the QT interval varies with heart rate, a formula (Bazet's formula) was derived to correct for heart rate variation.

$$\text{Bazet's formula} \qquad \textbf{QTc} = \frac{\text{QT interval in seconds}}{\sqrt{\text{R} - \text{R interval in seconds}}}$$

QTc is the abbreviation utilized for a heart-rate corrected QT interval. Fortunately, QTc calculators are programmed into 12 lead EKG machines!

Another measure, QT dispersion (**QTd**) is used to determine variation in myocardial refractoriness. In this metric, the QT interval is measured on the same beat in all 12 EKG leads. The shortest QT interval measurement is subtracted from the longest QT interval measurement. The resulting difference is an indicator of the degree of variation (dispersion) in refractoriness. The greater the degree of dispersion, the presumed higher the risk for ventricular tachycardia or ventricular fibrillation associated with a proarrhythmic drug effect.

In general, patients presenting with a QT interval measurement of 600 milliseconds (0.06 seconds) or greater are presumed to have a higher risk. Unfortunately, a prolonged QT interval is only a moderate predictor of risk! To date, there are no absolute risk predictors.

Torsades de points is slightly more common in women than men. The dysrhythmia can be precipitated by ischemia, hypokalemia or hypomagnesemia (both conditions cause repolarization delay) or proarrhythmic drug effects (an arrhythmia worsens or a new arrhythmia appears). Some degree of TdP risk is associated with the proarrhythmia effects of the following antiarrhythmic drugs.

Class 1A drugs (procainamide, quinidine, disopyramide)
Class 1C drugs (encainide, flecainide)
Class III drugs (sotalol, amiodarone, ibutilide, dofetilide)

Additionally, albuterol (a bronchial dilator) and erythromycin have been associated with TdP.

The risk classification of drugs is continuously updated as clinical data are available. The most up-to-date information on drug induced arrhythmias can be found on the University of Arizona CERT International Registry for Drug Induced Arrhythmias. Information specific to QT interval prolongation can be accessed at www.qtdrugs.org/med-pros.

Treatment for TdP depends on the severity of symptoms. In paroxysmal TdP (sudden bursts), intravenous magnesium sulfate ($MgSO_4$) and potassium chloride (KCl) are typically the first treatment agents employed. Magnesium sulfate acts as an antiarrhythmic agent and can also be utilized to treat ventricular fibrillation unresponsive to other treatments. Sustained TdP requires immediate synchronized cardioversion.

That brings us to the lethal subject of *ventricular fibrillation*.

Ventricular fibrillation is chaotic, uncoordinated, ineffective, ventricular depolarization.

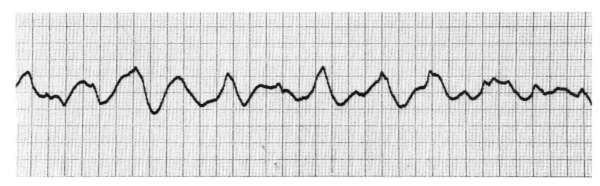

Coarse ventricular fibrillation

In ventricular fibrillation, there is *total irregularity* of electrical activity. There is usually constant variation in the amplitude. **No PQRST** can be seen, and the baseline appears to wander. Ventricular fibrillation may be *coarse* (large waves) as seen above. Or, ventricular fibrillatory waves may be *fine* (more or less like atrial fibrillatory waves without QRSs).

Since there is *no* coordinated ventricular electrical activity, there is *no significant ventricular muscle contraction*. If one were to directly view the fibrillating heart, it would appear to quiver. Because the pumping action of the heart is lost, death occurs within minutes.

Usually, ventricular fibrillation does not just appear. Characteristically, myocardial irritability will first be evident—such as P.V.C.s. However, it has been demonstrated that ventricular fibrillation may occur spontaneously when associated with acute myocardial infarction. In most instances, ventricular fibrillation is a *terminal event,* and is associated with ischemic heart disease. It may, however, be induced by digitalis toxicity—particularly if digitalis intoxication is associated with hypokalemia. Ventricular fibrillation may also occur with *severe hypothermia*—when the body temperature approaches 28° centigrade. Further, electrical shock may induce ventricular fibrillation.

The only treatment for ventricular fibrillation is electrical defibrillation. CPR should be instituted immediately. (Defibrillation will be discussed in Section 7.)

Commonly, one can anticipate successful defibrillation when the ventricular fibrillation occurs in a patient without heart failure or extensive myocardial damage and when the precordial shock is delivered within the first few minutes of the dysrhythmia. In the presence of fine ventricular fibrillatory waves unresponsive to initial defibrillation attempts, epinephrine may be administered. Epinephrine may convert fine fibrillatory waves to coarse waves, often more responsive to electrical shock.

* Precordial Shock

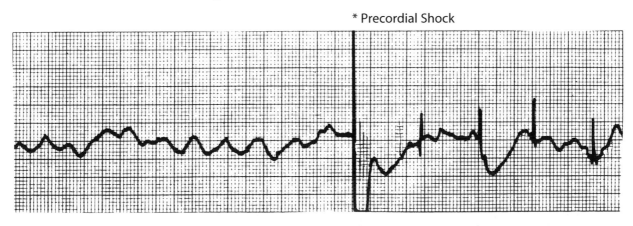

**The above strip demonstrates ventricular fibrillation. Non-synchronized precordial shock
(defibrillation) interrups the chaotic rhythm and a sinus rhythm resumes.**

Defibrillation may be unsuccessful in the patient with long-standing respiratory or cardiac disease. The efficacy of defibrillation is also comprised in morbidly obese persons.

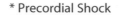
* Precordial Shock

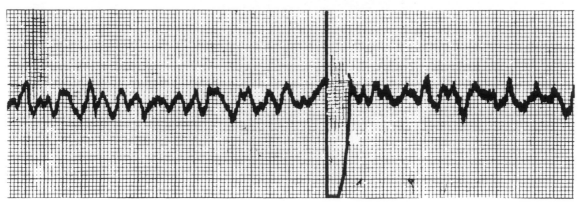

This strip demonstrates unsuccesful defibrillation.

One should bear in mind that the body *rapidly* converts to anaerobic metabolism with the cessation of circulation. There is a rapid buildup of lactic acid—resulting in metabolic acidosis. For this reason, buffering agents such as sodium bicarbonate may be administered following the establishment of adequate ventilation. Electrical intervention is more successful when the acidotic state has been corrected. *ACLS Guidelines* (American Heart Association) should be consulted for the latest, up-to-date treatments for code arrest.

Practice Exercise 6

Practice time again!

Describe these two rhythm strips in detail! Indicate the probable treatments or interventions.

A. _____

_____

_____

_____

_____

_____

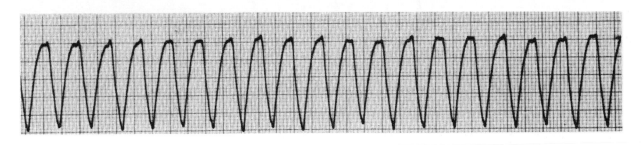

B. _____

_____

_____

_____

_____

_____

 For Feedback 6, refer to page 134.

input section 4.7 Pulseless Electrical Activity (PEA)

Yesteryear, Pulseless Electrical Activity (PEA) was known as electrical-mechanical dissociation (EMD). Either term is a descriptive designation of a phenomenon whereby electrical activity or electrical waveforms are visible on the monitor, but the patient or victim is pulseless. In other words, cardiac muscle contraction and perfusion do not follow electrical stimulation. PEA is a true cardiac emergency requiring immediate resuscitative measures, including CPR. In the presence of ventricular tachycardia (VT) or ventricular fibrillation (VF) wave forms, defibrillation is commonly the initial therapeutic intervention. When unsuccessful, intravenous epinephrine may be administered followed by further defibrillation attempts.

For rhythm patterns other than VT or VF, stimulating drugs such as epinephrine or atropine may be given in attempt to generate or speed up a slow pulse.

When the above measures fail to initiate a pulse, transcutaneous pacing is initiated.

In the adult patient, **hypoxia and respiratory failure** are the most common causes of pulseless electrical activity. Other causes include the following clinical conditions.

    severe acidosis
    severe hypovolemia
    marked electrolyte imbalances
    hypothermia
    pulmonary embolism
    tension pneumothorax

Beyond resuscitative measures, initial actions include diagnostic efforts to identify the precipitating cause of PEA. Once identified, therapeutic interventions are geared toward correcting or mitigating the underlying condition.

In summary of PEA, the patient is pulseless, despite the presence of electrical wave forms on the monitor. PEA represents a cardiac emergency requiring both life saving interventions as well as therapies to correct or improve the underlying clinical problem.

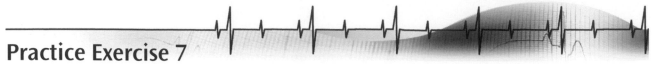

Practice Exercise 7

A. Indicate whether the following statements are True (T) or False (F)!

_____ Pulseless Electrical Activity conveys the same message as Electrical-Mechanical Dissociation.

_____ In PEA, rhythms or wave forms appear on the monitor.

_____ CPR is the first intervention to treat a pulseless patient.

_____ Treatment is focused on restoring adequate perfusion and correction of the underlying clinical disorder.

B. In the adult patient, _____ and _____ are the most common causes of PEA.

C. Write a one sentence description of PEA. _____

_____

_____

_____

_____

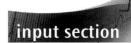 **For Feedback 7, refer to page 134.**

input section   4.8   Ventricular Escape Beats and Rhythms

This is the *last* exercise of this section, so we'll keep it brief!

Since we have more or less exhausted the subject of ectopic ventricular rhythms, we now need to explore ***ventricular escape rhythms***.

As previously discussed, the heart has many potential pacemakers, each with its own inherent rate of impulse formation. The more distant a pacemaker is located from the sinus node, the slower its inherent ability to pace or initiate impulses.

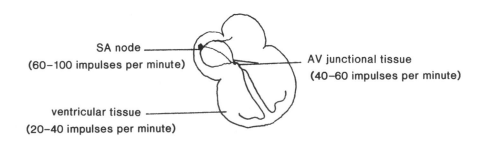

SA node
(60–100 impulses per minute)

AV junctional tissue
(40–60 impulses per minute)

ventricular tissue
(20–40 impulses per minute)

If the sinus node fails to discharge an impulse—or if the SA node discharges so slowly that the heart rate becomes inadequate—or if the sinus impulse fails to be transmitted, a lower (more distal) pacemaker may discharge spontaneously. That's a mouthful!

The SA node may be depressed by acute hypoxia, myocardial damage and/or reflex activity through the vagus nerve. In essence, an escape rhythm is a rhythm maintained by a pacemaker other than the sinus node, when the sinus node fails to activate the heart muscle or does so in an ineffective manner. Thus, an escape rhythm is never a primary phenomenon. An escape rhythm results *secondary* to another event or problem. Escape rhythms are *life saving mechanisms.* This should sound familiar (junctional escape rhythms were discussed on page 88)!

Escape rhythms are *generally* regular and may vary in rate from 10–100 beats per minute. If the escape rhythm is initiated in the AV junction it is called an idiojunctional rhythm (narrow QRS complex). If the escape rhythm originates in the ventricles (wide QRS, 0.12 seconds or greater) it is called an **idioventricular rhythm** or a **ventricular escape rhythm**.

Examine this example of an idioventricular rhythm.

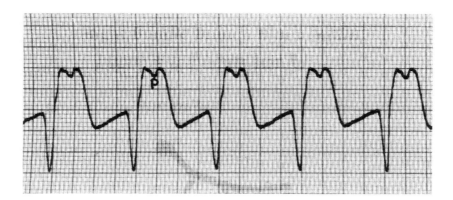

The previous rhythm strip demonstrates a probable idioventricular rhythm with a heart rate of approximately 75 beats per minute. The rate is somewhat faster than the inherent ventricular rate (20–40 beats per minute), so it would be appropriate to term this rhythm an *accelerated* idioventricular rhythm. You will notice that the rhythm is regular. Escape rhythms are *almost* always regular! There are no P waves preceding the QRS complexes. Rather, *retrograde* P waves are obvious following each QRS indicating atrial depolarization followed ventricular depolarization. (Retrograde P waves are not always obvious in an escape rhythm.) Because no P waves occur before the QRS complexes, this cannot be a sinus rhythm. This cannot be a junctional (escape) rhythm because the QRS duration measures 0.12 seconds. Therefore, the rhythm is assumed to be of ventricular origin.

Examine this next example of a ventricular escape rhythm.

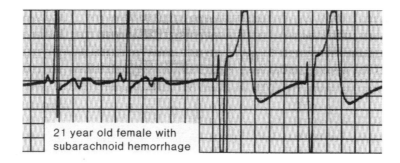

21 year old female with subarachnoid hemorrhage

The underlying rhythm here is a borderline sinus bradycardia. When the sinus pacemaker failed to initiate an impulse, a ventricular escape pacemaker assumed control of the rhythm. One might have expected an AV junctional pacemaker, rather than a ventricular pacemaker, to emerge thus commanding the escape rhythm. At times, however, a given pathology affects both the sinus and AV junction mechanisms, rendering them both incapable of effective impulse generation. Remember, escape rhythms never occur as primary disorders. When observed, escape beats or escape rhythms occur *late* in the cardiac cycle (as opposed to premature), coming *after* the next anticipated beat!

As with all ventricular impulses, *ventricular escape beats are widened, the QRS measuring 0.12 seconds or greater.* It simply takes a longer period of time for the ventricular escape impulses to depolarize the ventricles because they travel backward, outside the normal conduction system. Remember, moving horizontally across the EKG paper denotes time.

The patient with an *escape ventricular rhythm* may experience hemodynamic embarrassment owing to both the slow ventricular rate and the *loss of atrial kick*. In fact, persons with diseased myocardial tissue, particularly the patient with an acute myocardial infarction, may suffer greatly as a result of the ventricular escape rhythm, even if the heart rate is within a normal range. If the atrial contraction does not precede the ventricular contraction by the normal interval, one loses the *atrial kick*. The atrial kick is simply the residue of blood forced into the ventricles during atrial systole (contraction), just prior to ventricular systole (contraction). In other words, the atrial kick is an extra "umph" to the distended ventricles before they contract. This essentially *supercharges* the cardiac output. When heart muscle damage is present, the absence of atrial kick may reduce cardiac output by as much as 25%. So, when a patient with heart damage presents with an idioventricular rhythm, he may exhibit shock symptoms owing to both the loss of atrial kick and the slow ventricular rate.

Treatment is *always* supportive in nature and is aimed at speeding up the heart rate and restoring hemodynamic equillibrium. If the SA node fires too slowly allowing a lower pacemaker to take control, treatment is focused on speeding up the rate of SA impulse discharge. Atropine is most usually the drug of choice, but pacing may also be required.

If the sinus mechanism (or AV junctional tissues) cannot be successfully engaged as a higher order pacemaker, a transcutaneous pacemaker will likely be inserted until a transvenous pacemaker can be inserted under fluoroscopy. This is often necessary when an idioventricular rhythm is associated with extensive myocardial damage. (Myocardial damage associated with acute myocardial infarction will be discussed in Section 11.)

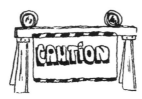

It is *important* to distinguish between ventricular escape beats or rhythms *and* P.V.C.s or ventricular tachycardia. Escape beats or escape rhythms are *life saving* while P.V.C.s or ventricular tachycardia may be *life threatening*.

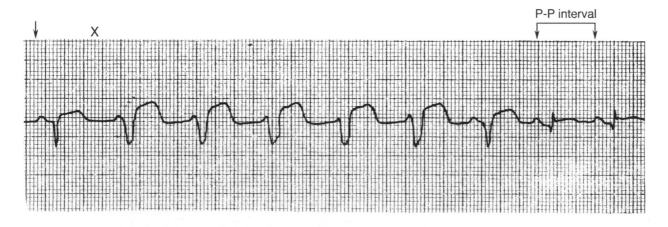

Above, a ventricular escape rhythm emerges when the sinus pacemaker fails to initiate a timely impulse. Measure the P-P interval (see arrows) of the two sinus beats occurring at the end of the strip. Then, apply that same P-P measure to the beginning of the strip. The X indicates the location of the next expected sinus impulse. When the sinus impulse fails to fire on time, a lower more distal (ventricular) pacemaker assumes control.

P.V.C.s (or ventricular tachycardia) on the other hand, interrupt the underlying rhythm and are, therefore, inscribed early (prematurely) in the cardiac cycle, before the next anticipated beat.

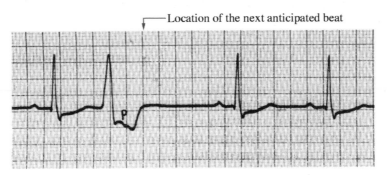

A P.V.C. interrupts the normal underlying rhythm.

The *appropriate* treatment depends upon recognizing whether the abnormal beats are "premature" or "delayed" beats!

Of course, some rhythms are *simply* complicated! See for yourself.

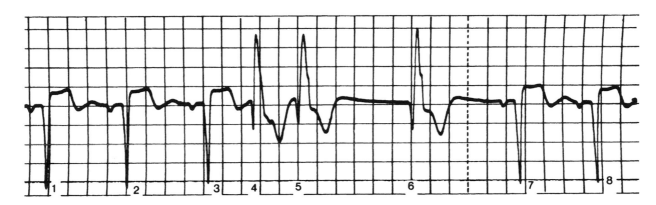

The previous rhythm strip belongs to a patient with an acute anteroseptal wall myocardial infarction. Notice that there is evidence of *both* "early" (*premature*) and "late" (*escape*) ventricular activity. Beats 4 and 5 are P.V.C.s; beat 6 is a ventricular escape beat. A situation like this is truly a *treatment dilemma!* Typically, amiodarone will be administered with a transcutaneous pacemaker available for backup.

Practice Exercise 8

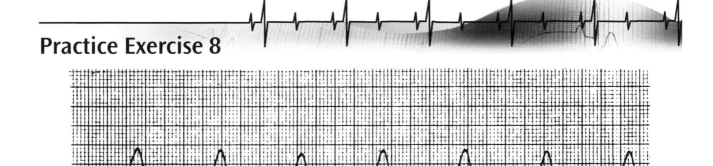

A. Examine the rhythm strip at the bottom of page 131 carefully—then describe all that you see! What treatment might be employed?

_____

_____

_____

_____

_____

_____

_____

 For Feedback 8, refer to page 135.

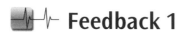 # Feedback 1

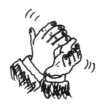

You're becoming a Pro!

A. This is a sinus rhythm with a heart rate of approximately 90 per minute. Beat 4 is premature, interrupting the normal rhythm. The P-R interval of normally conducted beats measures 0.16 seconds. The QRS of normally conducted beats measures approximately 0.08 seconds. There is a P wave in the premature complex that you can see in the S-T segment. The QRS of the premature beat measures greater than 0.12 seconds. This is a P.V.C. and it occurs on the T wave of the preceding beat. This could initiate ventricular fibrillation!

B. The underlying rhythm is a sinus rhythm with an approximate rate of 80 beats per minute. Beat 2 and 5 occur prematurely, interrupting the underlying rhythm. Both of the premature beats have QRSs that measure 0.12 seconds or greater. The premature beats are P.V.C.s—but they do *not* look alike. So, we could say that there are multifocal P.V.C.s interrupting a sinus rhythm. The QRS of normally conducted beats measures approximately 0.10 seconds. The P-R interval of these beats measures approximately 0.14 seconds.

C. In this rhythm strip, *every other beat* is a premature ventricular contraction. This is known as *bigeminal P.V.C.s or ventricular bigeminy!*

To review then, premature ventricular contractions have the following EKG characteristics.

Characteristics of Premature Ventricular Contractions
- They occur prematurely, interrupting the underlying rhythm.
- There may be a P wave following the QRS.
- The QRS complexes are wide and bizarre in appearance, measuring 0.12 seconds or greater.
- There may be a compensatory pause following the premature beat.

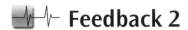 ## Feedback 2

We've got a winner folks!

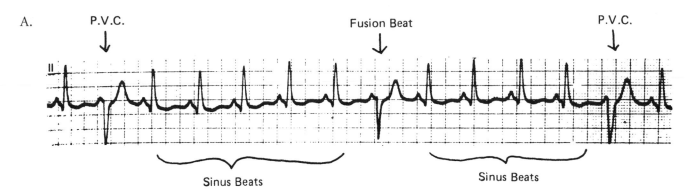

B. A fusion beat is an abnormal beat produced by a double stimulation. A sinus impulse is conducted normally through the atria (initiating atrial depolarization), through the AV junction, and into the ventricles initiating ventricular depolarization. At the same time, an ectopic ventricular focus fires (P.V.C.) initiating depolarization of the lower part of the ventricles. The sinus impulse and the ectopic ventricular impulses somewhere in the ventricles. Consequently, the QRS of the fusion beat looks somewhere in between the normal sinus QRS and the P.V.C.!

Whew!

Remember, to truly identify a fusion beat, there *must* be both a sinus beat and a P.V.C. for comparison purposes. Fusion can only take place if the atrial impulse has started to penetrate the ventricles from above— so, *a P wave will always precede the abnormal appearing QRS!*

Feedback 3

A. The underlying rhythm is probably sinus rhythm. The underlying rhythm is interrupted by frequent bursts of ventricular tachycardia! P.V.C.s fall on the vulnerable T waves (R on T phenomenon) initiating short "runs" of ventricular tachycardia. The QRSs of the ventricular tachycardia are wide and bizarre. Amiodarone would be the probable treatment of choice.

Dynamite!

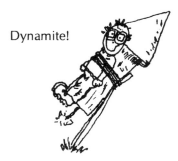

B. This strip demonstrates <u>ventricular tachycardia</u> with a heart rate of <u>150</u> beats per minute.

Criteria That Assist in Identifying Ventricular Tachycardia

- The ventricular rhythm is *basically* regular.
- The rate is usually rapid, between 140–200 beats per minute.
- The P waves are usually buried in the QRS complexes, making them obscure.
- The QRS complexes are wide and bizarre.
- The ventricles are directly stimulated by an ectopic ventricular focus firing repeatedly or through a reentry process. Ventricular action is independent of atrial activity.
- Fusion or capture beats may be evident.

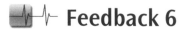 **Feedback 6**

Nice work!!

A. There is no coordinated electrical activity in this strip. The activity is totally irregular. No PQRST can be seen. The baseline appears to quiver or undulate. This is ventricular fibrillation. Treatment would consist of electrical defibrillation. Until electrical defibrillation is administered and a sustaining rhythm is established, full cardiopulmonary resuscitation must be continued!

B. The rhythm is regular at a rate of approximately 187 beats per minute. No P waves can be identified. The atrial activity is probably hidden in the QRS complexes. The QRS complexes are wide (0.12 seconds or greater) and bizarre in appearance. This is most likely ventricular tachycardia. Treatment likely would consist of amiodarone administration or synchronized cardioversion. If the patient is unconscious, defibrillation may be used.

Criteria for Identifying Ventricular Fibrillation

- No PQRST can be observed.
- Totally uncoordinated electrical activity.
- The baseline appears to quiver.
- The waveforms may be coarse or fine.*

---

* The rhythm strip on page 125 demonstrates a "coarse" ventricular fibrillation. The first practice exercise strip on page 126 demonstrates a "fine" ventricular fibrillation.

Feedback 7

A. The following statements are all True (T)!

___T___ Pulseless Electrical Activity conveys the same message as Electrical-Mechanical Dissociation.

___T___ In PEA, rhythms or wave forms appear on the monitor.

___T___ CPR is the first line of intervention to treat a pulseless patient.

___T___ Treatment is focused on restoring adequate perfusion and correction of the underlying clinical disorder.

B. In the adult patient, <u>hypoxia</u> and <u>respiratory failure</u> are the most common causes of PEA.

C. <u>PEA is a descriptive classification where wave forms are present on the monitor, but the patient is pulseless.</u>

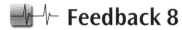 **Feedback 8**

How are you doing? Sometimes it's difficult to grasp ESCAPE rhythms . . . so, you may want to reread Input 9 one more time.

A. The rhythm is regular with a heart rate of approximately 70 per minute. There are no P waves preceding the QRS complexes. The QRS complexes are wide, measuring greater than 0.12 seconds. This must be a ventricular escape rhythm! (One only sees an escape rhythm when higher pacemakers fail!) Typically, a ventricular escape rhythm will be slow, 20–40 beats per minute. One might call this rhythm an accelerated ventricular escape rhythm since the rate is 70 beats per minute.

   The treatment for this rhythm would depend on the cause. Any suppressant drugs (i.e., digitalis) would be discontinued. Treatment would be aimed at restoring a normal rhythm. One might attempt to speed up the SA node with atropine—or speed up a slow ventricular response rate with Isuprel or a transvenous ventricular pacemaker.

   Remember, there are no pacemakers distal to the ventricles! If the ventricular escape pacemaker fails, the patient's monitor picture may look like this. . . .

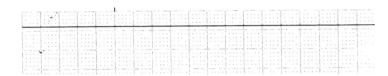

This straightline is referred to as *ventricular standstill* or *asystole*.

Notes

_____

_____

_____

_____

_____

_____

_____

_____

_____

_____

_____

_____

_____

_____

_____

_____

_____

_____

_____

Conduction Disturbances and Heart Block

Objectives

When you have completed Section 5, you will be able to describe or identify

1. sinus arrest (sinus pause) and sinus block
2. atrial tachycardia with block
3. relevant history
4. first degree AV block
5. second degree AV block
   a. Mobitz type I—Wenckebach
   b. Mobitz type II
6. complete heart block
7. bundle branch block

You've come a long way! 😊 I hope EKG interpretation has not become the focal point of your existence.

However . . . as was noted earlier, once you have a good grasp of the fundamentals, it is *repeated* practice that adds finesse!

We are now leaving the world of dysrhythmias to consider *conduction disturbances* and *heart block*. Before doing that, however, it is helpful to review the conduction system one more time.

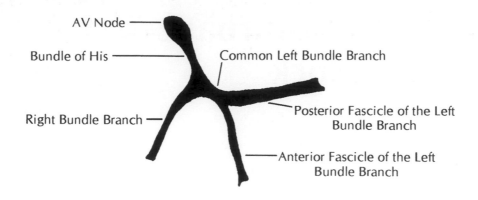

You will notice that the bundle branch system looks somewhat different than in earlier drawings. That is because *in reality,* the left bundle branch has both an anterior and posterior division. Thus, the bundle branch system is composed of three fascicles (or little bundles) . . . the right bundle branch, the anterior fascicle of the left bundle branch, and the left posterior fascicle of the left bundle branch.

The important point to be made here is that *disease* or *toxic drug manifestations* may delay normal sinus impulse transmission or result in failure of impulse transmission from the atria to the ventricles (thus, the term *block*). This delay or interruption may occur anywhere within the conduction system!

Conduction disturbances and heart blocks are sometimes a bit confusing, so read carefully and proceed fearlessly!

Proceed Ahead . . .

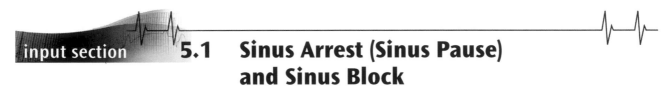

input section **5.1   Sinus Arrest (Sinus Pause) and Sinus Block**

Occasionally excessive vagal tone, ischemic damage of the AV node, degenerative disease of the sinus node or digitalis or other toxicity may interrupt the firing or conduction of the normal sinus impulse.

When this phenomenon occurs, a normal sinus rhythm may be interrupted by a pause or pauses.

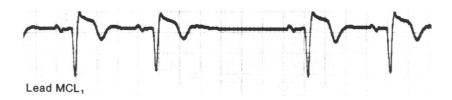

Lead MCL₁

Though there are many abnormalities in the above strip, notice the pause following two normally conducted sinus beats. The pause is thought to result from failure (arrest) of the sinus mechanism.

As you inspect the previous tracing, recognize that such pauses would serve to give the patient an irregular pulse . . . therefore, one would need to count the heart rate for one full minute. If you look closely, you will notice that the next *anticipated* event during the pause is a P wave followed by a QRS. Because that anticipated P wave did not occur in a timely fashion, we assume that the sinus pacemaker did not initiate an impulse, or, if it did, it did not cause atrial depolarization. (Remember . . . the presence of a P wave tells us the atria have depolarized . . . therefore, the *absence* of a P wave tells us the atria did *not* depolarize.) ☺

For purposes of definition, *sinus arrest* (or sinus pause) occurs when the sinus pacemaker fails to discharge an impulse at the expected time. The resulting pause is of *undetermined length,* as is demonstrated in the previous rhythm strip. Sinus arrest may be associated with degenerative disease of the sinus mechanism or drug toxicity. If the pauses are of significant duration, pacemaker therapy may be required.

Sinus block, on the other hand, exists when the sinus pacemaker initiates an impulse at the expected time, but that impulse is blocked within the sinus mechanism itself. In other words, the sinus impulse does not penetrate into the atria to initiate atrial depolarization. In this case, the resulting pause is usually predictable.

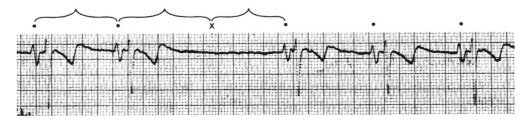

The X denotes the location of the next expected P wave.

Commonly, the pause associated with sinus block will be the same duration as the distance between two normally conducted sinus beats. SA block may be associated with vagotonia (athletes), digitalis administration, and rarely with hypokalemia. Usually, no specific treatment is required.

Interestingly enough, a true differential diagnosis between sinus arrest and sinus block cannot be established on the basis of an EKG alone . . . because all one observes is a pause (the absence of a P wave)!

Probably the best way to describe a strip like the one above is to call it a *sinus pause,* reporting the duration of that pause. (Remember, each small square represents 0.04 seconds!) In the above strip, 2.2 seconds elapse between the R wave prior to, and the R wave following, the pause.

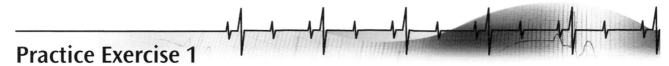

Practice Exercise 1

Look at this strip closely . . . then describe all that you see!

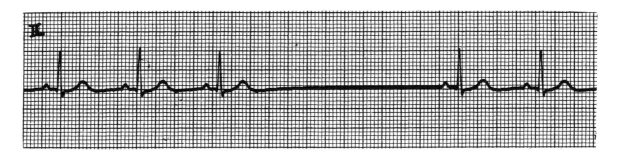

For Feedback 1, refer to page 165.

input section   5.2   Atrial Tachycardia with Block

Remember atrial tachycardia? . . . We discussed this dysrhythmia on page 59. You will recall that atrial tachycardia is a rapid ectopic atrial dysrhythmia with an atrial rate of 160–220 per minute. Well, atrial tachycardia with rapid rates may be complicated by second degree AV block, the *physiologic* variety. This is the same *physiologic block* that we discussed earlier (page 66) . . . a protective mechanism that guards the ventricles from the effects of rapid stimulation.

Here is an artist's rendering of atrial tachycardia with block. Notice that there are two P waves for every QRS.

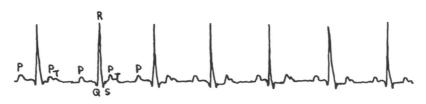

Atrial tachycardia with 2:1 AV block.
Ventricular rate = 100 (regular)
Atrial rate = 200 (regular)

Frequently, *atrial tachycardia with block* occurs as a manifestation of digitalis toxicity, and is therefore a contraindication for the continued administration of digitalis preparations.

Much like atrial flutter, the atrial rate in atrial tachycardia with block is described as a ratio to ventricular conduction, e.g., 2:1, 3:1, etc. In other words, there are two P waves for every QRS, three P waves for every QRS, and so forth.

In the event that you are wondering how atrial tachycardia with block differs from atrial flutter . . . remember, it's *ALL* in the atrial rate! By definition, if the atrial rate is regular at a rate of 160–220, the rhythm is atrial tachycardia. If, however, the atrial rate is regular at a rate of 220–350, the rhythm is atrial flutter!

Additionally, P waves become "saw toothed" in appearance at more rapid rates. Simple enough, right?

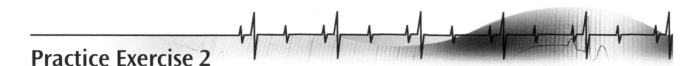

Practice Exercise 2

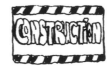

Draw an example of 2:1 atrial tachycardia or atrial tachycardia with 2:1 block.

For Feedback 2, refer to page 165.

In the early days of electrocardiography, most conduction disorders were thought to occur primarily in the AV node. You will remember though that impulse transmission from the atria to the Purkinje system is electrically silent on the EKG. In other words, the P-R interval is electrically silent, representing impulse "travel time" from the atria to the Purkinje system.

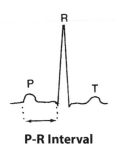

P-R Interval

Looking only at the P-R interval, it is impossible to detect where in the conduction system a delay or block is occurring. In 1969, a technique to study impulse conduction was introduced—the His bundle electrogram (HBE).

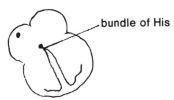
bundle of His

Anatomically, the bundle of His lies under the membranous portion of the intraventricular septum. By positioning a catheter electrode in this area, actual depolarization of the bundle of His was recorded—allowing determinations to be made about the location of a block or delay. In other words, the delay was determined to occur either above or below the bundle of His.

However, that was then, and this is now. Today sophisticated intracardiac electrophysiology (EP) studies utilize multiple wires and techniques to identify questionable conduction anomalies.

In any event, the early His Bundle Electrogram studies demonstrated that conduction defects or blocks occurring above the bundle of His were usually *benign,* seldom progressing to complete heart block. Conduction defects or blocks originating below the bundle of His were more commonly associated with a *grave* prognosis!

Thus, the early HBE procedure refined the classification of heart blocks, and that knowledge continues to assist the modern practitioner. For the most part, heart (conduction) blocks can be classified in the following manner:

5

Heart blocks located above the bundle of His

- First degree AV block
- Mobitz Type I (Wenckebach) second degree AV block
- Complete AV block with a QRS of normal duration (less than 0.12 seconds)

Heart blocks located below the bundle of His

- Mobitz Type II second degree AV block
- Complete AV block with a widened QRS (0.12 seconds or greater)

Usually, AV conduction delays or blocks occurring *above* the bundle of His are *benign* (non-life-threatening) in nature and are frequently associated with ischemia or toxic drug effects. Conduction delays or blocks occurring *below* the bundle of His are *commonly* associated with extensive myocardial damage and therefore have poorer prognoses.

The above chart will be a useful reference as we continue on. In the event that you are confused, be assured you are progressing in a normal fashion!

Practice Exercise 3

How about some practice?

A. Label the parts of the conduction system.

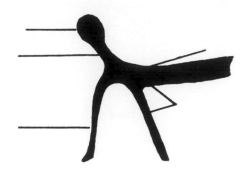

B. Atrial depolarization is represented on the EKG as a _____ wave.

The P-R interval represents _____

_____

_____

_____

C. The QRS represents _____

> **NOTE:** Remember, the P-R interval is electrically silent!

 For Feedback 3, refer to page 166.

Input Section 5.4 First Degree AV Block

First degree heart block is the terminology used to signify that the *P-R interval is greater than* the upper limits of normal.

Your long-term memory should now be registering that the duration of a normal P-R interval is between 0.12–0.20 seconds, or 3–5 small EKG squares. The P-R interval represents the time it takes for the pacemaker impulse to travel across the atria, through the AV junction, down the bundle branches to the Purkinje system. Remember?

When the P-R interval is prolonged (measuring greater than 0.20 seconds) it is impossible by EKG to determine where in the AV conduction system the delay is occuring since the P-R interval is electrically silent. However, the prolongation indicates that something is holding up the show!!!

Here, it is helpful to understand earlier studies which demonstrated that first degree heart block (an abnormally long P-R interval) is *usually* due to a block somewhere *above* the bundle of His. First degree heart block is most usually a benign dysrhythmia.

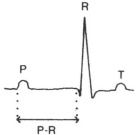

Examine this rhythm strip.

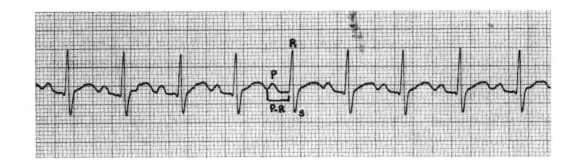

You will notice that the P-R interval measures greater than 0.20 seconds (greater than five small squares). Specifically, the P-R interval measures 0.24 seconds. The P waves are of normal shape. The QRS is of normal configuration and duration (less than 0.12 seconds). *All* sinus impulses reach and activate the ventricles. The sinus impulses are merely taking longer time than expected to reach and activate ventricular depolarization. So, this is a sinus rhythm with a first degree heart block.

That's all it takes to identify a **first degree heart block**!

Because first degree heart block is usually benign (non-life-threatening), it needs only to be watched. However, *an increasing P-R interval should always be reported*. First degree heart block is most frequently associated with coronary artery disease, digitalis administration, and all types of acute myocardial infarction.

On this next strip, notice that the P-R interval measures 0.28 seconds or 7 small squares. (There is other pathology as well, but that will be discussed in later sections). Notice that due to the prolonged PR interval, the P's are very close to the T waves.

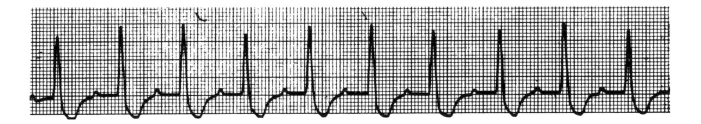

The above rhythm strip demonstrates a sinus rhythm with a first degree heart block. Most authorities note that a P-R interval may be as long as one second and still conduct!

Now review this next strip.

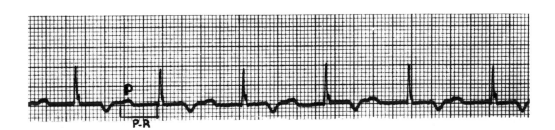

This strip demonstrates a sinus rhythm, rate approximately 70 per minute, with a prolonged P-R interval. The P-R interval measures *almost* two large squares, or 0.4 seconds! Thus, we have a sinus rhythm with a first degree AV block. It is always important to measure the duration of the P-R interval!

To review then, first degree heart block manifests as a *prolonged P-R interval!*

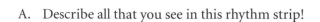

Practice Exercise 4

See what you can do with this!

A. Describe all that you see in this rhythm strip!

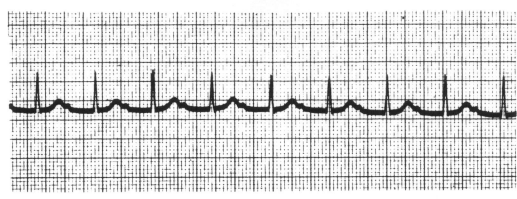

_____

_____

_____

_____

_____

_____

B. The P-R interval in the rhythm strip below measures approximately _____ small squares or

_____ seconds.

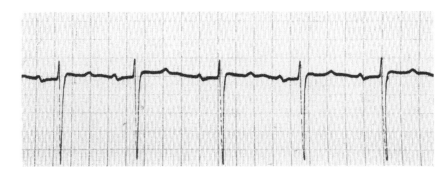

C. First degree heart block is usually benign and needs only _____.

 For Feedback 4, refer to page 166.

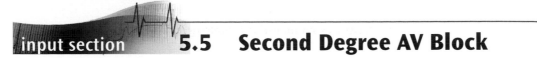

input section 5.5 Second Degree AV Block

That brings us to the subject of *Second Degree Heart Block.*

The very *best* description that I've ever heard of second degree AV block went something like this . . .

. . . "Some P's make it and some don't; those that don't, should!"

Very simple and to the point!

To complicate the understanding of second degree heart block, there are two types, Mobitz type I (Wenckebach) and Mobitz type II.

Mobitz Type I—Wenckebach

Mobitz type I, also known as *Wenckebach,* is a fun rhythm . . . **honest!**

In Wenckebach, one finds a *progressive prolongation of the P-R interval until a P wave is finally blocked* or not conducted, as demonstrated in the following strip.

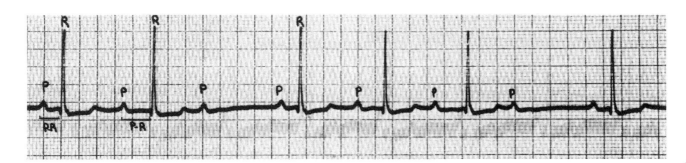

In the above strip, notice that the P-R interval gets progressively longer until *finally,* the third P wave on the strip fails to conduct. Then, the P-R interval progression begins again.

Because the P-R interval progressively becomes longer, the ventricular response is irregular—or, one could say that there is a *varying R-R interval* . . . (the distance between any two R waves varies). In Wenckebach, or Mobitz type I, the **P-R interval lengthens**, while the **R-R interval shortens**.

The Wenckebach rhythm is usually described as a ratio, the number of P waves to QRS complexes per cycle. The following tracing would be described as a "5:4 Wenckebach" (five P waves for four QRS complexes).

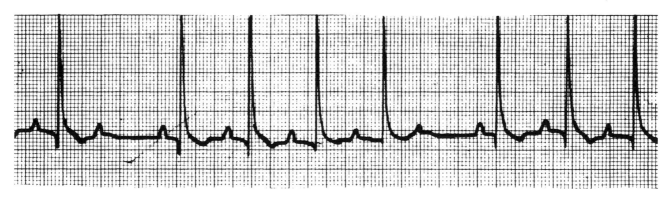

A 5:4 Wenckebach pattern

A Wenckebach type of second degree heart block is most frequently associated with acute inferior wall myocardial infarction, and is probably due to ischemic damage of the AV node. The AV junctional artery fills from the right coronary artery—and it is commonly the right coronary artery involved in the inferior wall infarction. Wenckebach may also be a manifestation of digitalis toxicity since digitalis increases block in the AV junction.

Electrophysiologic studies have shown that this conduction disturbance is usually located above the bundle of His. *If associated with acute inferior wall myocardial infarction, Wenckebach will usually develop within the first 24-hours after the infarction, and usually will not persist beyond the third day.* Since we expect it to disappear within 72 hours, we merely observe it. If Wenckebach occurs secondary to digitalis toxicity, the administration of digitalis should be discontinued.

Mobitz type I, or Wenckebach, is thought to occur because of progressive fatigue in the AV junctional tissues. In other words, a sinus beat is conducted normally through the AV junction. The next impulse conducts more slowly because the AV junction is tired. Each additional impulse tends to be conducted progressively slower—until *finally,* the AV junction says, "I'm going to sit this one out boys!" When associated with myocardial infarction, the fatigue occurs secondary to ischemic changes along the conduction pathway. The AV junctional tissues become so fatigued that they are incapable of transmitting the impulse. Thus, an atrial impulse finds the AV junctional tissues *refractory* (unable to receive the next impulse), and the impulse is blocked. This gives the AV junctional conducting tissues a rest! Then, the whole process begins again!

With Wenckebach, the cycle of dropped beats may vary, giving the patient a varying radial pulse.

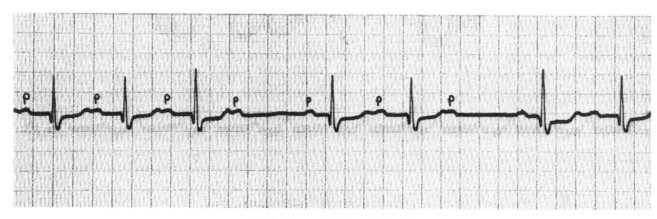

Variable cycle Wenckebach

P.S. If you need review of junctional escape beats, refer to page 88.

That about wraps up the subject of Mobitz type I (Wenckebach). So let's explore Mobitz type II.

Mobitz Type II

Most always, Mobitz type II blocks originate below the level of the bundle of His (in the bundle branches or the Purkinje system) and are of organic origin. Frequently, Mobitz type II is associated with acute anterior wall myocardial infarction (extensive myocardial damage).

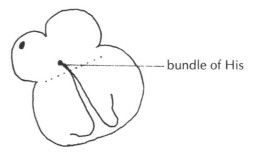

bundle of His

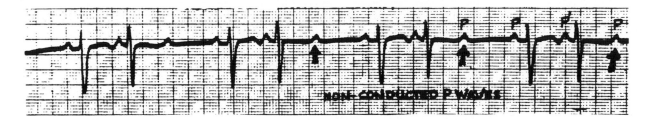

On EKG, one sees, without warning, a *suddenly* blocked P wave. The P-R interval of all conducted beats is constant. The P wave that fails to conduct is neither premature nor late . . . *it occurs in rhythmic sequence with the other P waves.* Thus, throughout the rhythm strip, the P-P interval remains unchanged. The ventricular response is irregular owing to the non-conducted P waves. The duration of the QRS complexes are usually within normal limits, though the QRS may be widened depending upon the underlying pathology.

To definitely identify Mobitz II, there must be *two or more consecutively conducted* sinus impulses with a constant P-R interval before the blocked P wave.

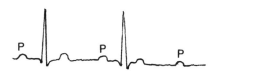

Notice the constant P-R interval of the two consecutively conducted sinus beats in the above drawing.

In Mobitz type II, the impulse transmission failure occurs distal to or below the bundle of His. Since the impulse never reaches the ventricles, the problem is due to intermittent bilateral blockage of the bundle branches!

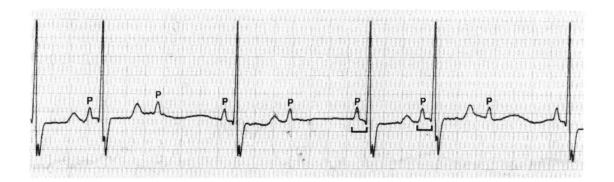

The above strip demonstrates a Mobitz type II block. Notice that the P-R interval of all conducted beats is constant and measures approximately 0.14 seconds. The nonconducted P waves occur in rhythmic sequence with the other P waves. Thus, the P-P interval remains constant. The QRS complexes are widened, measuring almost 0.16 seconds.

REMEMBER: To definitely identify Mobitz type II heart block, one must observe two or more consecutively conducted sinus impulses in order to determine a constant P-R interval.

The patient with Mobitz type II must be monitored closely and constantly. At any point, a Mobitz type II rhythm could progress to complete heart block or ventricular standstill secondary to sustained bilateral bundle branch block.

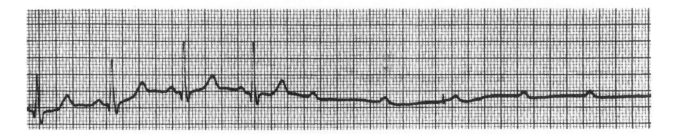

The above strip demonstrates a Mobitz Type II rhythm that progresses (without warning) to ventricular standstill. In ventricular standstill, none of the P waves conduct. The P waves are *suddenly* blocked resulting in the absence of cardiac output. Ventricular standstill is a medical emergency that requires immediate CPR.

In the presence of a confirmed or suspected Mobitz type II rhythm, a transcutaneous pacemaker will be kept on standby. Depending on the underlying pathology and patient prognosis, consideration may be given to the insertion of a ventricular pacing wire.

You will remember from the first part of this section, the prognosis for a patient with Mobitz type II second degree AV block is usually grave. Mobitz type II is *most usually* associated with extensive myocardial damage. It is the *extent of myocardial damage* that ultimately determines the prognosis or outcome.

To review then, to *definitely* identify Mobitz type II, there must be two or more consecutive sinus impulses with the same P-R interval conducted to the ventricles before a blocked impulse occurs. The blocked sinus impulse is neither premature nor delayed.

Owing to the fact that Mobitz type II is commonly associated with extensive myocardial damage, there is usually evidence of intraventricular conduction defects. In other words, even when the sinus impulses are conducted normally, there may be some delay in ventricular activation. Therefore, the QRSs associated with Mobitz type II rhythms are *commonly* widened, measuring 0.12 seconds or greater.

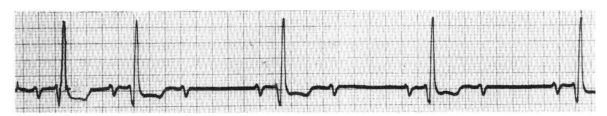

Mobitz type II second degree AV block with widened QRSs measuring approximately 0.18 seconds.

2:1 AV Conduction

This "cookbook method" of looking at EKGs is not always a sure method. A patient's heart rhythm may not perfectly conform to our rules!

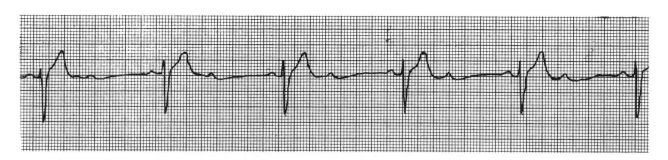

The above rhythm strip demonstrates a 2:1 conduction pattern, two P waves for every QRS. One cannot determine whether the P-R interval increases or stays constant because *only* one conducted beat occurs before each blocked beat. In this case, one would simply describe what is observed . . . there are *two* P waves for every QRS (2:1 conduction). The QRS complexes measure 0.12 seconds and the ventricular rate is 38 per minute! Because the P-R interval of the conducted beats is constant, we know that the atrial and ventricular activity are related.

REMEMBER, two consecutively conducted P waves must occur in order to distinguish between Mobitz type I (Wenckebach) or Mobitz type II. Although the above rhythm is a form of second degree heart block, it is *unclear* which type, since there are *never* two consecutive impulses conducted through to the ventricles.

The following rhythm strip also demonstrates a 2:1 conduction pattern. The QRS complexes are widened, measuring 0.12 seconds.

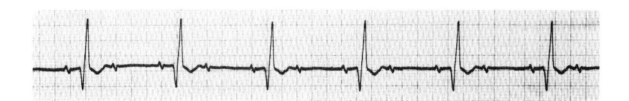

A 2:1 AV conduction pattern associated with *narrow* QRS complexes *usually* represents a form of Wenckebach. A 2:1 AV conduction pattern associated with wide QRS complexes (0.12 seconds or greater) is *commonly* associated with a delay in conduction below the bundle of His—thus, it is *usually* a Mobitz type II block.

If only the 2:1 conduction pattern is observed, further study may be warranted to identify the origin of the block. Oftentimes, if one continues to observe a 2:1 conduction pattern, there may be a point where two sinus impulses are *consecutively conducted* to the ventricles. When this occurs, the P-R of the two consecutively conducted beats can be measured. If the P-R interval *increases,* you are *no doubt* looking at a Wenckebach rhythm! On the other hand, if the P-R interval of the two consecutively conducted beats *remains the same,* the rhythm is *probably* Mobitz type II.

In either instance, a slow ventricular rate may require augmentation. Since the sinus mechanism is healthy, atropine may serve to increase the sinus rate. Although atropine will not reduce the block, it may serve to increase overall rate of those beats which are conducted. Whew!

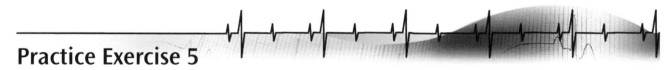

Practice Exercise 5

It's funny how it **always** seems to be practice time!

A. Study the rhythm strip at the top of page 150, then describe what you see!

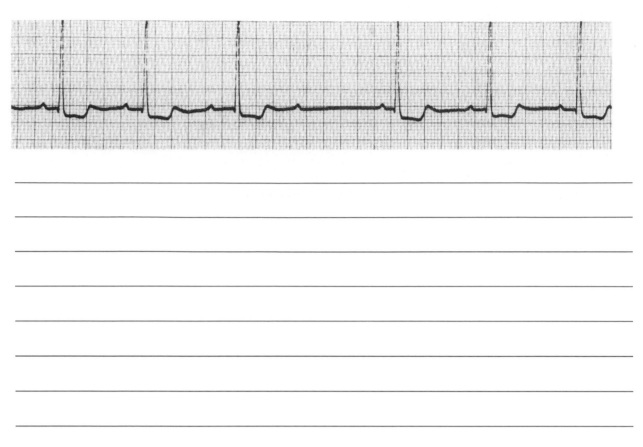

_____

_____

_____

_____

_____

_____

_____

_____

B.   Describe this rhythm strip in detail!

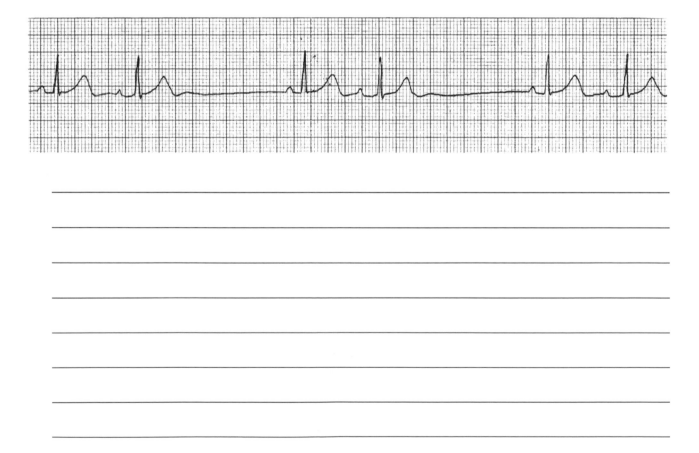

_____

_____

_____

_____

_____

_____

_____

_____

C. What would you say about this rhythm?

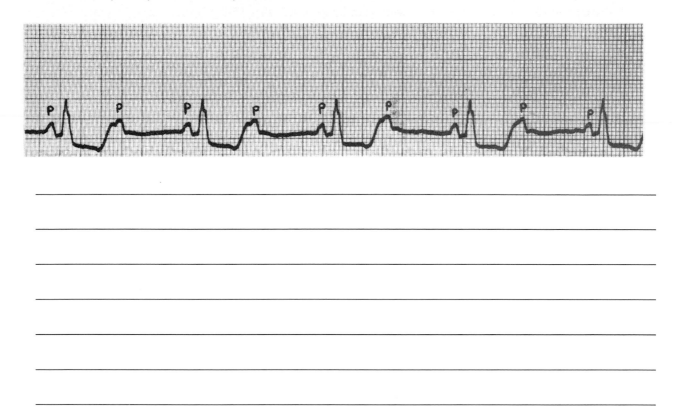

 For Feedback 5, refer to page 167.

 input section 5.6 Complete Heart Block (CHB)

Now that you have an appreciation for first and second degree heart blocks, it is time to explore third degree, or complete heart block.

Complete heart block (CHB) is a good descriptive term. It simply means that none of the atrial impulses conduct through to ventricles to initiate ventricular depolarization.

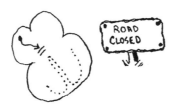

In other words, while the sinus pacemaker discharges normally (60–100 per minute) causing atrial depolarization, none of the impulses conduct through to the ventricles.

Thus, the patient's EKG *could* look like this!

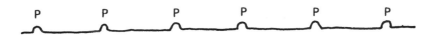

However, you will remember . . . if a sinus impulse fails to discharge or *fails to be transmitted,* a lower (more distal) pacemaker will usually take control of heart beat! Hurray for escape pacemakers!

And, that is exactly what happens in complete heart block! Because none of the sinus impulses are conducted through to the ventricles, a more distal pacemaker initiates ventricular activation.

When the AV junction is healthy (uninvolved in the underlying pathology), it will initiate the escape rhythm. Remember at idiojunctional or junction escape rhythms from Section 3?

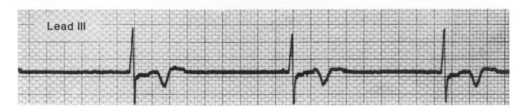

A junctional escape rhythm with no obvious P waves.

An idiojunctional rhythm is regular with a heart rate usually 40 to 60 beats per minute. A P wave may occur before, during, or after the QRS complex. The QRS complexes are narrow, measuring less than 0.12 seconds!

When the AV junction is diseased or damaged, it may be unable to take over as the escape or safety pacemaker. When this occurs, the next lower (more distal) pacemaker located within the ventricles assumes the ventricular pacing role (ventricular escape rhythm).

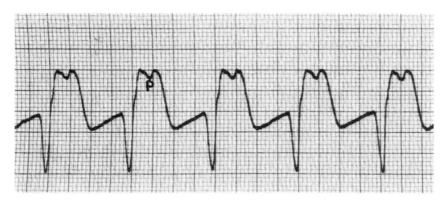

Accelerated ventricular escape rhythm.

You will recall that idioventricular or ventricular escape rhythms are usually regular and slow (20–40 beats per minute), though rates may vary from 10–100 beats per minute. Ventricular escape rhythms have no P waves preceding the QRS complexes. However, P waves may be hidden in, or follow, the QRS complexes. Ventricular impulses are *widened,* measuring 0.12 seconds or greater, owing to the fact that ventricular activation is outside the normal conduction pathway.

(If you need review of idioventricular rhythms, turn back to page 129.)

 In complete heart block, none of the sinus impulses are conducted through to the ventricles . . . so, a lower (more distal) pacemaker initiates ventricular depolarization.

There is one thing you need to remember . . . both the sinus P waves and the escape rhythm will be obvious on the EKG recording. There is no failure of the sinus pacemaker or atrial activation, only a failure of impulse transmission to the ventricles. Thus, P waves will be present!

Closely examine this next strip.

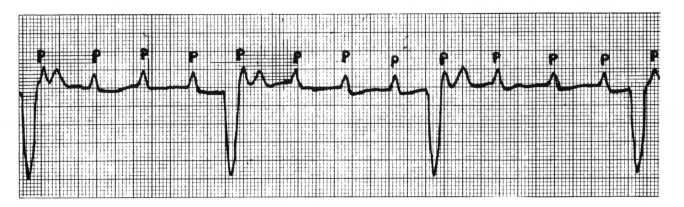

First, locate all the P waves and evaluate atrial activation. Atrial activation is occurring at a rate of approximately 107 per minute (count the number of small squares between P waves . . . there are 14 small squares between P waves. So, I looked back to the chart on page 39 and found that 14 small squares yields a rate of 107 per minute).

Next, evaluate ventricular activity. The QRSs are occurring regularly and slowly at a rate of less than 30 per minute. If I wanted to know the exact rate, I could count the number of small squares between the QRS complexes . . . that comes to 55 small squares. The chart on page 39 does not give the rate for 55 small squares, so I could do the calculation myself! Divide 55 into 1500 . . . there are 1500 small squares in a one minute time interval.

$$55\overline{)1500} ^{27}$$

So, the ventricular rate in this strip is about 27 beats per minute. *Ugh!*

The QRS complexes measure 0.16 seconds in duration. Thus, we know the escape rhythm is most likely of ventricular origin.

Now comes the important question, *Are atrial and ventricular activity related? No!* The P-R interval is *never* constant in complete heart block.

There are two *independent*, or asynchronous, pacemakers (atrial and ventricular) bearing no relationship to one another! Thus, the two pacemakers are dissociated. Hence, we have a new term . . . *AV dissociation*.

Criteria for Complete Heart Block

- The atrial and ventricular rates are different—the atrial activity is independent of, or dissociated from, ventricular activity (*AV dissociation*)
- The atrial rate (P waves) is faster. No sinus impulses are conducted through to the ventricles
- The ventricular rate (QRS complexes) is slow and regular
- The QRS complexes may be narrow (less than 0.12 seconds) or wide (0.12 seconds or greater)

    Junctional escape rhythms have narrow (less than 0.12 seconds) QRS complexes; ventricular escape rhythms have widened QRS complexes (0.12 seconds or greater).

- The P-R interval is never constant

IMPORTANT NOTE: The term *AV dissociation* is a nonspecific generic term that may be applied to any rhythm where the atria and ventricles are activated independently. This independent activation will be evidenced as a varying P-R interval. AV dissociation is never a primary disorder; rather, it is a descriptive term.

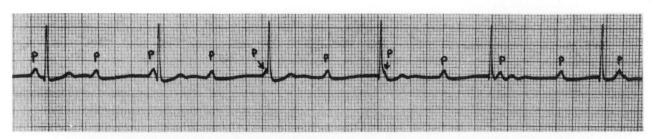

Complete heart block with QRS complexes of normal duration (less than 0.12 seconds).

Sometimes, in a complete heart block, the P waves are hidden in other wave forms. We assume they are really there! *P waves are said to be "marching" through the rhythm.* (Personally, I didn't know that P waves marched . . . but I bet John Phillip Sousa would have been happy to know that.) ☺

When QRS complexes measure within normal limits (less than 0.12 seconds), the defect in complete heart block is *usually* in the AV node. In this case, complete heart block usually develops *gradually* as a *progression* from *Wenckebach, Mobitz type I.* Commonly, ischemia resulting from an inferior wall myocardial infarction or digitalis toxicity are the *culprits* responsible for this rhythm! When complete heart block is intranodal in origin, the QRS complexes are narrow and the ventricular rate generally averages 40–60 per minute. Past studies have indicated that complete heart block of intranodal origin has a lower mortality rate than any other form of complete heart block.

Complete heart block associated with widened QRS complexes (0.12 or greater) is usually a manifestation of bilateral bundle branch block (Mobitz type II) and is almost always associated with *extensive* myocardial damage. The ventricular rate in this instance is usually less than 40 per minute. This type of complete heart block can lead to ventricular standstill with dramatic suddenness. The mortality rate has been estimated to be 80%.

Treatment for complete heart block is aimed at managing the underlying condition and supporting or augmenting the ventricular rate.

Complete heart block of intranodal origin (QRSs measuring less than 0.12 seconds) may be observed and not treated if the ventricular rate is adequate for perfusion. This is often the case when associated with inferior wall myocardial infarctions. If necessary, atrophine may be administered to increase the rate of the junctional escape pacemaker. When digitalis toxicity is the causative culprit (as confirmed by a serum digitalis level), digitalis administration is discontinued.

Complete heart block resulting from a blockage below the bundle of His (QRSs measuring 0.12 seconds or greater) poses a greater mortality risk owing to its common association with extensive myocardiam damage. In addition to therapeutic interventions aimed at reducing myocardial workload (to be discussed later in this text), a transvenous pacemaker may be inserted to augment ventricular activation and/or serve as a backup should ventricular activiation fail (ventricular standstill).

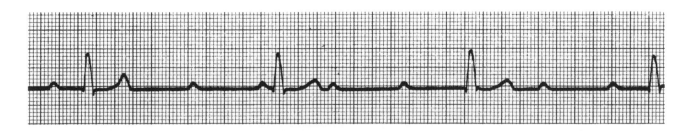

The above strip demonstrates complete heart block with a QRS duration of 0.13 seconds. The ventricular rate is 29 beats per minute! Note that the P-R interval is never constant and the P waves *march* through the rhythm. The atrial and ventricular pacemakers are functioning independently.

This next rhythm strip demonstrates ventricular standstill.

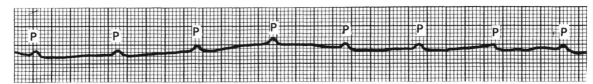

Ventricular Standstill (no evidence of ventricular activity).

In ventricular standstill, none of the atrial impulses reach and activate the ventricles, and a lower more distal pacemaker fails to emerge. This is an extreme emergency warranting immediate C.P.R. and the application of a transcutaneous pacemaker (TCP). TCP will be discussed in Section 8.

> **NOTE:** When looking at rhythm strips, a *general rule* to remember is . . . if the P-R interval is *never* constant, the rhythm can only be *Wenckebach* or *complete heart block* (CHB). Wenckebach has a *varying* R-R interval or irregularly occurring QRS complexes. CHB usually has a *regular* R-R interval—the QRSs occur in a regular pattern.

Bonus: Remember atrial fibrillation, the irregularly irregular rhythm with an undulating baseline? (If you need review, turn back to Section 2.)

There is *one* instance where one will find an atrial fibrillation with a ***regular*** ventricular response. When a complete heart block exists, all chaotic atrial impulses will be blocked. A lower more distal pacemaker will then assume the role of pacemaker. Thus, the monitor tracing will show undulating atrial activity and a slow, regular ventricular response!

Let's try some practice!

Practice Exercise 6

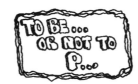

A. Complete heart block means that _____

_____

_____

_____

B. When atrial impulses are blocked or fail to conduct to the ventricles, a lower more distal pacemaker will usually take over, initiating ventricular activation. This back-up mechanism for ventricular activation is known as an _____.

C. If an escape rhythm has QRS complexes measuring less than 0.12 seconds and a rate of 40–60 beats per minute, it is probably a/an _____ rhythm. If an escape rhythm has a slow rate (20–40 beats per minute) and widened QRS complexes, it is usually a/an _____ rhythm.

D. Describe this next rhythm strip in detail. Evaluate both atrial and ventricular activity. Then, determine if there is a relationship between the two activities.

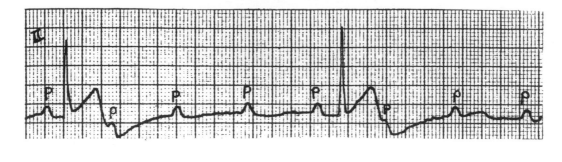

_____

_____

_____

_____

 For Feedback 6, refer to page 167. Nice work!

input section 5.7 Bundle Branch Block

Blocks, blocks and more blocks!

You will probably be happy to know that this is the last exercise in this section!

We now need to think about **Bundle Branch Blocks** (BBB).

When one speaks of bundle branch blocks, he or she is actually referring to a trifascicular system. You will remember that the left bundle branch has two branches or fascicles. So, the two bundle branches (right and left) have three conducting segments or fascicles (little bundles). That's where we get the term *trifascicular!*

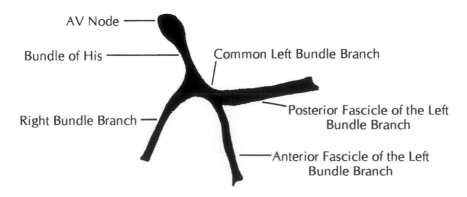

As seen above, the common left bundle branch divides into two separate fascicles early in its course through the ventricles. The anterior fascicle is longer, thinner, and has a single blood supply. In contrast, the posterior fascicle is shorter, thicker, and has a double blood supply.

Using these three fascicles, there are *11* types of block which could exist: bundle branch blocks, hemiblocks, bifascicular blocks, and trifascicular block! To *simplify* this matter, we will concentrate on right bundle branch block (RBBB) and complete left bundle branch block (LBBB)!

Bundle branch block implies that for some reason, conduction through either of the main bundle branches (right or common left) has been delayed or interrupted. This delay causes ventricular activation and depolarization to occur more slowly, causing the QRS to widen, measuring 0.12 seconds or greater.

Bundle branch blocks have a *multitude* of causes. The more *frequent* causative factors include coronary artery disease, myocardial infarction, hypertensive heart disease, excessive potassium intake, rapid tachycardia, and pronestyl or digitalis toxicities. Treatment of either right or left bundle branch block consists of managing the *underlying* disorder.

We will first consider right bundle branch block (RBBB) since it occurs twice as commonly as left bundle branch block.

Right Bundle Branch Block (RBBB)

Right bundle branch block (RBBB) occurs when conduction through the right bundle branch is delayed or interrupted. This delay or interruption may be associated with almost any variety of heart disease, hypertensive cardiovascular disease, right ventricular hypertrophy, or congenital lesions involving the septum. Occasionally, RBBB may be found in an otherwise healthy individual!

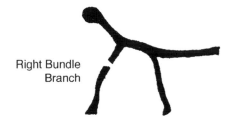

Right Bundle Branch

In RBBB, an atrial impulse is conducted normally through the atria and through the AV junction. A blockage in the right bundle branch, however, causes right ventricular activation to occur more slowly. And, you now know that slow ventricular depolarization is recorded as a widened QRS, 0.12 seconds or greater.

So, on the monitor, one would see a P wave and a normal P-R interval because the defect is confined only to the right bundle branch. The left ventricle is activated in a normal fashion. The right ventricle is stimulated by an impulse from the left bundle branch which passes to the right side of the septum below the block. This *abnormal* activation of the right ventricle requires a greater duration of time . . . thus, the QRS is widened.

Let's see if we can put that into perspective.

1. Septal activation occurs normally, from right to left. If we are monitoring from a right chest lead V_1, the force of septal depolarization moves toward the positive electrode. Thus, the initial part of the QRS is directed upward. You will recall the R wave is the first *upward* or *positive* deflection of a QRS complex. If a second positive deflection is observed in the QRS, it is also an R wave (the larger of the R waves is designated as R9; the smaller R wave is designated by a lower case r).

2. Next, the free wall of the left ventricle depolarizes. This time, the direction of depolarization is away from the positive electrode, so the next part of the QRS is directed negatively.

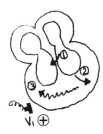

3. Last, the right ventricle is stimulated abnormally, with the direction of depolarization moving toward the positive electrode.

So, what does the QRS look like . . . you guessed it! In lead V_1, there are two R waves! Two R waves can produce a QRS complex that looks like an "M" or rabbit ears. And, because of the abnormal right ventricular activation, the QRS is widened! Neat, huh! Remember, when the force of depolarization moves

Lead V_1 ⊕

toward a positive electrode, the resulting deflection is *upright,* or positive. Likewise, when the force of depolarization moves *away from* a positive electrode (toward a negative electrode) the resulting deflection is *downward,* or negative. If you need a quick review of leads, turn back to Section 1! ☺

One can identify a bundle branch block on a monitor tracing by the widened QRS. Everything else about the rhythm is usually normal (at least in "textbook" cases)!

In order to *distinguish* right from left bundle branch block, however, it is necessary to look at the V leads. V leads (V_1–V_6) are the positive chest leads that look directly at the heart.

EKG Criteria for RBBB

- QRS measures 0.12 seconds or greater.
- Wide and slurred S waves in lead I, V_5, and V_6
- rsR′ (M pattern or "rabbit ears") in V_1 and V_2.

Right Bundle Branch Block Lead Patterns

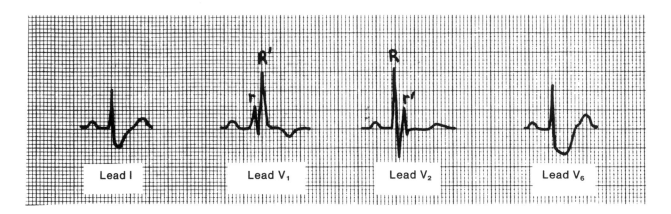

Remember, to distinguish right from left bundle branch block, one must look at the V leads! I have difficulty remembering all of that, so I just remember . . .

> In RBBB, the QRS in lead V_1 will appear wide and positive . . . (more or less of an "M" pattern).

No matter which lead one observes, the QRS will be widened, at least 0.12 seconds. This next strip is a lead V_1 monitor trace demonstrating RBBB.

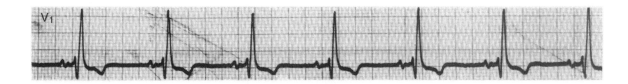

The rhythm is regular at a rate of approximately 80 beats per minute. P waves precede each QRS complex. All P waves are uniform. The P-R interval is of normal duration. The QRS complexes are uniform, occur regularly, and measure approximately 0.16 seconds. The QRS is widened and positive. In lead V₁ a positive, wide QRS characterizes right bundle branch block.

So, this is a sinus rhythm with RBBB!

Right bundle branch block occurs twice as commonly as left bundle branch block and frequently develops with changes in heart rate—especially tachycardias. If the bundles are diseased or suppressed by drugs, as heart rate increases, the bundles may fail to conduct. RBBB is *generally* a consequence of occlusion of the anterior descending coronary artery, and is generally associated with extensive myocardial damage. Most authorities agree it is probably the extent of myocardial damage that determines the patient's prognosis. Treatment is supportive.

Rate Dependent Bundle Branch Block

Now, rate dependent bundle branch blocks will be explored. Conducting tissues that are diseased may only be capable of conducting normally when the heart rate is slow. If that rate is speeded up, there may be delayed conduction or no conduction at all. The involved conducting tissue must have time to recover from its refractory period if it is to conduct normally. If recovery time is insufficient, conduction will be delayed. When conduction through a bundle branch is delayed, the monitor shows a widened QRS complex (a bundle branch block pattern). The delay in a bundle branch is due to unequal refractoriness of the bundle branches.

In a rate dependent bundle branch block, a patient will present with a normal rhythm. If his heart rate increases over a certain point, he will exhibit a bundle branch block pattern. The diseased conducting tissues are unable to recover as quickly at faster rates, so conduction occurs abnormally (wide QRS complexes). When the heart rate slows, conduction will again be normal. This is known as *rate related* or *rate dependent bundle branch block.* Most commonly, the defect in rate related bundle branch blocks occurs in the right bundle branch. That's a mouthful.

Examine this monitor tracing.

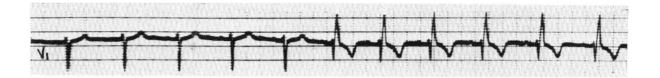

The first five complexes demonstrate a sinus rhythm with a heart rate of 75. When the heart rate increases to 80 beats per minute, conduction is *abnormal*. When this patient's heart rate approaches 80 beats per minute, his diseased conducting system requires *more* time for recovery. Notice that at the faster rate, the QRS is widened and positive. Since this is lead V₁, we are looking at a rate related right bundle branch block. Neat huh?

Left Bundle Branch Block (LBBB)

Left bundle branch block (LBBB) occurs when conduction through both segments or both fascicles of the common left bundle is *delayed* or *interrupted* as demonstrated below. This delay or interruption is often associated with coronary artery disease, left ventricular hypertrophy, and congenital lesions involving the septum.

LBBB may be associated with either inferior or anterior wall infarction depending upon the coronary vessel supplying the common left bundle branch.

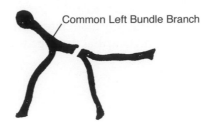

Common Left Bundle Branch

In LBBB, atrial impulses conduct normally through the atria and through the AV junction. A blockage in the common left bundle branch causes depolarization of the septum and left ventricle to occur *more slowly.* In left bundle branch block, the right ventricle is activated in a normal fashion. The left ventricle is then activated by an impulse from the right bundle branch which passes to the left side of the septum below the block. Thus, activation of the left ventricle is delayed causing a widening of the QRS.

Again, let's put this into perspective as seen from a right chest lead, V_1 ⊕

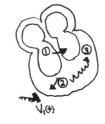

1. Septal activation is abnormal, moving left to right. The force of septal depolarization moves away from the positive V_1 electrode. Thus, the initial part of the QRS is directed negatively.
2. The right ventricle depolarizes normally, with the direction of depolarization moving toward the positive electrode. So, the second part of the QRS will be upwardly directed.
3. Left ventricular activation occurs abnormally, moving away from the positive electrode, thus taking additional time.

The "textbook" picture of LBBB in a V_1 lead is that of a *distorted* W. Usually, however, the W is not well defined, appearing more as a V. See for yourself!

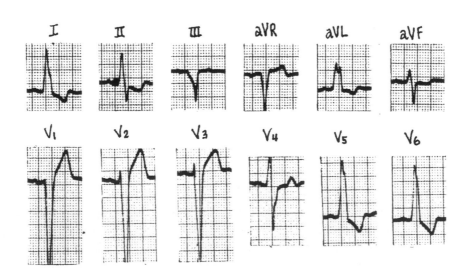

To distinguish left from right bundle branch block, one must look at the V leads.

EKG Criteria for LBBB

- QRS measures 0.12 seconds or greater.
- QRS is wide and may be notched—the T wave deflection is usually in the opposite direction to the R wave in most leads.
- W or V pattern seen in leads V_1 and V_2.

If this is complicated, just remember . . .

In LBBB, the QRS in lead V_1 will appear wide and negative.

No matter which lead one observes, the QRS will be widened . . . measuring 0.12 seconds or greater. Here is a V_1 monitor tracing showing LBBB. Notice that the widened QRS measures almost 0.16 seconds. Also notice the distortion (elevation) of the ST segment. The ST segment distortion results from the delayed activation of the left ventricle. In other words, altered activation of the left ventricle causes repolarization (ST segment) to be altered, as well.

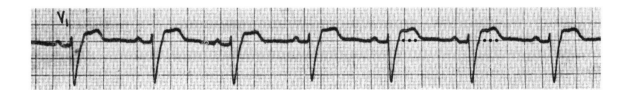

In the above strip, the rhythm is regular at a rate of 62 beats per minute. P waves precede each QRS complex. All P waves appear uniform. The P-R interval is of normal duration. The QRS complexes are uniform, occur regularly, and measure almost 0.16 seconds. The QRS is wide and negative. In lead V_1, a widened and negative QRS characterizes left bundle branch block. So, this is a sinus rhythm with LBBB! Also note that there is S-T elevation suggesting injury. The LBBB may indeed be due to injury of conduction tissue.

Though *rate dependent* bundle branch block is usually the result of delayed right bundle branch conduction, it occasionally occurs because of delayed left bundle branch conduction! See for yourself! Following is a rate dependent left bundle branch block. The first two complexes demonstrate a LBBB pattern, with a heart rate of approximately 62. When the heart rate slows to approximately 52 (as demonstrated in the remaining complexes), the LBBB pattern disappears.

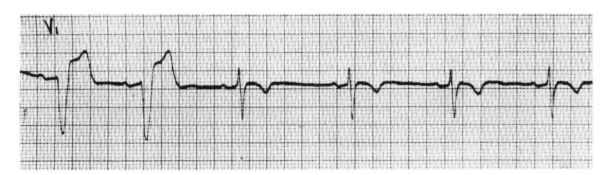

Rate dependent left bundle branch block.

It is easy to be fooled by widened QRSs . . . always look for preceding P waves! If a single P wave occurs before each widened QRS and the P-R remains constant, a bundle branch block exists. If no P wave is observed before the widened QRS, the beat is likely of ventricular origin!

To clarify any confusion . . . . . . *Remember* . . .

If a rhythm appears normal except for a widened QRS (measuring 0.12 seconds or greater), the patient has a bundle branch block. To distinguish between a right and left bundle branch block, inspect lead V_1.

> LBBB = QRS is wide and negative in lead V_1
> RBBB = QRS is wide and positive in lead V_1

It is the extent of myocardial damage or physiologic concern causing a bundle branch block that determines the patient prognosis. Treatment is aimed at the underlying pathology.

Practice Exercise 7

Are you ready for more practice? **Practice, practice, practice** . . . this is worse than piano lessons!

A.   This is lead II patient monitor tracing.

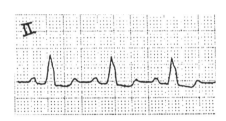

The rhythm is regular with a heart rate of approximately 88 beats per minute. The P-R interval is constant (0.19 seconds). Each QRS complex is preceded by a P wave, and all P waves appear uniform. The QRS complexes, however, are widened, measuring slightly greater than 0.12 seconds.

> Generally speaking . . .
>   There are only two types of rhythm patterns that demonstrate widened QRSs . . . ventricular rhythms and rhythms associated with bundle branch block. Ventricular rhythms **do not have P waves preceding the widened QRSs**.

So, since there are definitive P waves in the above monitor tracing, this must be bundle branch block.

But which type . . . right or left????

Turn to the next page to solve the mystery.

To determine whether this rhythm is a right or left bundle branch block, one must inspect the V leads—particularly V_1 and V_6. Remember, all V leads (V_1–V_6) are $\oplus$ leads.

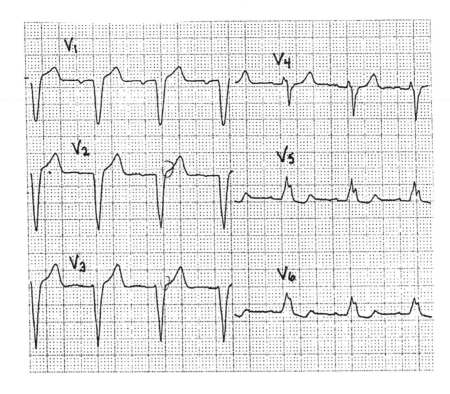

Here are the V leads—all six of them! *Determine whether this rhythm is a right or left bundle branch block and explain your logic.*

_____

_____

_____

_____

_____

_____

_____

_____

_____

_____

_____

B. Another patient has the following lead II monitor tracing.

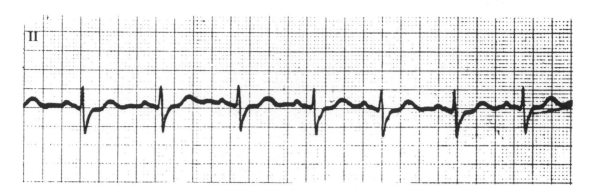

Everything appears normal—**except** that the QRSs measure 0.14 seconds. To be within normal limits, the QRS duration must be less than 0.12 seconds!

Because you are a *suspicious* creature, you review both the patient's chart and a recent 12-lead EKG. Following are the EKG precordial or V leads! Use the lines provided below to present your analysis and conclusion(s).

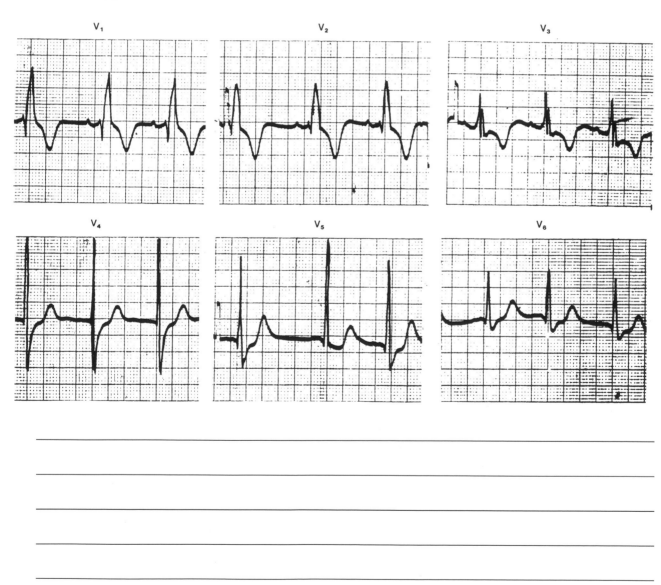

_____

_____

_____

_____

_____

C. The following rhythm strip "belongs" to a 78 year old female and demonstrates a rate-related or rate dependent right/left (circle one) bundle branch block.

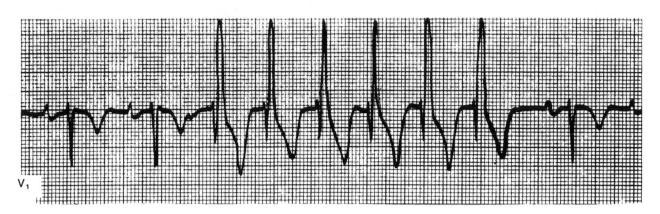

V₁

Describe the above rhythm strip and justify your conclusion. What do you think might have precipitated the rhythm change?

_____

_____

_____

_____

_____

_____

 For Feedback 7, refer to page 168.

For Feedback 7, refer to page 168.

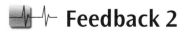 Feedback 1

How did you do? Hope your interpretation resembles mine!

The rhythm is irregular owing to an obvious pause! The rhythm is a sinus rhythm with P waves preceding each QRS and a constant P-R interval, measuring slightly greater than 0.16 seconds. The QRS duration is within normal limits measuring 0.8 seconds. There is a pronounced pause in the sinus mechanism. A P wave fails to occur at the expected time. The sinus pause measures 2.52 seconds!

Feedback 2

Good work!

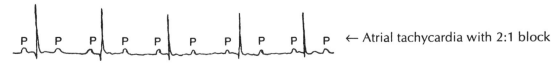

← Atrial tachycardia with 2:1 block

Atrial rate regular between 160-200 per minute.
I flattened out T waves so that P waves would be more prominent. (Don't forget, the P-R is always constant!)

⚡ Feedback 3

A.

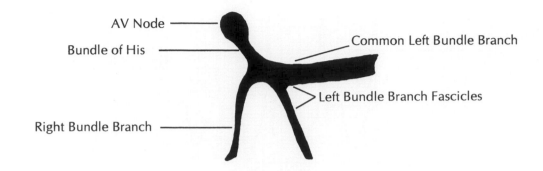

- AV Node
- Bundle of His
- Common Left Bundle Branch
- Left Bundle Branch Fascicles
- Right Bundle Branch

B. Atrial depolarization is represented on the EKG as a P wave. The P-R interval represents <u>the transmission of the pacemaker impulse from the atria to the AV node</u>.

C. The QRS represents <u>ventricular depolarization</u>.

⚡ Feedback 4

Excellent work!

A. The rhythm is regular with a heart rate of approximately 100 beats per minute. P waves precede each QRS. The P waves are uniform in appearance, sitting near the previous T waves. The QRS complexes are narrow, less than 0.12 seconds. But, voila! The P-R interval is prolonged. The P-R interval measures approximately 7 ½ small squares or approximately 0.30 seconds. The QRS measures 0.08 seconds. So, this is a borderline sinus tachycardia with a first degree heart block!

$$\begin{array}{r} 0.04 \\ \times\ 7.5 \\ \hline 0.30 \end{array}$$

B. The P-R interval in this rhythm strip measures approximately <u>6</u> little squares or <u>0.24</u> seconds. The QRS measures approximately 0.08 seconds.

$$\begin{array}{r} 0.04 \\ \times\ 6 \\ \hline 0.24 \end{array}$$

C. First degree heart block is usually benign and needs only <u>to be watched</u>. However, if the P-R interval is increasing, digitalis preparations should be withheld.

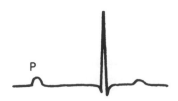

P

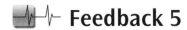 **Feedback 5**

Great Job . . .

If your answers look something like mine!

A. The rhythm is irregular. One of the P waves is not followed by a QRS complex. The P-R interval of the conducted beats gradually lengthens until finally a P wave is not conducted. The R-R interval shortens. The cycle then begins to repeat. This is "our friend" **Wenckebach**, usually a <u>benign</u> arrhythmia.

B. This rhythm is irregular and one must become a detective to discover why. There are three cycles that appear identical. The P-R interval of the first beat (first cycle) measures 0.20 seconds. The P-R interval of the second beat (first cycle) measures almost 0.24 seconds. This same pattern is evident in complexes 3 and 4 (the second cycle), and 5 and 6 (third cycle). This is a Wenckebach (Mobitz type I) rhythm. The P wave that fails to conduct (after beats 2, 4 and 6) is somewhat obscured, though it follows the T wave and is "flat" in appearance.

C. The rhythm is regular with a heart rate of approximately 45. There are two P waves for every QRS. Atrial activity is regular. The QRS complexes are widened, measuring approximately 0.12 seconds. This is a 2:1 AV conduction with widened QRS complexes. This may be a Mobitz type II AV block, so it should be observed *closely!* **In order to distinguish between a Mobitz type I and type II, two beats must be conducted consecutively so one can determine the constancy or progressive lengthening of the P-R interval.**

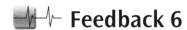 **Feedback 6**

Nice work.

Awesome!

A. Complete heart block means that <u>none of the sinus impulses are being conducted to the ventricles to initiate ventricular depolarization</u>.

B. When atrial impulses are blocked or fail to conduct to the ventricles, a lower more distal pacemaker will usually initiate ventricular activation. This back-up mechanism for ventricular activation is known as an <u>escape rhythm</u>.

C. If an escape rhythm has QRS complexes measuring less than 0.12 seconds and a rate of 40–60 beats per minute, it is probably an <u>idiojunctional or junctional escape rhythm</u>. If an escape rhythm has a slow rate (20–40 beats per minute) and widened QRS complexes, it is usually an <u>idioventricular or ventricular escape rhythm</u>.

D. P waves are occurring in a regular pattern at a rate of 83 per minute. The P waves appear to be "marching" through the rhythm strip. Two QRSs are apparent at a rate of approximately 28 per minute. The QRS complexes are narrow, measuring less than 0.12 seconds. There is no relationship between the P waves and the QRS complexes. The P-R interval is <u>not</u> constant. The P-R interval of the two conducted beats measures 0.24 and 0.28 seconds, respectively. This is complete heart block with an idiojunctional escape rhythm.

> **Complete heart block has the following features:**
>
> - Atrial and ventricular rates are different.
> - The atrial rate is faster.
> - The ventricular rate is slow and regular.
> - The QRS complexes may be narrow or widened.
> - The P-R interval is *never* constant—the P waves appear to be "marching" through the rhythm

Feedback 7

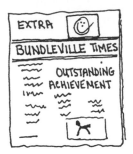

A. This is a left bundle branch block. The QRS in V$_1$ is wide (measuring slightly greater than 0.12 seconds) and negative.

B. This is a sinus rhythm (rate approximately 70 beats per minute) with right bundle branch block! The QRS measures approximately 0.14 seconds and V$_1$ demonstrate a wide, positively directed QRS.

C. The rhythm strip demonstrates a rate-related (right)/left bundle branch block. The underlying rhythm is a sinus rhythm. The first two complexes occur at a rate of 68 per minute and are conducted normally (QRS measures less than 0.12 seconds). When the heart rate increases to near 100 per minute, a widened QRS is evident. In lead V$_1$, the widened QRS has a crude M pattern. When the heart rate again slows, normal conduction is evident. An unsuccessful attempt to climb over the side rails precipitated this event!

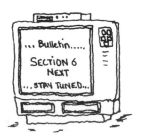

Notes

Notes

Artifact . . . To Be, or Not To Be . . .

Objectives

When you have completed Section 6, you will be able to describe or identify

1. electrical artifact encountered in monitoring
2. appearances and sources of artifact
   a. 60-cycle interference
   b. motion artifact
   c. signals from therapeutic electrical devices
   d. "off the monitor"
3. concerns associated with artifact
4. principles of artifact recognition
5. steps to reduce or eliminate artifact

Text by:
Delores D. Schultz

6.1   Introduction to Artifact

Now that you have been through most of all of the basic dysrhythmias, you may need a change of pace.

Sometimes you will observe "things" on a monitor that have nothing whatsoever to do with electrical conductivity of the heart. These unusual patterns are commonly known as *artifact* or *electrical interference*. Other popular words are "glitches" or "noise." Artifact is an electrical signal which appears on the tracing and which originates from sources other than the heart!

Let's try another simple analogy.

This is a kid watching cartoons on Saturday morning.

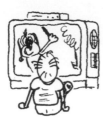

Here is the mother in the next room cleaning . . . and . . . she turns on the vacuum.

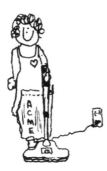

Instantly, above the noise of the vacuum, the mother hears, "**okay, what's wrong with this picture?**" The picture looks like this:

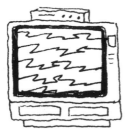

What is a mother to do???

   a. Kick the television.

   b. Send it off for repair.

   c. Turn off the vacuum.

Fortunately, this mother chose alternative c. The restored picture now looks like this.

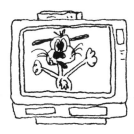

And the kid looks like this.

In this case, there was nothing wrong with the television *and* there was nothing wrong with the vacuum. Simply stated, *the impulses generated by one electrical device in operation interfered with the correct operation of a second electrical device.* The precise electrical theory behind all of this is very complicated . . . at least, *I* think so.

If the mother plugs the vacuum into a different outlet, she may discover that the T.V. is working fine and the kid still looks like this . . .

. . . or, she may elect to finish vacuuming at some later time!

A monitoring system attached to a patient acts much like the television. The monitoring system picks up electrical signals from the heart and transmits them to an oscilloscope. If another electrical device is in operation nearby, electrical signals generated from that device may be picked up by the monitoring system as well, thus interfering with the monitor picture. What you see on the monitor might look like this.

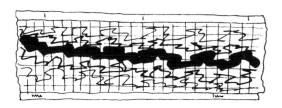

Like the T.V. and the vacuum, the patient's heart *and* the electrical device are probably operating correctly . . . it's just that the electrical device is altering the monitor picture. *Whew!*

To expertly monitor a patient, one needs to recognize artifact when it appears, distinguish it from a patient's rhythm, and take appropriate steps to minimize the artifact.

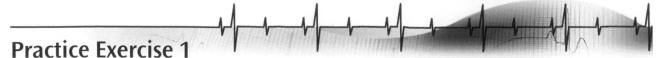

Practice Exercise 1

Now for a short practice session.

Fill in the blank

A. "Glitches" or "noise" on the monitor tracing are known as _____, or electrical interference.

True or False (Use a T or F to correctly answer Questions B. and C.)

B. _____ The presence of artifact is a signal that there is a disturbance in the heart's electrical activity.

C. _____ The presence of artifact is an indication that an electrical device in proximity to the patient is malfunctioning.

Fill in the blank

D. To monitor a patient's rhythm effectively, one needs to _____ artifact when it appears, _____ it from the patient's rhythm, and take appropriate steps to _____ it.

Not too difficult so far, huh?

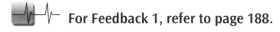 **For Feedback 1, refer to page 188.**

input section 6.2 Sixty-Cycle Interference

There are several different types of artifact commonly encountered in monitoring. This tracing shows 60-cycle interference.

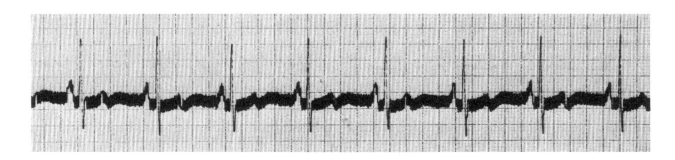

Sixty-cycle interference is characterized by a *wide, fuzzy baseline* which often makes atrial activity difficult to recognize. A "good" tracing should have a narrow, distinct baseline. Monitors may normally show a few seconds of 60-cycle interference when they are first turned on. If the interference persists, it is usually related to *faulty electrode contact*. Poor electrode contact is usually the result of inadequate skin preparation techniques, dried electrode gel, or defective wires or patient cable. Of course, if the patient is using an electric razor, turning the shaver off may resolve the problem!

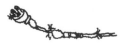

The source of 60-cycle interference is the current which supplies power to the electrical wall outlets.

 The 60-cycle energy is given off by the electrical wiring in the patient's room and is picked up by both the lead wires and the patient. This is *normal*, and this radiant energy *cannot be eliminated*. Although monitors are designed to reduce 60-cycle interference, there must still be good contact along the path from the patient skin to the monitor, and the electrical path must be well shielded.

Specific interventions (*anti-artifact techniques*) include checking to see that the EKG cable is not draped across, or parallel to, other cables (such as call-light, electric bed, or transducer cables). Also, the EKG cable must not touch the metal parts of other electrical equipment such as side rails of electric beds or metal portions of ventilators. Make certain there are no loose connections in the monitoring system. It may be helpful to apply new electrode patches (using correct skin prep) and/or replacing the cable. If these techniques are unsuccessful, biomedical personnel should be called to evaluate and correct the problem.

Now, it's your turn. You are officially commissioned as a "troubleshooter" or a detective. This is a patient's monitor tracing. Notice the broad baseline.

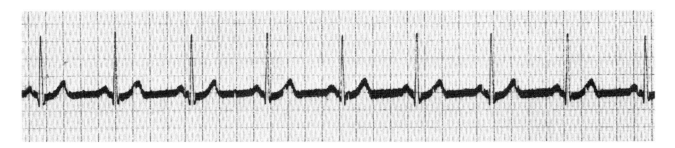

And, here is the patient.

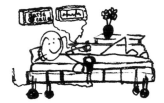

What should one do?

    a. Nothing.

    b. Notify the *managing* physician regarding a rhythm change.

    c. Try moving the cable away from the call light cable.

If you chose c, the patient's tracing now looks like this:

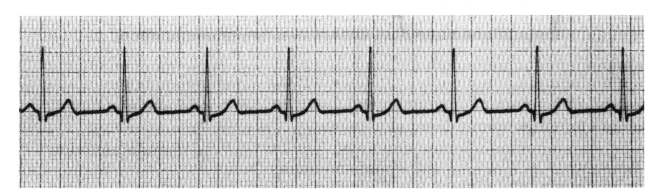

Nice work!

Practice Exercise 2

A. Sixty-cycle interference is characterized by a _____ baseline.

B. Identify at least five ways to reduce 60-cycle interference:

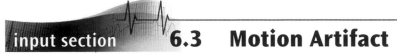

1. _____

2. _____

3. _____

4. _____

5. _____

For Feedback 2, refer to page 194.

input section **6.3   Motion Artifact**

Following is an example of motion artifact.

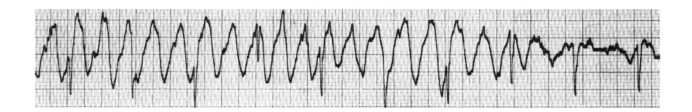

    A Fairy Tale: Long, long ago in a CCU far away, a nurse saw the previous tracing on a monitor. Mr. Jones, the patient, had not been looking too well prior to this "picture." The nurse raced to the room and administered a resounding thump on the patient's chest. Mr. Jones stopped brushing his teeth, leaped from the bed, and was out of the door in a flash, never to be seen again. (☺)—The End

    The moral of the story . . . *look* (before) *the patient leaps!*

    Motion artifact can be the *most troublesome* and *confusing* type of artifact, even for the "so-called" experts! Many patients have undeservedly been thumped on the chest or given antiarrhythmic drugs for this kind of tracing. If the nurse had examined the patient before thumping, (she) would have had the first clue that this was artifact rather than ventricular tachycardia. If the nurse had checked the patient's pulse, (she) would have noted that (his) pulse was regular at a rate of approximately 80.

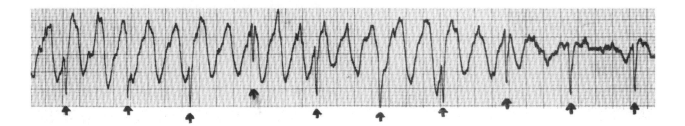

In the previous monitor tracing, you will notice (see arrows) sharp deflections throughout the entire tracing (which just happen to coincide with the patient's pulse). These deflections are QRS complexes. Since ventricular contraction follows ventricular depolarization (QRS), and ventricular contraction results in a pulse, you can usually verify the presence or absence of QRS complexes by checking the patient's pulse.

Believe it or not, the skin is the source of the small electrical signals which produce motion artifact. A voltage of several millivolts can be generated by stretching the outer layer of skin, the epidermis. It is the stretching which results in the artifact. *Large baseline shifts* occur when the patient turns over in bed, brushes his teeth, taps an electrode, etc.

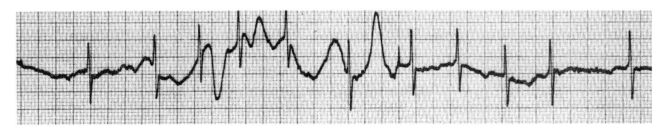

The above strip demonstrates an example of a shifting baseline. If an electrode is placed close to the diaphragm, even the skin movement produced by breathing will cause artifact!

Following are some examples of motion artifact.

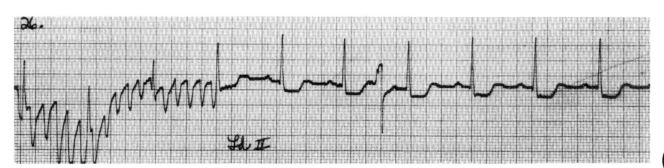

The notorious toothbrush artifact

In the above strip, the artifact might be mistaken for atrial flutter. Did you notice, though, that the R-R interval (the distance between any two R waves) remains precisely the same when the "supposed flutter" converts to sinus rhythm? In other words, measure the R-R interval at the beginning of the strip and compare that to an R-R interval at the end of the strip. Voila! It's the same! This would *seldom* occur if an actual atrial flutter were converting to a sinus rhythm! There is usually a pause when atrial flutter stops, and then, a different ventricular rate when the sinus node takes over. Makes sense, right?

Following is another patient (like the one in the fairy tale), brushing his teeth. This monitor tracing sent a "rescue squad" rushing to the patient's room in belief that the patient was in ventricular tachycardia. Can you find the narrow spikes appearing in the tracing at a rate of approximately 95 per minute? Those are the patient's normal QRS complexes . . . and correspond to the patient's pulse. When in doubt, check the patient's pulse. If the patient is alert and in no distress, it is highly unlikely that he or she has a heart rate of 300!

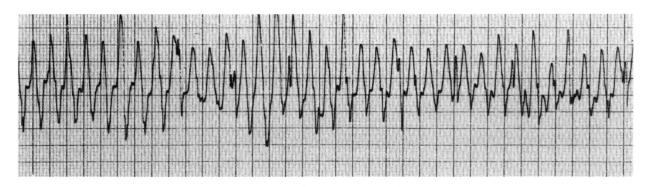

This is the same patient a few seconds later still brushing his teeth, but now his underlying rhythm is more visible! Notice that there is no change in the QRS rate from the previous strip. This constant rate strongly suggests that the underlying rhythm is the same as in the previous strip. If there is any doubt in your mind about a rhythm, always assess the patient. *It is especially important to compare the patient's pulse with the monitor picture.*

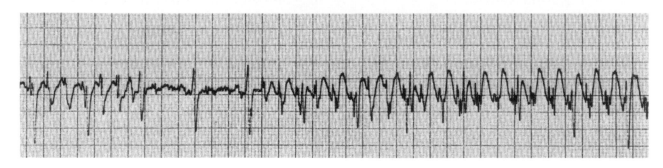

Following are two other tracings displaying artifact mimicing ventricular dysrhythmias. In strip A, the patient is swinging his monitor cable. In strip B, an electrode is being tapped. (*Some smart patients learn that if they tap an electrode, someone will appear immediately.*) By now, you can easily discern artifact! The narrow electrical spikes "walk through" the artifact and correspond to the normal QRS complexes.

A.

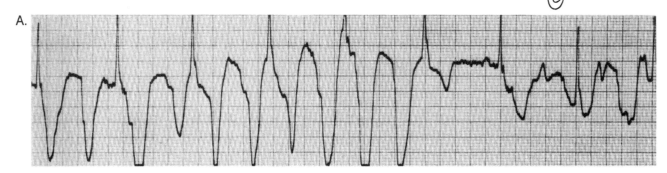

B.

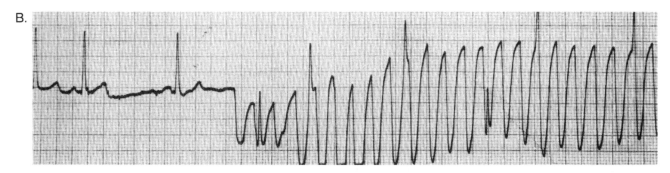

The next strip is more difficult! See for yourself below.

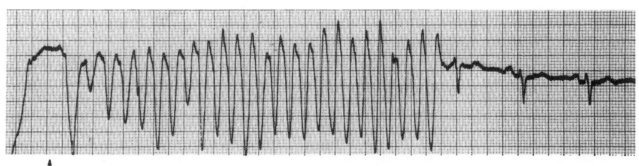

↑
Baseline shift

The previous tracing would send almost anyone running for "the antidysrhythmic drug dujour," *including me*. There are two clues that indicate this might possibly be artifact. The first clue is the shift in the baseline that occurs before the onset of what appears to be "ventricular tachycardia." This shifting baseline strongly suggests patient movement. The second clue relates to the termination of the "ventricular tachycardia." When a patient converts from a ventricular tachycardia to a sinus rhythm, there is *almost always a pause* before the sinus pacemaker resumes. It is important to note that in this tracing, the ventricles would not have sufficient time to repolarize before we see the first normal QRS. If this were a true ventricular tachycardia, the sinus beat following the termination of the ventricular ectopic rhythm would *usually* be widened since the ventricular recovery period is incomplete.

What should one do if unable to decide between artifact and what might be a run of ventricular tachycardia or flutter? Here are four *possible* actions, although step 1 is most important.

1. Check with the patient. He may admit to the fact that he was idly *tapping* his electrode . . . or you might catch him brushing his teeth!
2. Get another opinion. Two or three, or more, heads are often better than one when it comes to deciphering a puzzling strip.
3. Consult with the patient's *managing* physician and let him or her diagnose the rhythm and determine the treatment.
4. Monitor the patient closely!

Following are more examples of motion artifact.

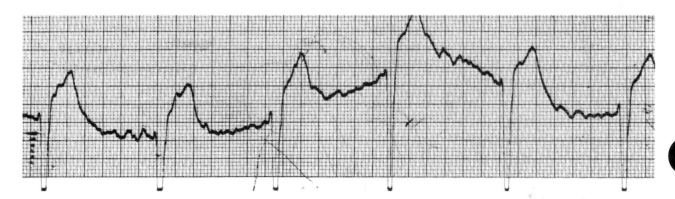

The above monitor pattern demonstrates a *wandering baseline*. It is the result of pronounced, slow patient movements, such as stretching, turning over in bed, and so forth.

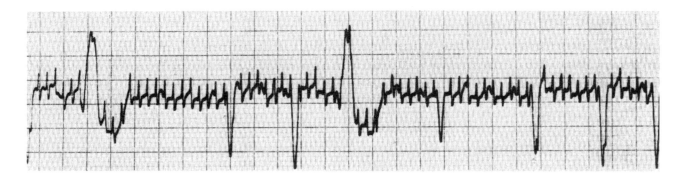

The patient above is receiving *chest percussion* and drainage (for respiratory disorders). *Motion* from seizure activity or muscle tremor could also produce this pattern. It is usually impossible to diagnose atrial dysrhythmias with this type of artifact. (Brilliant, right?!)

This next tracing demonstrates one type of respiratory artifact.

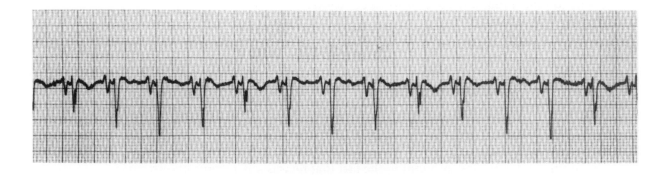

Notice the *cyclic* variation in the QRS amplitude and configuration, as well as in the T waves. Chest wall movement during normal respiration and mechanical ventilation can produce cyclic changes in the baseline, the QRS amplitude, and the T wave appearance! When assessing a patient, one can usually correlate (his) respiratory cycle with the changes that appear on the monitor.

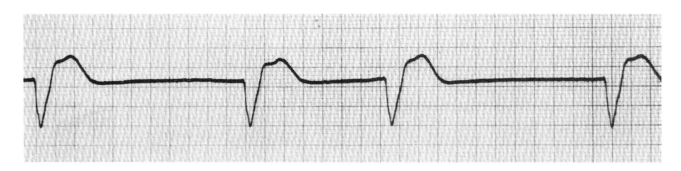

The above tracing is an example of what may be observed when a patient is coding. The artifact is produced by chest compression, or CPR. In order to visualize the underlying rhythm, compression must be stopped momentarily. The underlying rhythm is obvious when chest compression is momentarily interrupted, as evident on the rhythm strip below.

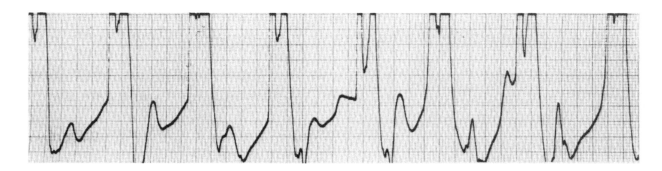

(Just in case your memory has failed, this is an idioventricular rhythm!)

The foremost responsibility in dealing with motion artifact is to *recognize it* as artifact! Accurate analysis will prevent unnecessary patient treatment and will prompt one to take steps to eliminate the artifact. *It is important to eliminate the artifact so that any underlying dysrhythmias will not be masked.*

Some of the same *principles* for eliminating 60-cycle interference also apply to motion artifact. Correct skin preparation and ample gel on the electrode patches can effectively reduce motion artifact. To prevent cable and wire movement, clip the cable to the patient's clothing. Perhaps there is an underlying clinical problem which may need medical treatment. Check to see if the patient is having tremors, seizure activity, or an increase in movement because of discomfort or confusion. Ask the patient to lie quietly or assist (him) in doing so to better analyze the underlying rhythm. Respiratory artifact can be minimized by monitoring on a lead where the positive electrode is not directly over the diaphragm, for example, lead I. Motion artifact can generally be reduced by *attaching the electrodes over bony areas* rather than over skin folds, large muscle masses, joints, or large amounts of fatty tissue.

Always check the patient before treating any dysrhythmia. Remember, one should . . .

> Treat the patient, not the monitor

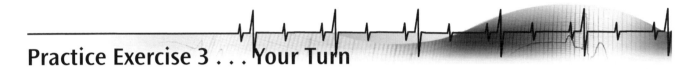

Practice Exercise 3 . . . Your Turn

A. Motion artifact commonly results from electrical signals produced by the _____.

B. Describe how you can determine this tracing demonstrates motion artifact rather than ventricular tachycardia.

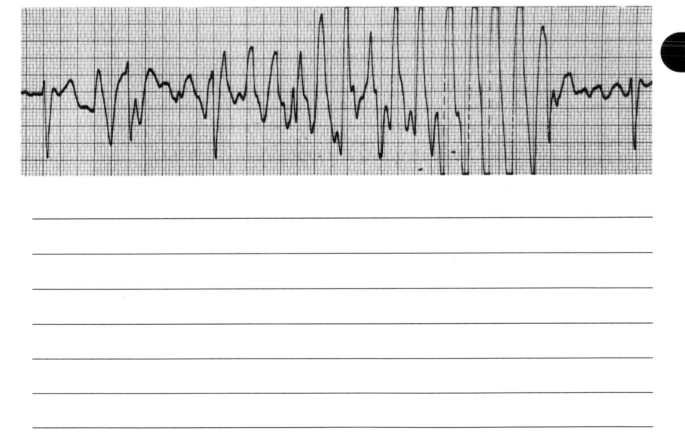

_____

_____

_____

_____

_____

_____

_____

C. List at least three steps one could take to reduce the motion artifact in this tracing.

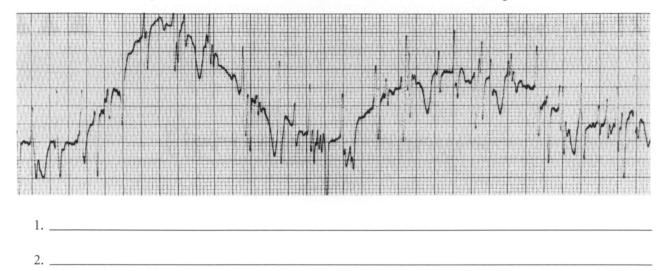

1. _____

2. _____

3. _____

For Feedback 3, refer to page 188.

For Feedback 3, refer to page 188.

input section 6.4 Artifact Produced by Electrical Devices

More artifact . . . ugh!

The next type of artifact to be discussed originates from *signals* produced by therapeutic *electrical devices*. This artifact appears as little "blips" on the monitor tracing. Two types of electrical devices, *pacemakers* and *pain control devices* (TENS), may produce these little blips!

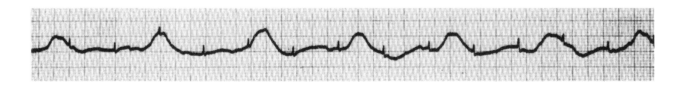

Note the "spikes" throughout this EKG. Spikes are usually the artifact caused by a pacemaker (see discussion in Section 8). So first establish if the patient has a pacemaker. If the patient does not have a pacer, look for other sources of artifact such as chest compressions or interference from medical devices.

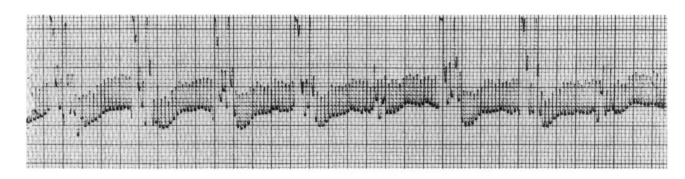

When the patient with the previous EKG was admitted to a monitored stepdown unit, the artifact present on his tracings caused quite an uproar until the staff became aware that the patient had a *TENS* unit. *TENS* stands for a *transcutaneous electrical nerve stimulator*. People who suffer from various types of chronic pain may experience pain reduction or elimination by wearing this electrical device. Whenever this TENS unit was turned on, the monitor tracing appeared normal. In order to obtain a meaningful 12 lead EKG and monitor tracing, the TENS unit had to be turned off periodically.

How about a simple practice exercise?

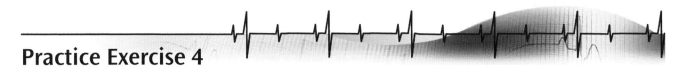

Practice Exercise 4

A. Little "blips" or spikes occurring on a monitor tracing usually originate from adjacent electrical equipment. Two of the *most*-frequent electrical equipment culprits are _____ and

_____ .

B. Pacemaker spikes may be nearly invisible or they may have a larger amplitude than the patient's QRS complexes. This variation in amplitude often depends on the _____ .

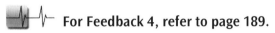 **For Feedback 4, refer to page 189.**

input section   6.5   "Off the Monitor"

The following tracing is from a patient who is "off the monitor." The straight line, indicating the absence of rhythm, may be mistaken for asystole. If you have experience with monitors, you already know that the most common cause of an "asystole-appearing" tracing is a loose electrode. Rarely do patients go directly from a normal rhythm to the complete absence of any rhythm! Reattaching the wire or electrode will restore the normal rhythm to the scope. ☺

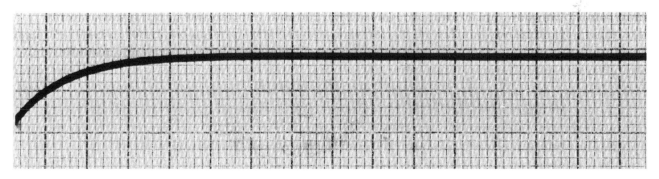

"Off the monitor"

At this point, however, I am reminded of a little lady who, in fact, did go into asystole (the absence of rhythm) from her normal rhythm. The "rescue squad" went to her room immediately to reattach the electrode and found themselves calling a code. Here the maxim is, "*look at the patient—immediately.*"

In most monitoring systems, all of the electrodes must be attached to the patient in order for a tracing to be present. If the wires come loose at either end, if an electrode patch comes loose, or if a wire is broken internally, the tracing will disappear.

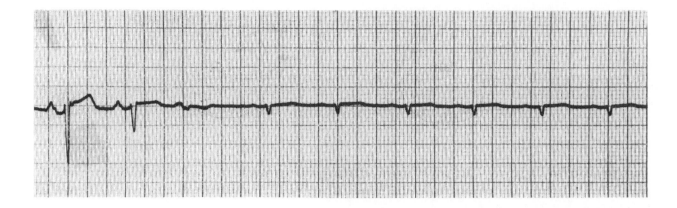

In the above strip, the amplitude setting (gain) was decreased causing the tracing to nearly disappear. When a monitor can no longer "sense" the QRS complexes, a rate alarm may be activated.

When a patient looks like this . . .

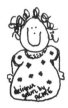

and her tracing looks like this . . .

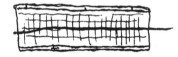

there are several steps one may take to solve the problem.

Steps for Correcting "Off the Monitor"

- Reattach any disconnected wires
- Check to see that the cable is attached to the monitor
- Check electrode patches for intactness and replace any loose patches, making certain than an ample amount of gel is present
- Replace lead wires
- Check for a defective cable by replacing the cable
- Check the amplitude setting to see if the amplitude is set correctly

Sometimes a patient intermittently goes "off the monitor" and the tracing looks like this!

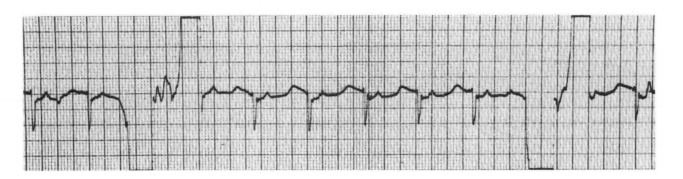

This type of tracing is produced by intermittent interruption of the continuous path from the patient to the monitor. It may be remedied by all the same actions that one might take if the patient were completely "off the monitor."

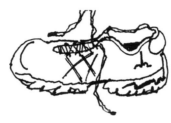

Practice Exercise 5

Make a run at this one!

A. Describe what has happened in this tracing:

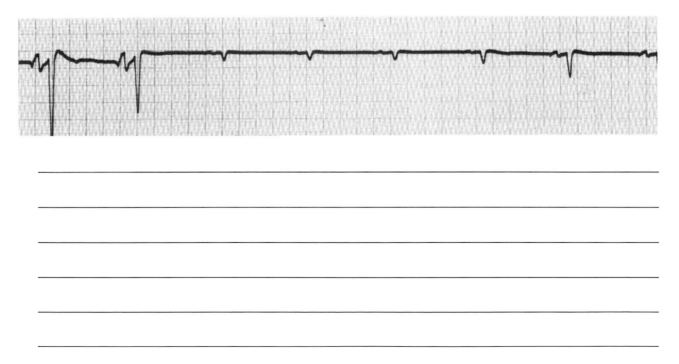

_____

_____

_____

_____

_____

_____

B. Name at least three steps one can take to correct "off the monitor."

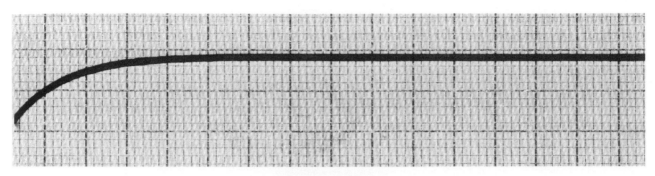

"Off the monitor"

_____

_____

_____

For Feedback 5, refer to page 189.

input section 6.6 Concerns Associated with Artifact

There are two major concerns associated with artifact. The **first** is that artifact may _mimic_ atrial or ventricular dysrhythmias and cause treatment to be initiated unnecessarily. (Even if one does not treat the patient, it may cause you unnecessary worry.) With a little practice you will be able to look at a tracing and recognize that something is "wrong with the picture," rather than the patient.

Here is a list of _clues_ that may assist you in _determining_ the presence of artifact.

Clues for Identifying Artifact

- Baseline should be fine, narrow lines
- QRS complexes _must_ be followed by T waves. Whenever ventricular depolarization occurs, ventricular repolarization must follow. A T wave is always preceded by a QRS complex. If one observes a T wave in the middle of nowhere, chances are, this is an artifact
- A change in supraventricular rhythm, e.g., atrial flutter to sinus rhythm or vice versa, is usually accompanied by a change in ventricular rate
- Cells in the heart cannot be depolarized by two impulses simultaneously. They must repolarize after the first impulse before they can be depolarized by a second. If one observes portions of normal QRS complexes superimposed on a run of "ventricular tachycardia," the "V tach" is probably artifact. Whew! 😊
- P waves should have an established rhythm and a logical configuration. P waves do not usually appear out of nowhere, except sometimes in digitalis toxicity or sick sinus syndrome. If P waves occur prematurely in the cardiac cycle, there should be a pause before the next P wave is observed
- Patients rarely go from a normal rhythm to a straight line rhythm. Usually, "off the monitor" relates to a disconnected electrode or patch. However, **always** check the patient

---

If you are still uncertain after considering all of the above points, obtain a second opinion, and remember—look at the patient!

The **second** major concern is that artifact may *mask* underlying dysrhythmias which deserve or warrant treatment. With experience, you will be able to determine the cause of the artifact and then proceed with appropriate measures to reduce or eliminate it. For troubleshooting steps, refer back to the specific type of artifact covered in this section.

Prevention

There are two simple actions one can take to prevent or reduce artifact and the associated problems. The *first* is assuring the presence of conductive gel. (If electrode gel is partially dry, problems with 60-cycle interference and motion artifact will be magnified and intermittent loss of tracing may occur. Completely dry gel will result in the *absence* of any tracing.) To prevent drying, store the electrodes in their original foil package until ready for use. Keep the package tightly closed and avoid storing the container in warm areas. Use the electrodes prior to the expiration date on the package and check each one for adequate gel before applying it to the patient.

A *second action* to help prevent artifact is correct skin preparation before electrode application or reapplication. To defat the skin, that is, to remove oils, rub the skin with an alcohol gauze pad prior to electrode application. Avoid using acetone which is more irritating, produces less contact, and is a fire hazard!

Preventing, recognizing and coping with the various kinds of artifact is an ongoing function of cardiac monitoring. The ability to recognize and eliminate artifact is a skill which will assist one in monitoring patients safely, effectively, and efficiently. However, *recognizing artifact is a function of monitoring experience! I* do not expect you to remember all the details in this section, though a periodic review of this material may be helpful. (Personal note from the management!)

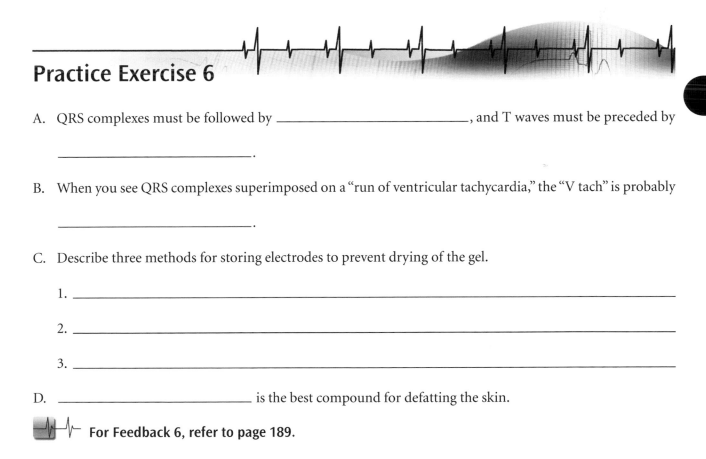

Practice Exercise 6

A. QRS complexes must be followed by _____, and T waves must be preceded by

_____.

B. When you see QRS complexes superimposed on a "run of ventricular tachycardia," the "V tach" is probably

_____.

C. Describe three methods for storing electrodes to prevent drying of the gel.

1. _____

2. _____

3. _____

D. _____ is the best compound for defatting the skin.

For Feedback 6, refer to page 189.

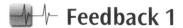 **Feedback 1**

You probably have answered all the practice exercises correctly. If so . . . ***Hooray!***

A. "Glitches" or "noise" on the monitor tracing are known as <u>artifact</u>, or electrical interference.

B. False. (The presence of artifact is *NOT* a signal that there is a disturbance in the heart's electrical activity.)

C. False. (The presence of artifact is *NOT* an indication that an electrical device in proximity to the patient is malfunctioning.)

D. To monitor a patient's rhythm effectively, one needs to <u>recognize</u> artifact when it appears, <u>distinguish</u> it from the patient's rhythm, and take appropriate steps to <u>minimize</u> it.

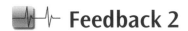 **Feedback 2**

You are quickly becoming an expert! 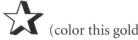 (color this gold)

A. Sixty-cycle interference is characterized by a <u>wide</u>, <u>fuzzy</u> baseline.

B. Any of these are acceptable answers:

1. Make certain that the EKG cable is not draped across, or parallel to, other cables such as call-light, electric bed, or transducer cables.

2. Make certain that the EKG cable is not touching the metal parts of other electrical equipment.

3. If possible, try momentarily pulling the plug of any other electrical equipment in contact with the patient to see if the artifact disappears.

4. Tighten any loose connections in the monitoring system.

5. Apply new electrode patches using correct skin preparation.

6. Check the gel on the electrode patches and replace if gel is dry.

7. Replace any defective wires.

8. Try a different monitor cable.

Feedback 3

You are becoming more skillful at coping with artifact!

A. Motion artifact commonly results from electrical signals produced by the <u>skin</u>.

B. This is a bit more difficult!

1. The beginning of the strip demonstrates motion artifact that is fairly obvious and does not look like ventricular tachycardia. This gives one a clue that the patient is moving.

2. During the portion that looks like "V tach," one can still walk the normal QRS complexes through the strip, and in most cases, one can see portions of the normal QRS.

3. A QRS complex occurs immediately after the cessation of "V tach." In true ventricular tachycardia, there is usually a pause before a normal QRS appears.

C. Any of the following responses are correct.

    1. Check with the patient to see if you can help reduce excessive patient motion.

    2. Make certain all the electrode patches are secure and that sufficient gel is present.

    3. Secure loose wires.

    4. Replace defective wires.

    5. The wandering baseline could be due to respirations. Try changing the location of the positive electrode slightly or try switching to a lead I.

    (Perhaps you can think of others that I neglected to mention!)

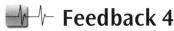 ## Feedback 4

You' re doing super!

A. Little "blips" or spikes occurring on a monitor tracing usually originate from electrical equipment. Two of the *most* frequent electrical equipment culprits are <u>pacemakers</u> and <u>pain control devices</u>.

B. The variation in amplitude often depends on the <u>lead</u>.

Feedback 5

You know almost everything there is to know about artifact!

A. Someone has decreased and then increased the amplitude setting. (Sometimes your *tricky* cohorts may try to fool you.)

B. Any three of these actions can be considered:

    1. Make certain that all electrodes are intact.

    2. Make certain that the monitor cable is plugged in.

    3. Check for defective wires and replace if necessary.

    4. Check for a defective cable by replacing the cable.

    5. Check the amplitude setting and adjust if necessary.

Feedback 6

You are truly an expert! (If you have not *absolutely* mastered this material, do not panic.) You may wish to refer back to this chapter for future help when problems with artifact develop.

A. QRS complexes must be followed by <u>T waves</u> and T waves must be preceded by <u>QRS complexes</u>.

B. When you see QRS complexes superimposed on a "run of ventricular tachycardia," the "V tach" is probably <u>artifact</u>.

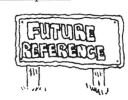

C. Methods for storing electrodes to prevent drying of the gel include:

    1. Keeping the electrodes in their original foil package.

    2. Closing the package tightly.

    3. Avoiding storage in warm areas.

    4. Using the electrodes prior to their expiration date.

D. <u>Alcohol</u> is the best compound for defatting the skin.

Notes

Cardioversion and Defibrillation

Objectives

When you have completed Section 7, you will be able to describe or identify

1. refractory and vulnerable phases of the cardiac cycle
2. synchronized precordial shock or cardioversion
3. nonsynchronized precordial shock or defibrillation
4. automatic external defibrillator (AED) functioning

7

7.1: Refractory and Vulnerable Phases of the Cardiac Cycle

In previous sections, reference was made to *precordial shock* as a treatment option for uncontrolled rapid dysrhythmias producing hemodynamic imbalance. To appreciate precordial shock treatment, one must have an understanding of the cardiac cycle.

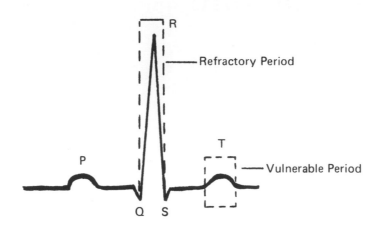

Each cardiac cycle has an **absolute refractory period** during which time the tissues are immune or resistant to further electrical stimulation. A brief **vulnerable period**, essentially encompassing the T wave, follows the refractory period. It is during the vulnerable period that an electrical stimulus (a shock from a live electrical source, lightening, a P.V.C. occurring in an ischemic heart, etc.) can induce ventricular fibrillation.

The vulnerable period, the T wave, can actually be thought of as having two parts. The first half of the T wave is relatively refractory to electrical stimulation, meaning that a sufficiently strong electrical current would be necessary to stimulate action. The middle and latter half of the T wave is truly the vulnerable period, requiring only a minimal electrical stimulus to initiate a response.

Thus, when electrical stimulation (precordial shock) is used as a therapeutic intervention to disrupt rapid dysrhythmias, a method of delivery must prevent the shock from occurring during the vulnerable period (the T wave) to avoid the risk of ventricular fibrillation. Avoiding the vulnerable period is achieved by synchronizing the timing of the electrical shock to the patient's rhythm, specifically to the R wave of the QRS (the refractory period). Precordial shock introduced during the refractory period will avoid the risk of ventricular fibrillation.

Synchronization of the defibrillator unit to the patient's rhythm is achieved by connecting a cable from the patient's EKG recording device (EKG machine or monitor) to the defibrillator unit. Once connected, a *synchronization option* (or button) is selected on the defibrillator unit. The defibrillator unit is then able to *sense* the tall R wave of the QRS cycle. Occasionally, the gain or amplitude setting will need to be increased for the R waves to be sensed.

The defibrillator unit will have an indicator (usually a blinking light) that signals the sensing of R waves. Each time the light blinks, it's saying "I see an R wave, I see an R wave" . . . etc.

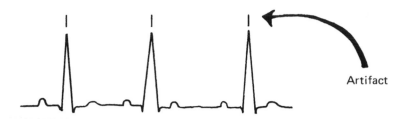

Artifact

In addition, the monitoring device will show an artifact above each R wave. The artifact also indicates that the defibrillator unit is reading or sensing the R wave of each QRS complex. Now, no matter when in the cardiac cycle the buttons for releasing the electrical energy are pressed, the defibrillator unit will not deliver the energy until it senses the R wave! The synchronized defibrillator does *all* the work.

In essence then, this synchronization prevents the electrical shock from occurring during the vulnerable period (T wave).

There are two types of precordial shock, *synchronized* and *unsynchronized*. Synchronized precordial shock is most usually referred to as **cardioversion**. Unsynchronized precordial shock is referred to as **defibrillation**.

Defibrillation is the treatment of choice for ventricular fibrillation, the chaotic, uncoordinated, ineffective depolarization of the ventricles and for pulseless ventricular tachycardia. Remember, CPR must be instituted immediately upon the recognition of ventricular fibrillation or the determination of pulselessness unless an automatic external defibrillator (AED) is immediately available.

Both synchronized cardioversion and defibrillation work on the same principle. Electrical energy of brief duration is delivered through the chest wall. This shock causes depolarization (release of energy) of a critical mass of myocardial cells, thus halting or disrupting the chaotic or ectopic activity, and hopefully allowing the sinus pacemaker to resume control of the rhythm.

Review the following rhythm strips demonstrating ventricular fibrillation.

1.

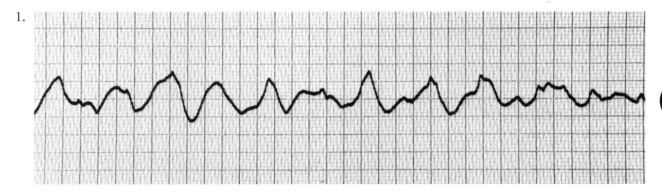

2.

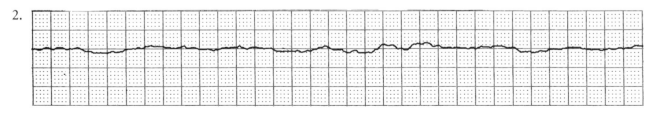

The first strip depicts a *coarse* ventricular fibrillation; the second strip displays a *fine* ventricular fibrillation. To interrupt the chaotic ectopic activity, precordial shock must be instituted. . . .

. . . but which kind?

synchronized, or unsynchronized?
cardioversion, or defibrillation?

Ah-ha! Since no QRSs are present, it is *impossible* to use synchronized precordial shock! As a matter of fact, if one set or programmed the defibrillator unit to deliver synchronized shock, the machine would **never** release the energy through the paddles. It would hold the energy until it "sensed" an *R wave* . . . which would never appear! Thus, because QRS complexes are absent, non-synchronized precordial shock or defibrillation would be used.

With non-synchronized precordial shock or defibrillation, the energy is delivered through the paddles at any point during the chaotic rhythm, as soon as the "energy delivery" button(s) is pressed. Usually, a high energy shock is used—between 200 and 400 watt/seconds or joules of energy (depending upon the patient's size and chest wall thickness).

It should be noted that there are two *general* types of defibrillators. Hospital defibrillator units have three capabilities: defibrillation; synchronized cardioversion; and, external pacing.

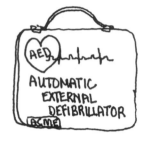

A second type of defibrillator unit, an **automatic external defibrillator (AED)** is a "grab and go" unit used by fire departments, airlines, rescue squads and certain large businesses for the treatment of cardiac emergencies. An AED is a battery-powered portable unit equipped with adhesive electrodes, electrical circuitry, and an internal microprocessor for interpreting rhythms. The AED unit includes diagrams for guiding the placement of electrodes and usually has both visual and audio prompts. Essentially, the AED senses and analyzes the underlying cardiac rhythm, then advises (prompts) the operator whether electric shock is needed (shock/no shock). When electrical shock is needed (ventricular fibrillation/ventricular tachycardia), the AED automatically calculates and delivers a pre-determined amount of energy (joules), though most units allow a manual override for alternate current settings. In the presence of ventricular tachycardia, the AED senses the QRS configuration and synchronizes the timing of energy release to avoid current delivery during the vulnerable phase of a cardiac cycle. AED units come with treatment algorithms and can both record and print monitor tracings.

As this text goes to press, the FDA is evaluating a foreign AED (FRED easyport) that is small enough to be worn on the belt. The unit is light weight and uses a pulsed biphasic waveform, allowing the same efficiency using less energy.

Additionally, the FDA approved *over-the-counter* sales of an in-home defibrillator with programmed audio directions.

> **CRITICAL NOTE:** Owing to variation in defibrillator equipment, the practitioner is strongly cautioned to become familiar with devices available for use. Initial training and periodic "hands-on" reviews are required to maintain competency. In cardiac emergencies, speed is critical. In the face of ventricular fibrillation (pulselessness), chances of survival decrease approximately 7–10% each passing minute. Defibrillation within the first 3–4 minutes affords the best chance for survival. Immediate CPR is required for any pulseless event and should be continued until the "all standback for defibrillation" command is given. If defibrillation is unsuccessful, CPR should be reinstituted immediately. Clinicians and *field-warriors,* alike, should stay abreast of current resuscitation guidelines published by the American Heart Association (ACLS and PALS Guidelines).

Practice Exercise 1

Let's see how much you remember!

A. Here is a QRS complex. Draw and label the refractory and vulnerable periods.

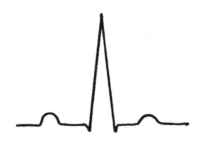

B. Refractory means that _____

_____

_____

_____

_____

C. Vulnerable implies that _____

_____

_____

D. In synchronized precordial shock, or _____ the defibrillator unit will deliver its energy *only* on _____ of the EKG cycle.

E. When defibrillation or non-synchronized precordial shock is used, the defibrillator unit will deliver its energy _____

_____

_____

F. Following is a rhythm strip of a patient experiencing severe chest pain and a falling blood pressure.

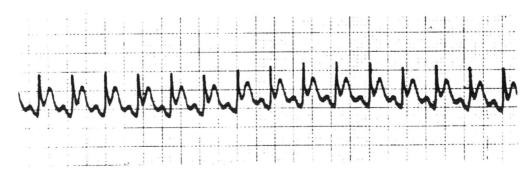

This rhythm is an _____. Because the clinical condition is deteriorating rapidly, it has been decided to administer precordial shock to terminate the ectopic rhythm.

Cardioversion / defibrillation (circle one) would be used because _____

_____

_____

_____

G.

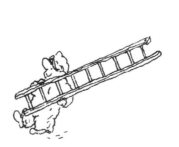

The rhythm strip above is that of a code arrest victim. _____ precordial shock would be administered because there are no _____ complexes present!

H. The abbreviation AED stands for _____.

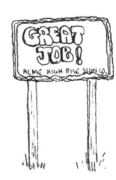 For Feedback 1, see page 197.

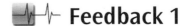 **Feedback 1**

A.

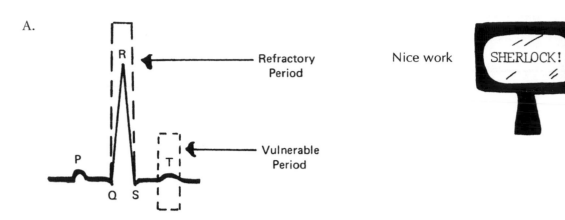

Nice work   SHERLOCK!

B. Refractory means that <u>this phase in the cardiac cycle (the QRS) is immune to any additional electrical stimulation</u>.

C. Vulnerable implies that <u>this phase in the cardiac cycle (the T wave) is sensitive to electrical stimulation. Electrical stimulation during the vulnerable period may induce ventricular fibrillation</u>.

D. In synchronized precordial shock, or **cardioversion**, the defibrillator unit will deliver its energy <u>only</u> on the **R Wave** of the EKG cycle.

E. When defibrillation or non-synchronized precordial shock is used, the defibrillator unit will deliver its energy <u>as soon as the energy delivery buttons are pressed anywhere in the chaotic rhythm</u>.

F. This rhythm is <u>supra-ventricular tachycardia</u>.

<u>Cardioversion</u> would be used because <u>QRS complexes are present and principally to avoid the risk of inducing ventricular fibrillation</u>.

G. <u>Unsynchronized</u> precordial shock or defibrillation would be administered because there are no <u>QRS</u> complexes present!

H. The abbreviation AED stands for <u>automatic external defibrillator</u>.

7

Notes

Pacemaker Basics

Objectives

When you have completed Section 8, you will be able to describe, identify or define

1. the purpose of pacemaking
2. indications for pacemaker support
3. pacemaker generated heart rhythms
4. pacemaker sensing and capture
5. pacemaker identification codes
6. common pacemaker modes

8

Text by:
Stephanie L. Woods, Ph.D., R.N.

Section 8 is included to provide a *basic* overview of cardiac pacemakers. Pacemakers can be used temporarily or permanently to pace the heart when the normal conduction tissue is unable to generate a normal or adequate rhythm. Pacemaker technology has become very sophisticated over the past many years. Pacers have evolved from simple ventricular demand mode to multi-programmability. This chapter will briefly overview the principles of pacemaking. Further study will be required to understand the many different types of pacemakers.

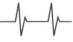

input section   8.1   Pacemaker Fundamentals

Cardiac pacemakers, often called pacers, are small battery powered generators used to deliver electrical stimulation to the myocardial muscle when the normal conduction tissue of the heart fails to generate adequate beats per minute. The functions of the pacer depend upon the type of pacemaker inserted and the programmability of the generator.

General Purposes for Pacemakers

- To provide electrical stimulation when the SA node has failed and the AV node or Purkinje fibers cannot provide an adequate back-up rhythm
- To generate a heart rate that creates an adequate cardiac output and stable blood pressure
- To generate atrial contractability in lower generated pacer rhythms (junctional and ventricular), improving ventricular filling
- To override (outpace) ectopic tachycardic rhythms

Types of Pacemakers

There are two basic types of pacemakers: temporary and permanent.

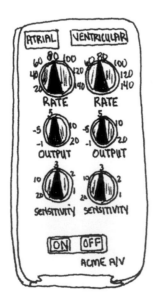

Temporary pacemaker generator

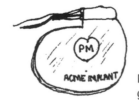

Permanent pacemaker generator

Temporary pacemaker

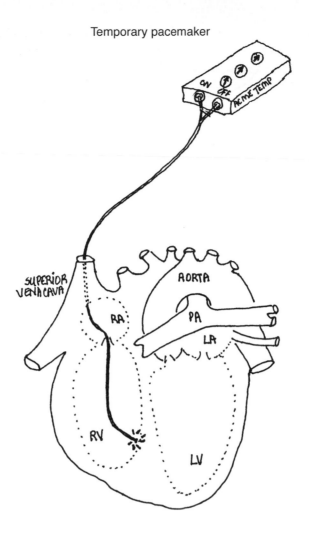

Temporary pacing can be accomplished by:

- Inserting a pacing wire (pacing catheter) into the right atrium and into the right ventricle via the subclavian vein. The end of the pacing catheter is visible outside of the patient's body and is attached to an external generator. This is called **transvenous pacemaking**.

- Applying a large electrode patch to the anterior and the posterior chest surfaces over the heart. Pacing wires are attached to each patch and a pacing module that is part of a defibrillator unit acts as the generator. An electrical impulse is applied directly to the skin over the heart and conducts from the anterior to the posterior patch, thereby stimulating contraction of the heart muscle. **This is called transcutaneous pacing. This type of pacing is used for minutes to hours until a transvenous or permanent pacemaker is inserted.**

- During heart surgery, temporary pacing wires can be applied directly to the epicardium (the outer surface of the heart). One wire can be placed directly onto the right atrium, and another wire directly onto the right ventricle. These wires are brought out through the skin and usually coiled up and taped to the patient's chest. They can be attached to an external pacing generator if the need arises. **This is called epicardial pacing.**

Permanent pacing is accomplished by inserting a pacing wire into the right atrium and into the right ventricle via the subclavian vein, as well. However, the permanent pacing wire is much shorter than the temporary wire and is not visible outside the patient's body. The permanent pacing wire is attached to a small generator that is implanted underneath the patient's skin, usually below the clavicle, near the shoulder.

8

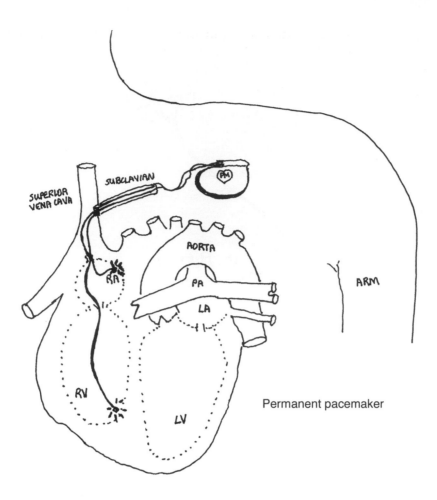

Permanent pacemaker

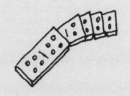

SPECIAL NOTE: In both temporary and permanently implanted pacemakers, the pacemaker wire(s) is placed in the right heart muscle wall. This is because the pacer wires are inserted transvenously, via the superior vena cava which enters the right atrium.

Temporary Pacemaker Lead Placement
• Right ventricular muscle wall

Permanent Pacemaker Lead Placement
• Right ventricular muscle wall (ventricular pacer only)
• Right atrial and right ventricular muscle wall (atrio-ventricular)
• Right atrial and right ventricle and coronary sinus (bi-ventricular)

Pacemaker stimulation induces cell depolarization in the placed chamber(s). Electrical impulse (mA) is delivered at the point of lead implant. That wave of depolarization then spreads outward, activating all myocardial muscle cells . . . more or less of a domino effect!

Anatomy of a Pacemaker

Both tempoorary and permanent pacemakers have the following standard parts:

• **Generator**—The generator is the power source for the pacer. Electrical energy or output is measured in milliamperes (mA). Electrical output can be varied from 0.1 to 20 mA. Pacemakers are powered by batteries. Temporary pacers can use simple 9 volt mercury zinc batteries where permanent pacemakers usually use lithium batteries. Lithium batteries can have a life span of ten years or greater.

- **Wires/Electrodes**—All pacemakers must have pacing wires with electrodes. Wires attach to a generator. The generator provides the electrical energy that flows down the pacer wire. The pacer wire is inserted into the heart until the pacer wire comes in contact with the myocardium. When energy flows down the pacer wire, the myocardial muscle should contract in response.

- **Rate setting**—Rates can be widely varied in pacers, depending upon the pacer's intended use. If the pacer is to be used to create an adequate ventricular rhythm the rates may be set between 40 and 80 beats per minute. If the pacer is to be used to overrride an etopic rhythm such as atrial tachycardia, the rate may vary between 150 and 350 beats per minute.

- **Mode**—The mode describes the primary function of the pacer. Most modern pacers are programmable, allowing for varying functions. The mode may be as simple as single chamber pacing or as complex as atrial and ventricular pacing with several programmed responses.

- **Sensivity**—Sensivity refers to the ability of the pacer to "sense" or see when the patient is having his own heart beat. When the patient is having his own beat, the pacer should not deliver a stimulus at the same time.

Indications for Pacing: Short-Term and Long-Term

Pacemakers can be used temporarily or permanently, depending upon the clinical problem or patient condition.

Temporary pacemakers are used for crisis intervention and anticipated short-term support.

- *Examples of crisis intervention:*
  —Third degree AV block
  —Symptomatic bradycardia
  —Cardiac arrest

- *Examples of short-term support:*
  —Second-degree AV block following cardiac surgery
  —Insertion of a temporary atrial pacing wire to override a patient's atrial tachycardia

Permanent pacemakers are inserted for long-term rhythm disturbances such as sinus bradycardia, sinus arrest, heart blocks, sick sinus (brady-tachy) syndrome, tachyarrythmias such as P.A.T., and atrial fibrillation with a slow ventricular rate.

Recognizing Pacemaker Rhythms

Pacemaker generated rhythms have three characteristics that distinguish them from normal rhythms. These characteristics are:

1. The presence of pacemaker artifact
2. Larger than normal atrial and ventricular wave formations
3. A rate not lower than the pacemaker "set" rate

Read on for detail!

1. **When a pacemaker fires an electrical impulse, one will typically see what is known as pacer spikes or pacer artifact on the EKG.** These spikes are usually about five boxes tall (5mm).

- If the pacemaker is an atrial pacer (single lead), one will see this spike just prior to the P wave (these are very rarely used!)

- If the pacemaker is a ventricular pacemaker (single lead), one will see this spike just prior to the QRS.

8

A Demand Ventricular Pacemaker

A demand pacemaker generates beats when the patient's heart rate falls below a set (programmed) number.

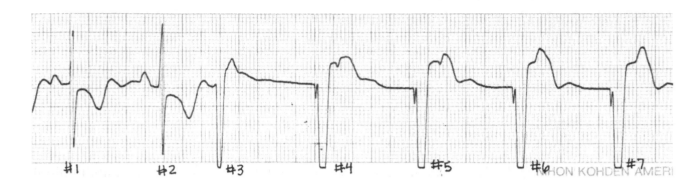

In the above strip, the pacemaker senses a patient's own ventricular activity (beats 1, 2, and 3). Thus, the pacemaker does not discharge a stimulus. When a ventricular beat fails to occur at the expected time (pause following premature beat 3), the pacemaker begins firing. Note the pacemaker spikes occurring before beats 4–7.

- If the pacemaker is an atrio-ventricular (AV sequential, dual lead) pacer, one will see spikes before both the P wave and the QRS.

When a patient requires atrial depolarization and contraction to increase ventricular filling in addition to ventricular pacing, an AV sequential pacer is inserted. The AV sequential pacemaker achieves synchronized atrial and ventricular functioning.

Dual Lead AV Sequential Pacing

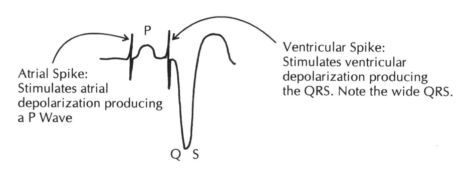

Atrial Spike: Stimulates atrial depolarization producing a P Wave

Ventricular Spike: Stimulates ventricular depolarization producing the QRS. Note the wide QRS.

In the above schematic, note both the atrial spike prior to the P wave and the ventricular spike prior to the QRS. An AV sequential pacer requires the placement of two leads.

An AV Sequential Pacemaker

The following strip is an example of an AV (atrial/ventricular) sequential pacemaker. Here the generator paces both the atrium and the ventricle, in sequence, and upon demand. In other words, when patient-generated atrial and ventricular activation fails to occur, the pacemaker initiates first an atrial, and then a ventricular (sequenced) stimulus. This dual sensing and pacing requires a two lead pacemaker system! The advantage of an A-V sequential pacemaker is that it allows complete atrial emptying and improved ventricular filling (a.k.a. "**atrial kick**") and therefore increases cardial output.

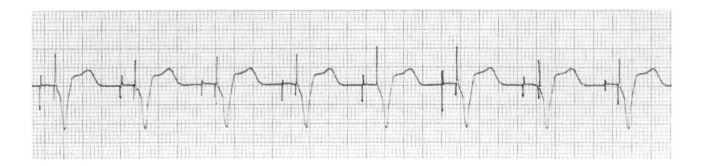

The interval between the atrial and ventricular spikes simulates a P-R interval, but in *pacer language* is called the *automatic interval*. A normal PR is 0.12–0.20 seconds. A normal automatic interval is approximately the same, but is measured in milliseconds. To convert seconds to milliseconds move the decimal point 3 places to the right. The normal automatic interval is usually 120ms.–160ms.

> **IMPORTANT TERMINOLOGY:** You will often hear people refer to pacer spikes as pacer artifact. **Pacer artifact** always means that a waveform is created by an outside or artificial source rather than by normal heart depolarization. Pacer artifact tells us that the pacer is discharging electrical impulses.

2. **A pacemaker spike is followed by a *larger than normal* P wave in atrial pacing, or a wider than normal QRS in ventricular pacing.** These larger or wider waveforms occur because the pacemaker is depolarizing the heart in an abnormal fashion.

> **IMPORTANT INFORMATION:** This larger than normal P wave or QRS following the pacer spike is referred to as capture. Capture means that the pacer has discharged an adequate electrical impulse (mA) and depolarization has occurred.

3. **The heart rate of the paced rhythm should not be lower than the lower rate limit set on the pacemaker.** A lower rate limit means, that the pacer is set to fire when the patient's heart rate falls below a set rate or limit. For instance, if the pacer is set to fire at 60 beats per minute, once the patient's heart rate falls below 60, the pacer should begin to pace the heart at 60 beats per minute. This is referred to as **demand pacing.**

> **IMPORTANT NOTE:** A **demand** type pacemaker setting is sometimes referred to as *synchronous* pacing meaning that the pacemaker generated impulse occurs on an *as needed* basis only. The demand pacemaker works in synchrony with the underlying rhythm. In contrast, a *triggered* or **non-demand** pacemaker setting programs the pacemaker to fire continuously at a fixed or set rate, regardless of the underlying rhythm. A triggered pacemaker response is often referred to as *asynchronous* pacing. It is the underlying rhythm pathology that determines the synchronous or asynchronous setting.

Practice Exercise 1

A.   List two indications for instituting pacemaker therapy.

1.   _____

_____

2.   _____

_____

B.   Temporary pacemakers are used to support *anticipated* short-term pathology or to correct crisis situations. List three underlying rhythm disturbances that may warrant temporary pacemaker insertion.

1.   _____

2.   _____

3.   _____

C.   List the three characteristics of paced rhythms.

1.   _____

2.   _____

3.   _____

D.   A demand pacemaker generator response means that

_____

_____

_____

_____

For Feedback 1, refer to page 213.

input section 8.2   Determining Pacemaker Rate

Determining the pacemaker rate on an EKG strip is a function of measuring the interval (small squares) between two consecutive pacer spikes. The trusty rate guide on page 39 can then be consulted, or one can divide 1500 (the number of small squares in one minute) by the number of small squares between the two pacer spikes.

Note the rate calculations on the following two strips.

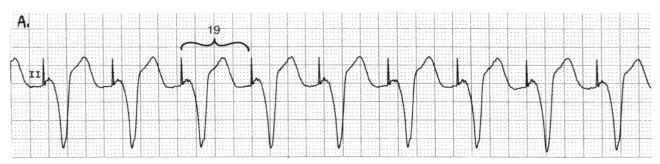

A ventricular pacemaker rhythm

$$\frac{79}{19\overline{)1500}} = \text{ventricular rate}$$

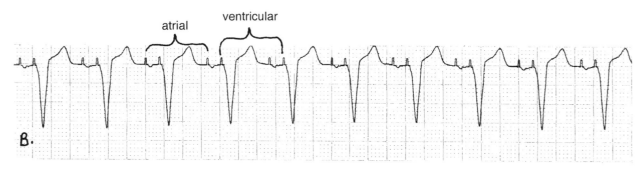

An atrio-ventricular (AV sequential) pacemaker

$$\frac{88}{17\overline{)1500}} = \text{atrial rate} \qquad \frac{88}{17\overline{)1500}} = \text{ventricular rate}$$

Practice Exercise 2

Calculate the heart rate in the following AV sequential pacemaker rhythm.

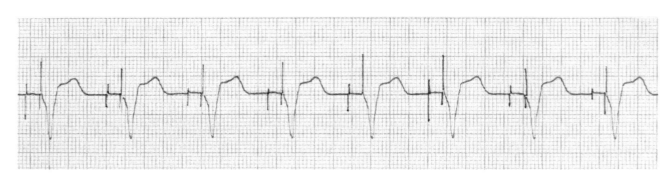

Atrial rate = _____.

Ventricular rate = _____.

For Feedback 2, refer to page 213.

input section   8.3   More about Capture

Earlier, the term *capture* was introduced. Capture is the term used to describe depolarization occurring secondary to a pacemaker stimulus. Capture occurs when a pacemaker spike is followed by the appropriate cardiac complex (P wave or QRS). *Non-capture* is present when a pacemaker spike fails to produce the desired effect (atrial depolarization or ventricular depolarization). Non-capture may result from: pacemaker malfunction, too low an mA setting; lead placement in electrically inactive scar tissue; or, drifting of the lead wire(s) away from the muscle wall. When non-capture occurs, any of the following *medical* actions may be appropriate.

> ### Methods for "Fixing" Pacemaker Non-Capture
> • Increase energy output of generator (mA)
> • Check battery
> • Reposition the pacer wire (medical intervention)
> • Evaluate lead wire for fracture (by x-ray)

The significance of sustained non-capture is dependent upon the presence of an underlying rhythm and patient signs and symptoms.

The following strip demonstrates both pacemaker non-capture and failure to sense.

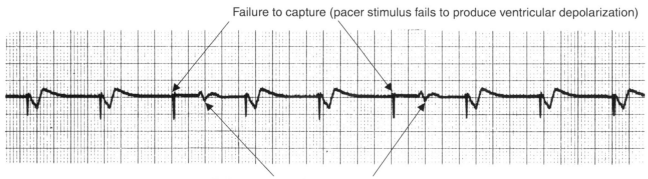

Failure to capture (pacer stimulus fails to produce ventricular depolarization)

Failure to sense (pacemaker fails to recognize patient's intrinsic electrical activity)

A quick "eyeball" analysis of the above strip reveals pacemaker spikes occurring regularly throughout the tracing. However, the pacemaker is not sensing the patient's underlying feeble rhythm and the pacemaker spikes are failing to capture. (This patient was scheduled for a "pacemaker replacement"!)

Practice Exercise 3

A. Pacemaker capture means

_____

_____

B. Pacemaker non-capture *may* be corrected by any of these three methods: (If uncertain, look above!) 🙂

1. _____

2. _____

3. _____

For Feedback 3, refer to page 213.

For Feedback 3, refer to page 213.

input section 8.4 Failure to Sense

When a pacemaker is programmed to *sense* electrical activity, it means that the pacer is "set" to detect a patient's *own* heart rhythm. Sensing can be programmed to recognize ventricular activity as well as atrial activity (in the case of dual leads.) In most cases, when the pacer senses the patient's own electrical activity, the pacer is inhibited from generating a pacer impulse. If the pacemaker fails to sense the patient's own cardiac rhythm and initiates an electrical impulse, the problem is referred to as *failure to sense.* The strips below are examples of failure to sense.

A.

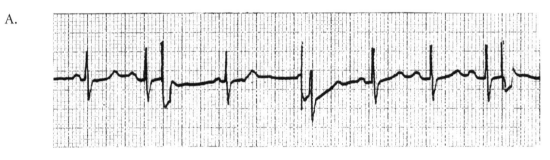

B.

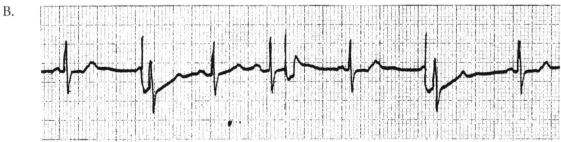

In the first strip (A), note the pacer spike that falls on the first part of the T wave following the second QRS. The pacer did not sense the patient's own beat and generated a paced beat. Luckily, the heart muscle was still in a refractory state; thus, the myocardium did not respond to the pacer impulse.

In the second strip (B), note the fourth QRS complex. Again, the pacer fired on the first part of the T wave. The pacer did not sense the patient's beat and generated a paced beat. This is much like the R on T phenomenon discussed earlier. There is a potential for the patient to experience ventricular tachycardia as a result. The pacer should be reprogrammed and sensitivity increased.

Another interesting phenomenon is observable in the above two strips. Notice the fourth QRS complex in strip A. Just prior to that complex, you will see a pacer spike. And, if you look very closely, you will see the beginnings of a P wave, just before the pacer spike. This particular set of waveforms and pacer spike is called a **fusion beat**. In this case, the patient generated a beat just as the pacer was generating a beat and the two fused together. This occurs again on strip B just before the second QRS, and again before the sixth QRS. When a patient is having frequent fusion beats, it is not a sensing problem, but rather a competition problem. When the patient's sinus node is firing at, or near, the same rate as the pacer, there will be competition for pacing the heart. In this case, the pacer should be reprogrammed or rate adjusted to a lower rate.

> **NOTE:** This brief section is informational with no associated practice exercise!

input section   **8.5   The Pacemaker Rhythm**

The pacemaker generator (temporary or permanent) generates a small electrical current (mA) intended to stimulate the cells at the point of pacemaker wire or lead contact with the muscle. This causes cellular depolarization which spreads across the myocardium, outside the normal conduction pathway. Again, if the mA is adequate, one will see capture. Sound familiar?

The exact functioning of the pacemaker is dependent upon the programming sequence or settings. There are five programming sequences:

- Rate
- Chamber(s) paced
- Response
- Programmability
- Anti-tachyarrhythmic

These programming sequences have been established by the North American Society of Pacing and Electrophysiology (NASPE) as indicated on the following table.

North American Society of Pacing and Electrophysiology (NASPE) Permanent Pacemaker Codes

Position	I	II	III	IV	V
Category	Chamber(s) paced	Chamber(s) sensed	Response to sensing	Programmability	Anti-tachyarrhythmic functions
	O = None A = Atrium V = Ventricle D = Dual (A-V)	O = None A = Atrium V = Ventricle D = Dual (A-V)	O = None T = Triggered I = Inhibited D = Dual (A-V)	O = None P = Simple Program. M = Multiprogram. C = Communicating R = Rate modulation	O = None P = Pacing (anti-tachyarrhythmia) S = Shock D = Dual (P + S)

Permanent pacemakers are identified by letter codes. The first letter in the code identifies the chamber(s) being paced. The second letter identifies chambers in which the pacer can sense the patient's electrical activity. The third letter tells one what the pacer does in response to sensing the patient's own electrical activity.

The fourth letter of the NASPE permanent pacemaker code tells one the sophistication of the pacer. Programmability refers to the ability of the pacemaker to have its functions changed. Some permanent pacers have only simple programmability for one or two functions, while other pacers have highly sophisticated multi-programmability, allowing virtually all functions to be programmed. These sophisticated programs and functions will be discussed in Section 9. Specially trained physicians, nurses, and technicians can use a pacemaker programmer (a hand-held device) held over the pacemaker to reprogram various functions.

Additionally a programmer can "interrogate" the pacemaker. Interrogation asks the pacer to identify current settings and functions. A printout is obtained listing the various settings and functions (see below). This is very helpful when a patient cannot find his or her pacer ID card with the original functions and settings listed, or if the medical records are not immediately accessible. Permanent pacemakers manufactured in the past ten years will have four letter codes like DDDR and VVIR. Permanent pacemakers used to override tachydysrhythmias (Anti-tachyarrhythmic functions) will have a five letter code such as DDDRD.

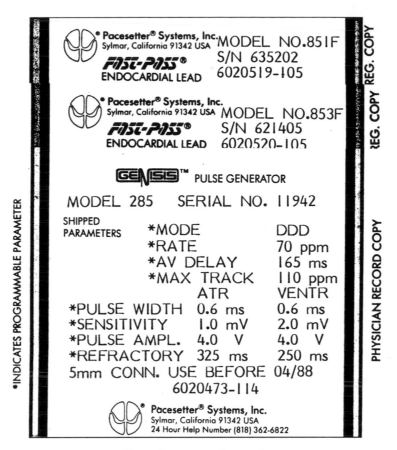

Pacer interrogation strip

Most implanted (permanent) pacemakers are of the ***AV sequential variety (dual lead)*** and are programmed on a ⅅ ⅅ ⅅ setting. However, when implanted in patients with chronic atrial fibrillation, AV sequential pacemakers are programmed to a Ⅴ Ⅴ Ⅰ setting. Because of the erratic firing of the atria in atrial fibrillation, a DDD pacer would be inhibited by sensed atrial activity. Anti-arrhythmic pacing will be discussed in detail in Section 9!

Less complicated temporary pacemakers are identified by a three letter code like VVI, AAI, DDD, as demonstrated in the following examples.

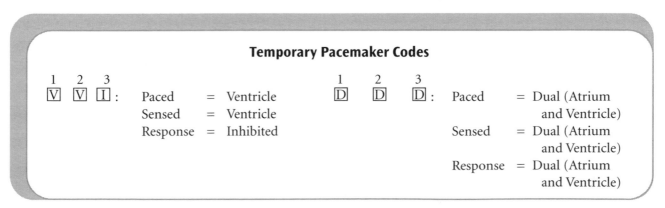

Temporary Pacemaker Codes

1 2 3				1 2 3		
Ⅴ Ⅴ Ⅰ :	Paced	= Ventricle		Ⅾ Ⅾ Ⅾ :	Paced	= Dual (Atrium and Ventricle)
	Sensed	= Ventricle			Sensed	= Dual (Atrium and Ventricle)
	Response	= Inhibited			Response	= Dual (Atrium and Ventricle)

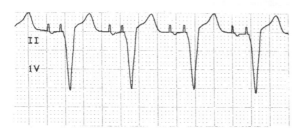

Practice Exercise 4

A. When assessing a pacemaker rhythm strip, one must know the pacemaker programming sequence which includes _____, _____, _____, _____ and _____.

B. Identify (circle) the atrial and ventricular spikes in the following strip and measure the automatic interval in milliseconds.

automatic interval = _____ ms.

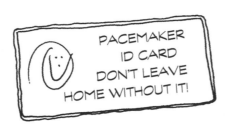

For Feedback 5, refer to page 214.

Message from Management

In order to determine correct pacemaker functioning, one must first know what the pacemaker is programmed to do! ALWAYS ask to see the patient's "PACEMAKER ID CARD" that details information about the pacemaker.

In summary, the indications for the various types and modes of pacing vary greatly depending upon the type and severity of the underlying dysrhythmia, the etiology of the dysrhythmia, and the extent of hemodynamic embarrassment.

This section was intended to be an introduction to pacemakers and a warm-up for Section 9!

Hope we captured your attention!

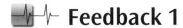 **Feedback 1**

A. Pacemaker therapy may be instituted for any of the following indications:

1. to increase slow or inadequate ventricular heart rates.

2. to stimulate atrial activity in the absence of a sinus pacemaker.

3. to stimulate ventricular activity in the absence of a ventricular or higher order pacemaker.

B. Any of the following rhythm disturbances may warrant temporary pacemaker insertion:

1. second degree AV block associated with acute myocardial infarction.

2. bradyarrhythmias associated with drug therapy.

3. third degree AV (complete) block.

4. symptomatic bradycardia.

C. Characteristics of a paced rhythm:

1. Pacer artifact or "spike"

2. Capture

3. Actual pacer rate equals pacer rate setting

D. A demand pacemaker generator response means <u>that the pacemaker fires only when the patient's own rate falls below the pacemaker setting</u>.

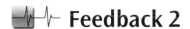 **Feedback 2**

The AV sequential paced heart rate is 60 per minute.

Atrial rate = 60 (Approximately)

Ventricular rate = 60 (Approximately)

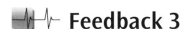 **Feedback 3**

A. Pacemaker capture means <u>that muscle depolarization is caused by the pacemaker stimulus. On the EKG strip, capture occurs when a pacemaker spike is followed by the appropriate cardiac complex (P wave or QRS)</u>.

B. Pacemaker non-capture *may* be corrected by

1. <u>increasing the energy output of the pacemaker generator</u>.

2. <u>changing the generator (battery)</u>.

3. <u>repositioning or replacing the pacer wire</u>.

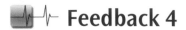 **Feedback 4**

There is no practice exercise associated with input 8.4.

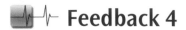 **Feedback 5**

A. When assessing a pacemaker rhythm strip, one must know the pacemaker programming sequence which includes: *rate; chamber(s) paced; response (demand* or *synchronous); programmability;* and, *anti-tachyarrhythmic.*

B.

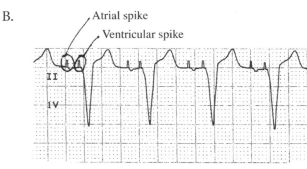

Automatic interval = 140 milliseconds

Need review? Please see page 207.

Bonus Points!

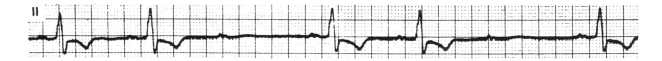

If you think the above symptomatic patient may need a pacemaker . . . You are doing GREAT!

Now that you have *captured* pacemaker basics, move on to the "Not So Basics" of pacemaker functioning in Section 9!

BASICS ➡ NOT SO BASICS
(completed)   (upcoming)

Notes

Advanced Pacemaker Features and Interventions (The *Not so Basics* of Pacemaker Function!)

Objectives

When you have completed Section 9, you will be able to describe or define

1. The **Who**, **What**, **When**, **Where** and **How** of common programmable pacing parameters:
   a. rate modulation
   b. hysteresis
   c. mode switching
   d. auto capture
   e. atrial arrhythmia suppression
   f. pacemaker mediated tachycardia
2. implantable devices for anti-tachy pacing, cardioversion and defibrillation
3. bi-ventricular pacing

9

Text by:
Victoria A. Paparelli, MSN, RN, CCNS-AS
Certified Cardiac Device Specialist
Heart Rhythm Society

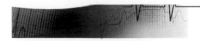 # Introduction

The *Not-So-Basic* pacemaker functions presented in this Section represent programmable options now considered part of basic dual-lead (or soon to be discussed bi-ventricular) pacemaker functioning. These topics build upon concepts presented in Section 8.

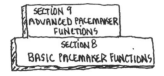

Review and Introduction of Some New Uses of Terms

A *"lead"* may represent a surface ECG lead or a portion of the permanent pacemaker that carries the electronic signals to and from the generator to the heart.

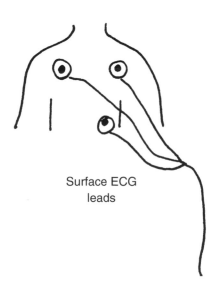

Surface ECG leads

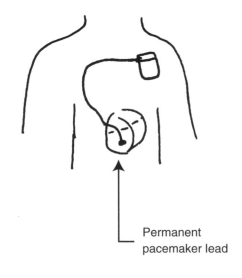

Permanent pacemaker lead

Many pacemaker options are programmed "**ON**" at the time of device implant. Other options may be added or changed in a *pacemaker follow up clinic*, as required by the patient. Options are selected or adjusted using a *manufacturer specific programmer* that communicates by telemetry with each device.

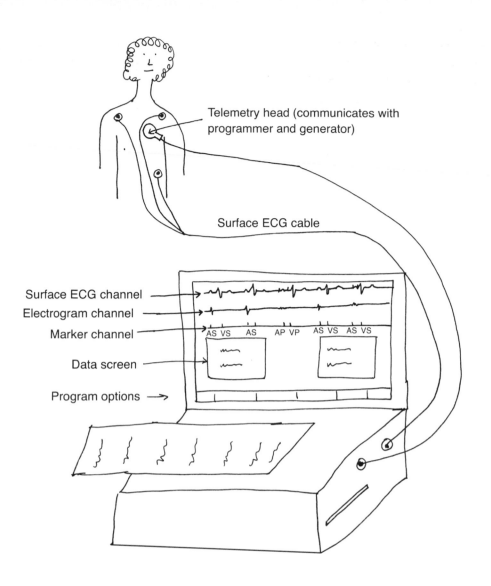

Telemetry head (communicates with programmer and generator)

Surface ECG cable

Surface ECG channel

Electrogram channel

Marker channel

AS VS AS AP VP AS VS AS VS

Data screen

Program options →

9.1 Rate Responsive or Rate Modulated Pacing

Chronotropy is defined as the ability to increase and decrease heart rate. *Chronotropic incompetence* is the inability of the heart to increase heart rate in response to increased oxygen demands. Chronotropic incompetence may occur in the following clinical conditions or situations:

WHO

- Persons with sinus node and conduction pathway disease
- Individuals requiring medications that decrease the ability of the conduction system to respond normally to increased physiologic requirements

When a healthy person exercises, is under psychologic stress, or is exposed to physiologic stressors (such as infection), heart rate increases in response. A person with chronotropic incompetence may have a slow heart rate, and lack the inherent ability to increase heart rate as required. Thus, activity tolerance is diminished.

Rate responsive pacing or *rate modulated pacing* is frequently the treatment option of choice for individuals with chronotropic incompetence. Rate responsive pacing is a dual lead pacemaker option that paces the heart at a rate faster than the base programmed pacemaker rate.

Rate responsive pacing is designated with a "**R**" (see NBG code below) as part of coding, i.e. DDD**R**

Rate response is programmable—**ON** or **OFF**, and varies in degree.

Following are NBG pacemaker codes. (For a review of *code interpretation,* refer back to Section 8.)

NBG Pacemaker Code				
I	II	III	IV	V
Chamber(s) Paced	Chamber(s) Sensed	Response to Sensing	Programmability Rate modulation	Antitachy Function
O = None	O = None	O = None	O = None	O = None
A = Atrium	A = Atrium	T = Triggered	P = Simple Prog.	P = Antitachy
V = Ventricle	V = Ventricle	I = Inhibited	M = Multiprog	Pacing
D = Dual	D = Dual	D = Dual	C = Communicating	S = Shock
			R = Rate Modulation	D = Dual

Bernstein AD, Camm AJ, Fletcher RD, et al. The **NASPE/BPEG** Defibrillator Generic Pacemaker Code for Antibradycardia and Adaptive-Rate Pacing and Antitachyarrhythmic Devices. PACE 1987; 10:794–799, Appendix II.

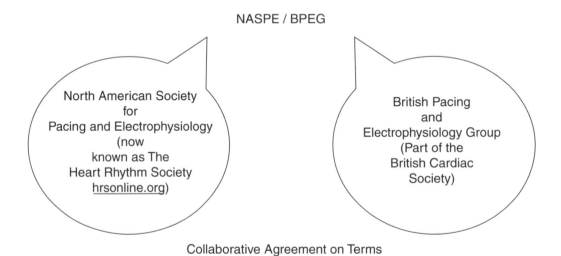

NASPE / BPEG

North American Society for Pacing and Electrophysiology (now known as The Heart Rhythm Society hrsonline.org)

British Pacing and Electrophysiology Group (Part of the British Cardiac Society)

Collaborative Agreement on Terms

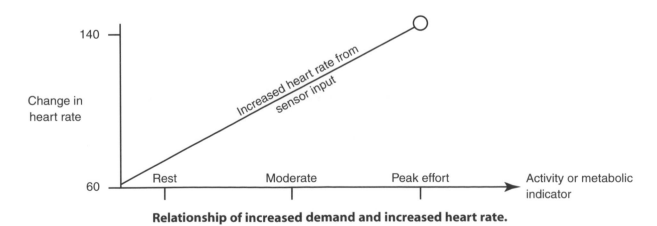

Relationship of increased demand and increased heart rate.

WHAT

Sensors built into the pacemaker device identify and respond to changes in heart rate.

- The *sensor* information is transmitted to the pacemaker to elicit the response of *change in rate*.
- The most common sensors are the piezoelectric (PE) crystal (A) and the accelerometer (B), both of which are inside the pacemaker and respond to movement, muscle motion and vibration. Increased movement, muscle motion and vibration are synonomous with increased demand for O_2, requiring increased heart rate (see graph at bottom of page).
- The response to movement is transformed into electrical signals. These signals are then transmitted to the pacemaker which increases or decreases the paced rate in accord with the pacemaker programming.

Two Most Common Sensors

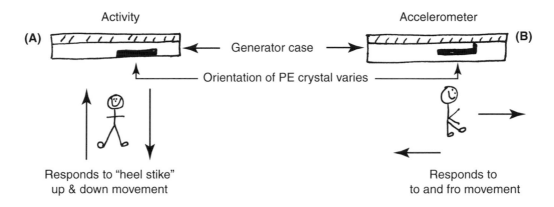

Concept of Blended Sensors

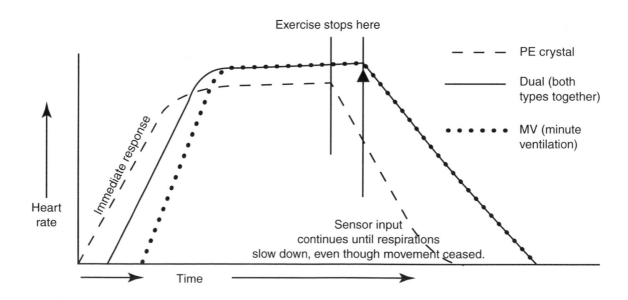

Thoracic impedance and minute ventilation sensors are also available; some require a specific lead. The sensors are programmable and may be used alone and or in combination.

Sensors for catecholamine levels, temperature, right ventricular pressure changes, and oxygen saturation are also available, but limited in use. These sensors require special leads and/or complicated algorithms. Further scientific development is needed to increase *user friendliness* for both the patient and clinician.

WHEN

Rate responsive sensors are most commonly used for *sinus bradycardia* with *chronotropic incompetence* or *drug induced rate suppression.* (Beta-blockers are the most commonly used drug producing this effect.) A sensor is indicated when the patient's ability to increase heart rate and meet metabolic requirements for physical activity is impaired (and there are no contraindications to rate response therapy.) If a patient has severe coronary disease, the demands of increased heart rate on the myocardium may be a *relative* contraindication for rate responsive pacing.

Pacing above the base programmed rate of the pacemaker is known as *sensor input* or *rate modulated* pacing.

A pacemaker programmed to DDDR at a set rate of 60, paces the atrium at a rate higher than 60 if there is *sensor input.* Pacing occurs in the ventricle only if the A-V delay is shorter than the patient's intrinsic P-R delay (P-R interval). In other words, the pacer senses the increased activity and increases the heart rate appropriately based on sensor input.

A *channel* is part of the programmer's monitoring system. Information is displayed on *channels* of the programmer. These *channels* may be selected to monitor different information (for example, the surface EKG, the atrial and ventricular recordings and the markers).

The diagram below demonstrates a pacemaker functioning at a rate *above* the programmed rate.

Device programmed DDDR at a rate of 60, A-V delay 150 msec

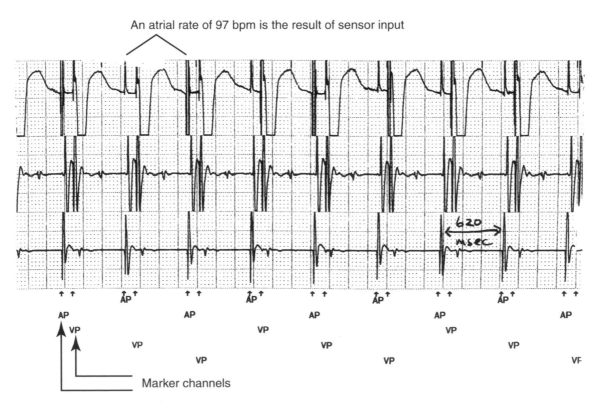

An atrial rate of 97 bpm is the result of sensor input

$$\text{Calculating Rate} = \frac{60,000 \text{ milliseconds/minute}}{\text{interval in milliseconds/beat}} \quad \textbf{or} \quad \frac{60,000 \text{ min}}{620 \text{ beat}} = 96.7 \text{ bpm}$$

Markers are a built-in *identity* mechanism. The pacemaker communicates to the operator the activity it senses, *identifying* and *labeling* activity as demonstrated in the graphics below.

It should be noted that markers are *manufacturer specific,* differing from one manufacturer to another. Following are example markers.

- The **P-R** designation identifies intrinsic (patient-generated) activity.
- **AP** indicates atrial pacing.
- **AS** refers to atrial *sensing.*
- **VP** indicates ventricular pacing.
- **VS** refers to ventricular *sensing.*

Marker Channel Connotations

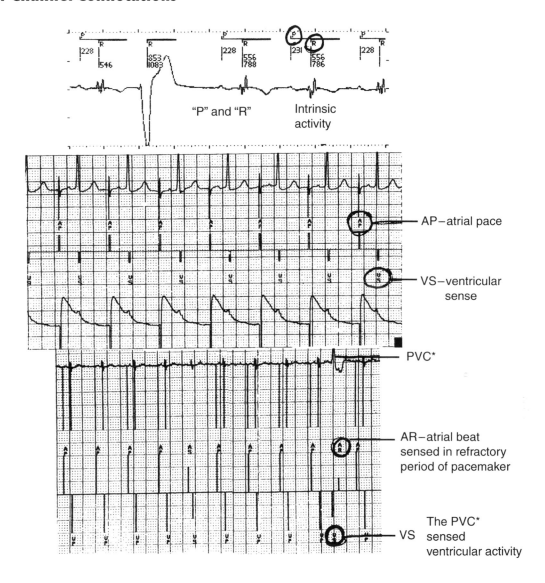

"P" and "R"

Intrinsic activity

AP – atrial pace

VS – ventricular sense

PVC*

AR – atrial beat sensed in refractory period of pacemaker

VS — The PVC* sensed ventricular activity

9

Atrial and Ventricular Electrograms

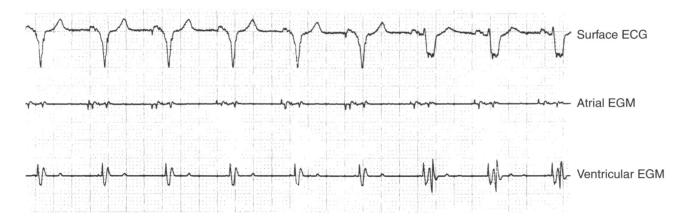

Surface ECG

Atrial EGM

Ventricular EGM

WHY

Rate modulated pacing helps to increase a patient's activity tolerance by augmenting heart rate, as necessary. However, providing for an increased heart rate *will not replace* conditioning and proper exercise regimes to improve cardiovascular health! Patients with extensive coronary artery disease *may* tolerate only limited rate modulation. These persons may experience episodes of angina or anginal equivalent associated with rate modulation.

Practice Exercise 1

A. Two common indications for rate modulated pacing are:

1. _____

2. _____

B. Electrograms (EGMs) are _____

_____.

C. Intrinsic atrial and ventricular activity are represented as _____ and

_____ on the EGM.

D. Atrial and ventricular pacing are represented as _____ and

_____ on the EGM.

For Feedback 1, refer to page 246.

9.2 Hysteresis, Mode-Switch and Auto Capture

Hysteresis, mode-switch and auto capture represent additional programmable options in permanent pacemakers.

Hysteresis

Hysteresis is a programmed option that allows a patient's heart rate to drop to a specific rate, lagging behind the base pacemaker set rate, before pacing is initiated.

WHO

Hysteresis is indicated for a patient with bradycardic episodes who occasionally needs to "catch-up." Stated differently, a patient who experiences a few episodes of bradycardia may require temporary help (a temporary boost) to recover. The patient feels better when the pacemaker is sensing and pacing only for support of a few bradycardic episodes.

> A pacemaker's function is something like a clock. The programming instructs the *clock* how long to wait for specific electrical events. The pacemaker response is based only on what it *senses or doesn't sense* in the programmed interval.

WHAT

The hysteresis program directs electrical pacing to *lag behind* the base pacemaker set rate. This *lag behind* function allows a patient's intrinsic activity to be maintained at a rate slower than the base pacing rate.

For example: Base pacing rate is 70 bpm (beats per minute)
Hysteresis rate is 60 bpm (beats per minute)

In this example, the pacemaker will not initiate pacing until the patient's heart rate falls below 60 beats per minute. The pacing is then initiated at a rate of 70 beats per minute. When the pacemaker *searches* and *senses* the patient's intrinsic activity occurring above 60 beats per minute, it will cease pacing until the intrinsic rate again falls below 60 beats per minute. In addition to preserving intrinsic activity and AV synchrony, the hysteresis function preserves pacemaker battery life.

The **thinking** definition of hysteresis is the *facilitation of a longer escape interval following a sensed beat* (intrinsic beat).

Example of a longer escape interval following a sensed beat

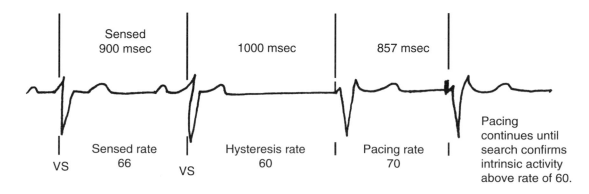

Sensed 900 msec	1000 msec	857 msec	
Sensed rate 66	Hysteresis rate 60	Pacing rate 70	Pacing continues until search confirms intrinsic activity above rate of 60.
VS	VS		

WHEN

Patients uncomfortable with the pacing sensation and those with certain types of syncope are candidates for hysteresis or *lagging behind* option.

HOW

Hysteresis is a programmable option in most pacemakers.

Mode-Switch or Atrial Tachy Response

Mode switch or **atrial tachycardia (tachy) response** is a programmable option in a dual chamber pacemaker that allows the pacemaker to respond to an abnormally fast atrial rhythm. Mode switch or atrial tachy response (**ATR**) is a specific program designed to change the pacemaker mode of function in response to a change in the patient's intrinsic rhythm.

WHO

Persons with paroxysmal supraventricular tachyarrhythmias including supraventricular tachycardia (SVT), atrial flutter and atrial fibrillation are candidates for the mode switching option.
(For a quick review of rapid atrial dysrhythmias, turn back to Section 2!)

WHAT

When a pacemaker senses no tachycardic or fast rhythm, the dual chamber pacing mode functions. However, when a rapid atrial rhythm occurs, the pacemaker will attempt to sense the rapid atrial activation and pace the ventricle accordingly. This may precipitate a rapid ventricular heart rate. Programming the *mode switch* or *atrial tachy response* function prevents rapid ventricular pacing. In essence, the mode switch option deactivates ventricular pacing in response to sensed atrial activity.
For example:

* Dual chamber pacing in the **DDD** mode at a rate of 70.
* Mode switch or ATR is turned **ON** for atrial rates >170
* The patient has an episode of atrial fibrillation (atrial rate >170).
* *Switch* occurs when atrial rates are >170 (this is a programmed selected rate).
* Ventricular pacing occurs in a mode that ignores the high atrial rate (DDI).
* After a *device specific* time period, the atrial channel is activated to search for atrial activity. If the atrial arrhythmia has terminated, the pacemaker *switches back* to the DDD mode. (See diagram on next page.)

SIDE BAR, AGAIN (AKA ANOTHER SPECIAL NOTE)

Device specific refers to pacemaker generator responses *specific to the device manufacturer.* These responses may or may not be programmable. For example, in the *switched mode,* the number of ventricular beats sensed or paced by the pacemaker before it begins searching for atrial activity is device specific. This feature differs by manufacturer, depending on the designed algorithm.

In *pacemaker thinking,* an algorithm directs the pacemaker to respond in a certain way to a specific physiologic event.

> **An algorithm is a set of precise rules.**

WHEN

If the atrial channel senses activity above the trigger rate (as in atrial fibrillation) the pacemaker is programmed to **CHANGE** its mode.

MODE SWITCH OR ATR

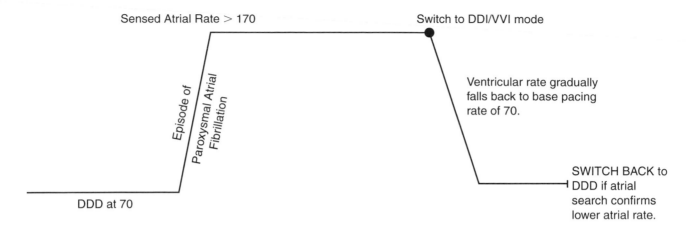

The specifics of this option are dependent on the manufacturer's design. All manufacturers include a method for selecting the sensed rate that will trigger the *switch*. Some devices have options allowing the selection of *mode switch* (for example: to **DVI** or **VVI**). The amount of time and manner of return to dual chamber pacing mode also varies by manufacturer and generation of device.

Auto-Capture

Auto-capture is another programmable option of some pacemakers, a safety feature to assure adequacy of the pacing stimulus. It also conserves battery energy, prolonging battery life.

WHAT

Auto-capture refers to the pacemaker's analysis of the pacing threshold, and adjustment of outputs according to the analysis. An interval algorithm provides for increased energy output if a pacemaker stimulus fails to elicit a paced response (failed capture).

Auto Capture Algorithm

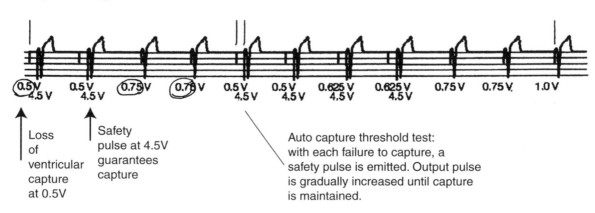

WHEN

The auto capture function is continuous and automatic if programmed "**ON**". Device specific algorithms determine frequency of capture analysis.

WHERE

The function is programmable and optional in some devices.

Auto-capture advantages include an analysis of the paced rhythm and a preserved pacemaker battery life. The disadvantages are: the option is limited to certain manufacturers; and, from a patient's perspective, some persons may feel an uncomfortable difference associated with higher energy outputs.

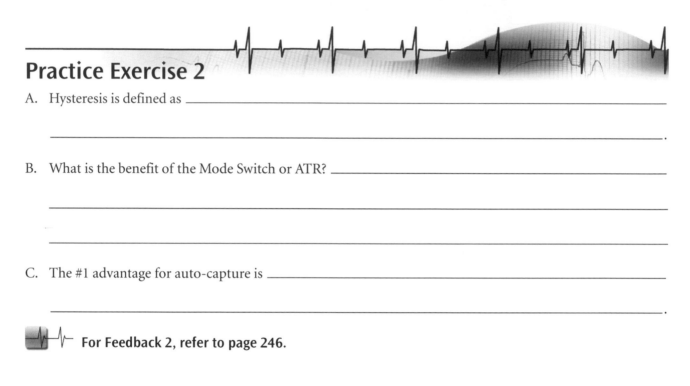

Practice Exercise 2

A. Hysteresis is defined as _____

_____.

B. What is the benefit of the Mode Switch or ATR? _____

_____

_____

C. The #1 advantage for auto-capture is _____

_____.

For Feedback 2, refer to page 246.

input section **9.3** **Atrial Dysrhythmia Suppression/Atrial Rate Stabilization (AKA Overdrive Pacing for Atrial Dysrhythmias)**

Atrial fibrillation is defined by *rapid, irregular atrial impulses occurring at a rate of 300–600 per minute.* Prevalence of atrial fibrillation in the general population is about 1%. This prevalence increases with age, up to 10% in those 80 years and older. Persons with cardiovascular disease, such as coronary artery disease and congestive heart failure, have an increased incidence of atrial fibrillation.

Atrial Fibrillation

Atrial flutter is defined by regular atrial contractions occurring at a rate of 250–350 times per minute. A consistent degree of physiologic block (2:1, 3:1, 4:1, etc.) will result in a regular, slower ventricular response. Varying degrees of physiologic block produces an irregular ventricular response. Atrial flutter is less common than atrial fibrillation and, at the outset, is not usually associated with structural heart disease. Without treatment, atrial flutter may deteriorate to atrial fibrillation.

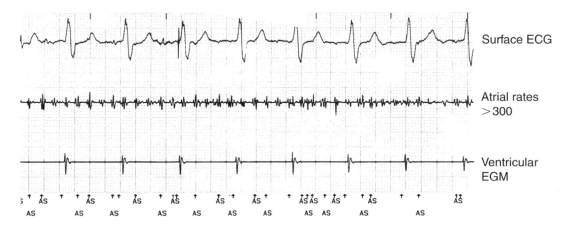

Surface ECG

Atrial rates
>300

Ventricular
EGM

AS † AS † † AS † AS † AS † AS † AS AS † AS † † AS † † AS
AS   AS   AS   AS   AS   AS   AS   AS AS   AS   AS

Atrial Flutter

Overdrive suppression is a therapeutic intervention for both rapid atrial and ventricular arrhythmias. As the name implies, the treatment overdrives the arrhythmia by attempting to *capture* the myocardium with a faster, stronger impulse than that of the existing arrhythmia. Here, the discussion focuses on atrial dysrhythmias.

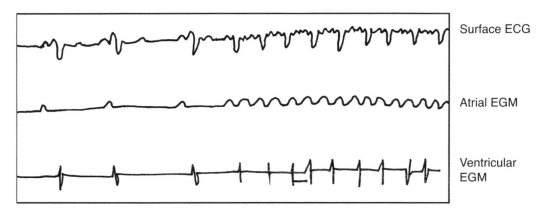

Surface ECG

Atrial EGM

Ventricular
EGM

As an example, a patient with atrial flutter (atrial rate of *250* beats per minute) is paced with a temporary atrial pacemaker. The action involves pacing the atria at a rate of *275* impulses per minute (slightly faster than the flutter rate) for 5 seconds with a high voltage stimulus, 5 mA (milliamphere). The atria is *captured* with the higher energy stimulus, *overdriving* the existing rate of 250. This is known as **entrainment** of the atria. In this situation, entrainment means the pacemaker is now controlling the rhythm rather than the intrinsic atrial flutter stimulus. Once the atria are captured, the quick termination of the pacing stimulus (275 bpm) results in the return to sinus rhythm.

Rapid Atrial Pacing

Rapid atrial pacing is now a programmable option in some permanent pacemaker devices.

A variation of this *atrial arrhythmia suppression* can sense isolated premature atrial contractions. These premature contractions or P.A.C.s are often the precursor to atrial tachyarrhythmias, such as atrial flutter and fibrillation. When the pacemaker senses a premature atrial contraction, an *overdrive (faster)* stimulus is emitted by the pacemaker to suppress other early beats. The faster pacemaker rate is short in duration, returning to the base pacing rate when early (premature) beats are no longer sensed on the atrial channel.

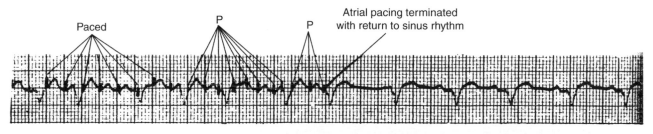

Paced

P

P

Atrial pacing terminated
with return to sinus rhythm

Overdrive Suppression

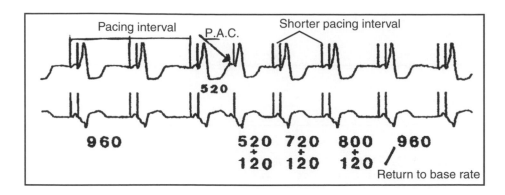

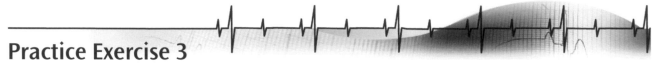

Practice Exercise 3

A. Another name for rapid pacing is _____.

B. Overdrive suppression is used to treat _____

_____.

For Feedback 3, refer to page 247.

input section 9.4   Pacemaker Mediated Tachycardia (PMT)

As its name implies, a pacemaker mediated tachycardia results when paced impulses create an anomalous conducting circuit. (You will recall, anomalous circuitry is responsible for most rapid, sustained ectopic rhythms!) Pacemaker mediated tachycardia (PMT) is a form of reentrant tachycardia that can occur in patients with dual- chamber pacemakers. When PMT occurs, the pacemaker serves as one leg (the antegrade leg) of the abnormal conducting circuit. The AV node serves as the other leg (the retrograde limb). PMT can be precipitated by electrical events which result in retrograde P waves.

The most common events than can precipitate PMT are: (1) P.V.C.s; or, (2) failure of atrial capture. These events produce retrograde P waves (indicating that ventricular activation precedes atrial activation) which can trigger pacemaker mediated tachycardia. A retrograde P wave may follow a P.V.C. owing to the timing of the backward activation of the atria. When an atrial pacemaker spike is not followed by atrial capture, the ventricular pacemaker fires (following the set AV delay). The paced ventricular stimulus initiates ventricular depolarization, followed by retrograde depolarization of the atria. This backward activation of the atria produces a retrograde P wave.

A pacemaker senses retrograde P waves as atrial events. When a pacemaker senses an atrial event, the AV delay clock starts. If no intrinsic (patient generated) ventricular activity occurs by the time the AV delay times out, a ventricular stimulus is emitted by the pacemaker. The paced ventricular stimulus produces ventricular depolarization and a backward activation of the atria, (retrograde P wave).

This backward activation of the atria (retrograde P) again starts the AV delay clock. When the AV clock times out, the pacemaker (once again) emits a ventricular pacing stimulus. This repeating process (retrograde P followed by a pacing ventricular stimulus) results in PMT. The PMT can continue until the atria becomes refractory or until the retrograde conduction is lost.

Following are examples to aid understanding.

A Retrograde P Wave Following a P.V.C.

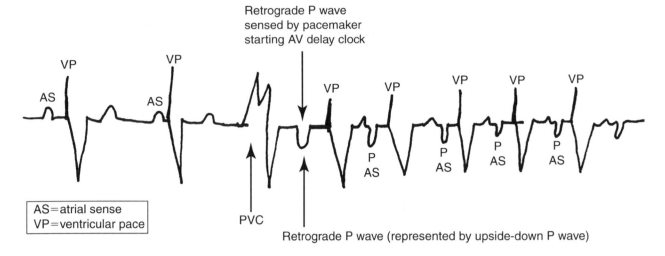

DDD pace with induction of PMT following a PVC with retrograde P wave

Retrograde P wave
sensed by pacemaker
starting AV delay clock

AS=atrial sense
VP=ventricular pace

PVC

Retrograde P wave (represented by upside-down P wave)

P.M.T. Initiated by a P.V.C.: Sequence of Events

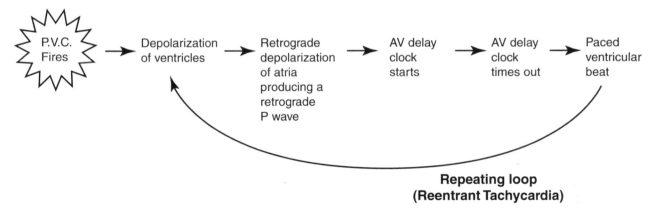

P.V.C. Fires → Depolarization of ventricles → Retrograde depolarization of atria producing a retrograde P wave → AV delay clock starts → AV delay clock times out → Paced ventricular beat

Repeating loop
(Reentrant Tachycardia)

Loss of Atrial Capture

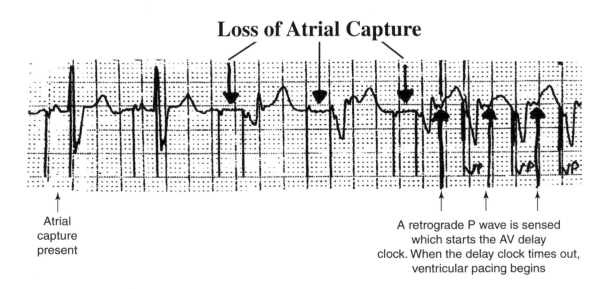

Atrial capture present

A retrograde P wave is sensed which starts the AV delay clock. When the delay clock times out, ventricular pacing begins

P.M.T. Initiated by Failed Atrial Capture: Sequence of Events

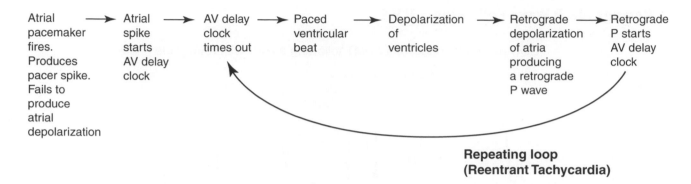

Atrial pacemaker fires. Produces pacer spike. Fails to produce atrial depolarization → Atrial spike starts AV delay clock → AV delay clock times out → Paced ventricular beat → Depolarization of ventricles → Retrograde depolarization of atria producing a retrograde P wave → Retrograde P starts AV delay clock

Repeating loop (Reentrant Tachycardia)

Pacemaker Mediated Tachycardia (PMT)

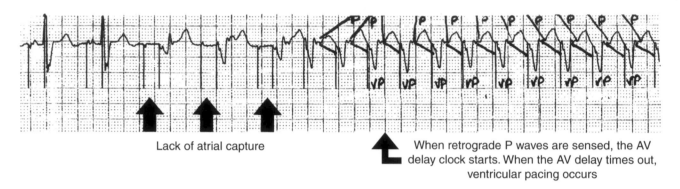

Lack of atrial capture

When retrograde P waves are sensed, the AV delay clock starts. When the AV delay times out, ventricular pacing occurs

NOTE: When a tachycardia occurs at the upper rate limit (**URL**) of the pacemaker, it suggests PMT!

Since the mid-1990s, most pacemakers have an algorithm to identify, record and terminate PMT. Older pacemakers do not have algorithms; thus, PMT may be encountered. There are, however, methods to prevent PMT by programming adjustments to **PVARP** (Post-Ventricular Atrial Refractory Period). In the following illustration, notice that PVARP programming prevents the sensing of retrograde P waves.

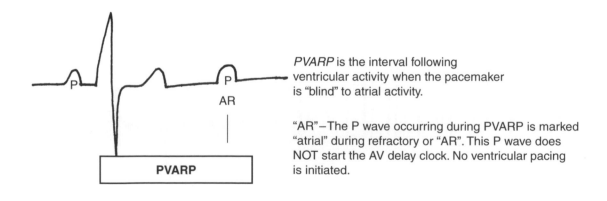

PVARP is the interval following ventricular activity when the pacemaker is "blind" to atrial activity.

"AR"—The P wave occurring during PVARP is marked "atrial" during refractory or "AR". This P wave does NOT start the AV delay clock. No ventricular pacing is initiated.

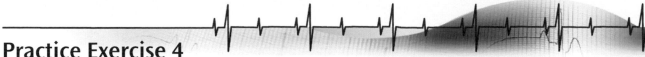

Practice Exercise 4

A. Two causes of PMT are:

1. _____

2. _____ .

For Feedback 4, refer to page 247.

For Feedback 4, refer to page 247.

input section   9.5   Implantable Devices for Overdrive Pacing and Defibrillation

Implantable devices for overdrive pacing *and* internal cardioversion or defibrillation are relatively young and *rapidly* changing technologies. Sophisticated capabilities now include

- Anti-tachycardia Pacing
- Automatic Internal Cardioversion
- Automatic Internal Defibrillation
- Criteria-based detection and treatment

Before moving on, several key terms and conditions deserve attention!

Some Key Terms and Conditions

- An **AICD** is an implantable Automatic Implantable Cardioverter, Defibrillator device
- A **PCD** is an older generation implantable Pacemaker, Cardioverter, Defibrillator device
- An **ICD** is an Implantable Cardioverter, Defibrillator Device

---

Originally both AICDs and PCDs were company proprietary terms for competing devices with similar functions. Now the *generic* ICD term is most often used.

For review, *defibrillation* is defined as the termination of an unsynchronized quivering of the ventricular muscle, using a high energy, asynchronous electrical stimulus delivered to the cardiac tissue. *Cardioversion* is defined as the termination of a tachyarrhythmia using a moderate electrical stimulus synchronized to the cardiac depolarization phase of a cardiac cycle (the R wave).

Here, it is helpful to again review NBG and NBD pacemaker codes and to consider the differences between *older* and *current* devices.

NBG Pacemaker Code				
I	II	III	IV	V
Chamber(s) Paced	Chamber(s) Sensed	Response to Sensing	Programmability Rate modulation	Antitachy Function
O = None	O = None	O = None	O = None	O = None
A = Atrium	A = Atrium	T = Triggered	P = Simple Program	P = Antitachy
V = Ventricle	V = Ventricle	I = Inhibited	M = Multiprogram	Pacing
D = Dual	D = Dual	D = Dual	C = Communicating	S = Shock
			R = Rate Modulation	D = Dual

Bernstein AD, Camm AJ, Fletcher RD, et al. The NASPE/BPEG Defibrillator Generic Pacemaker **Code for Antibradycardia and Adaptive-Rate Pacing and Antitachyarrhythmic Devices.** PACE **1987**; 10:794–799, Appendix II.

9

NBD Pacemaker Code			
I	II	III	IV
Shock Chamber	Antitachycardia Pacing Chamber	Tachycardia Detection	Antibradycardia Pacing Chamber
O = None A = Atrium V = Ventricle D = Dual (A+V)	O = None A = Atrium V = Ventricle D = Dual (A+V)	E = Electrogram H = Hemodynamics	O = None A = Atrium V = Ventricle D = Dual (A+V)

Bernstein AD, Camm AJ, Fisher JD, et al. **The NASPE/BPEG Defibrillator Code** PACE **1993**; 16:1776–1780, Appendix III.

The Similarities and Differences between *Older* and *Current* Implanted Defibrillator Devices

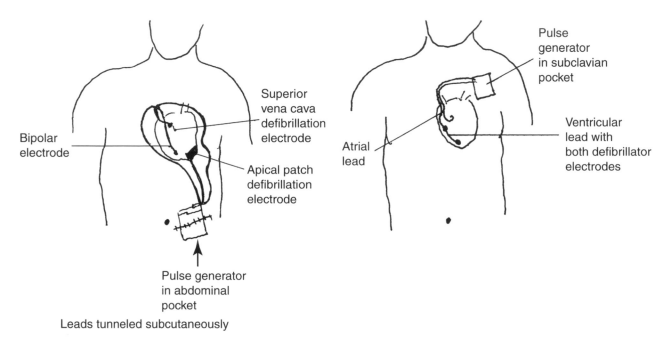

Bipolar electrode

Superior vena cava defibrillation electrode

Apical patch defibrillation electrode

Pulse generator in abdominal pocket

Leads tunneled subcutaneously

Pulse generator in subclavian pocket

Atrial lead

Ventricular lead with both defibrillator electrodes

Older devices (1980s)	*Newer* devices (1990s)
• Generator the size of a pack of cigarettes	• Generator the size of a pacemaker
• Implanted in the abdomen, due to weight and size	• Implanted in subclavian region
• Implanted with transthoracic approach	• Percutaneous, transvenous approach
• Leads placed **epicardially**	• Leads placed **transvenously**
• Recovery from open chest procedure	• IV sedation and minimal recovery
• Prolonged hospitalization	• 24–48 hours for initial implant

Anti-Tachycardia (Overdrive) Pacing

Anti-tachycardia or overdrive pacing is a treatment option for rapid, re-entry dysrhythmias. Anti-tachycardia pacing involves rapid electrical stimulation in attempt to entrain and interrupt a re-entrant tachycardia mechanism, as demonstrated below.

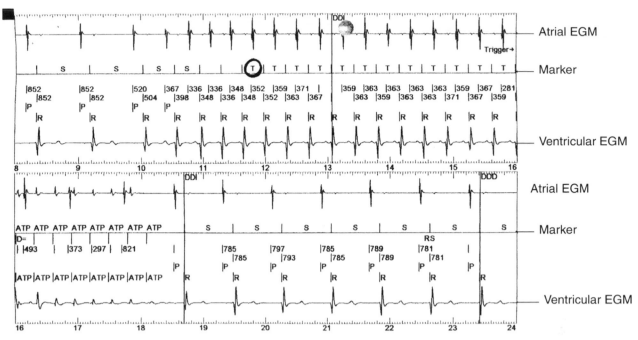

Markers

(T)—tachy interval

Trigger—tachy detection interval number has been met, so therapy begins

"ATP"—anti-tachy pacing therapy

Complex Arrhythmia Intervention

IMPLANTABLE DEFIBRILLATORS (ICDs)

An implantable defibrillator (ICD) is the therapy of choice for patients with lethal ectopic ventricular disorders and certain high risk conditions. It should be emphasized, however, clinical studies are ongoing to determine the specific clinical criteria warranting an implantable defibrillator.

WHO

Candidates for implantable defibrillator therapy include patients with the following disorders:

- documented episodes of *Sudden Cardiac Death*
- documented *inducible ventricular arrhythmias*
- high-risk conditions such as ischemic heart disease and low ejection fractions
- congenital cardiomyopathies and/or arrhythmogenic syndromes (such as long QT syndrome)

WHAT

Implantable defibrillators (ICDs) are multi-functional devices with the following capabilities.

- *Monitoring* constantly for both bradycardic and tachycardic rhythms.

- *Recording* information about the rhythm.

- *Pacing* for bradycardia.

- *Overdrive pacing* for tachyarrhythmias.

- *Cardioversion and defibrillation* for the interruption of tachyarrhythmias when specific criteria are met.

> **NOTE:** All implantable defibrillators have some pacemaker capability. The specific functions are dependent upon the device model and programming.

COUNTERS

Implantable defibrillators (ICDs) have **Counters** which identify and document rhythm events as demonstrated below.

Counters		

Recent Data Includes:	Episodes:		to	
	Dates:	06-MAR-2003	to	04-JUN-2003

	Since Last Cleared	Device Totals	
Episode Counters	06-MAR-2003		
Treated			
VF Therapy	0	③	← 3 therapies delivered for the lifetime of device.
VT Therapy	0	0	
VT-1 Therapy	0	0	
Commanded Therapy	0	0	
Nontreated			
No Therapy Programmed	0	0	
Nonsustained Episodes	0	②	← Non-sustained episodes are counted.
Total Episodes	0	5	
A-Tachy Response	0	0	
Therapy Counters			
Shocks Attempted	⓪	3	← No shock therapy this INTERVAL since 06-Mar-2003.
Delivered-Detection Met	0	3	
-Physician Commanded	0	0	
Diverted -Reconfirm	0	0	
-Physician Commanded	0	0	
ATP Schemes Attempted	0	0	
Delivered-Detection Met	0	0	
-Physician Commanded	0	0	

First-attempt Success Rate:				
	Delivered	Converted	Accelerated	% Success
VF Zone	0	0	—	0
VT Zone	0	0	0	0
VT-1 Zone	0	0	0	0

Electrogram are recorded for treatment purpose.

Parameters

describe the range of arrhythmia for this patient.
Defines the treatable rhythm

This patient's VF detection parameter is set to >200 bpm for a duration of 4.0 seconds. Redetect carried out in 1.0 second.

Pacing Parameters – ☆
Brady and Post Shock Brady

VF Zone

Initial Detection	
Rate	≥ 200 bpm
Interval	≤ 300 ms
Duration	4.0 sec

Redetection	
Redetect Duration	1.0 sec
Post-shock Duration	1.0 sec

Shock Therapy	
Shock 1	17 J ☆
Shock 2	31 J
Max Shocks	31 J

Brady Pacing

Normal Brady Pacing ☆	
Mode	DDDR
Lower Rate Limit	85 ppm
Maximum Tracking Rate	120 ppm
Adaptive Rate	
Maximum Sensor Rate	120 ppm
• Activity Threshold	Medium
• Reaction Time	30 sec
• Response Factor	8
• Recovery Time	5 min
Dynamic A-V Delay	OFF
A-V Delay	80 ms
Minimum Delay	— ms
Sensed A-V Offset	OFF ms
Hysteresis Rate	— ppm
Rate Smoothing	
Smoothing Up	OFF %
Smoothing Down	OFF %

Post-Shock Brady Pacing ☆	
Mode	DDD
Lower Rate Limit	85 ppm
Maximum Tracking Rate	120 ppm
Adaptive Rate	
Maximum Sensor Rate	— ppm
• Activity Threshold	—
• Reaction Time	— sec
• Response Factor	—
• Recovery Time	— min
Dynamic A-V Delay	OFF
A-V Delay	100 ms
Minimum Delay	— ms
Sensed A-V Offset	OFF ms
Hysteresis Rate	— pm
Rate Smoothing	
Smoothing up	OFF %
Smoothing Down	OFF %

Therapy Features

Shock	
Waveform	Biphasic
Polarity	INITIAL
Committed Shock	NO

ATP	
Atrial ATP Amplitude	5.0 V
• Atrial ATP Pulse Width	1.0 ms
Ventricular ATP Amplitude	7.5 V
Ventricular ATP Pulse Width	1.0 ms

• Only available during EP test

Therapy

describes the treatment regimen to be followed for a particular arrhythmia, defined by the parameters set in the device.
Shock Therapy set at 17 J once VF detect is met.

9

Automatic-Implantable-Pacer-Cardioverter-Defibrillators (ICDs) can "*think through*" rhythm analysis and therapy selection based on sophisticated algorithms and program selections.

- The ICD analyzes rhythms based on rate and morphology.
  Rate is a programmed detection number
      (i.e.-ventricular tachycardia detect rate 160 bpm)
  Morphology analyzes width, shape and size of the sensed electrogram.
      (This is a device specific algorithm and differs among manufacturers.)

- Therapy is delivered based on meeting programmed requirements for
  1. rate and/or morphology
  2. duration of the arrhythmia
  3. continuing rhythm disturbance (after the device charges and re-evaluates the rhythm)

Rate Identification with Marker Channels and Intervals of VT

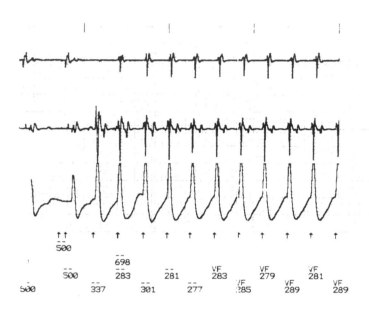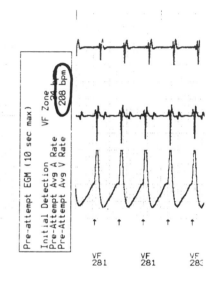

Therapy Initiated

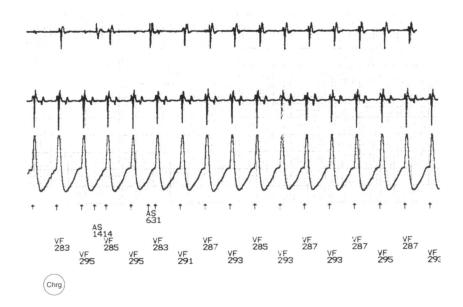

Confirmation Post Charge

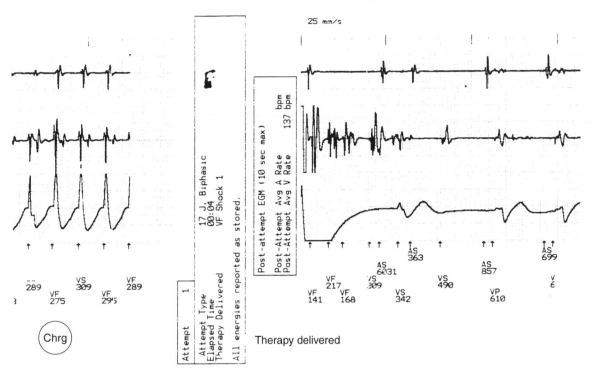

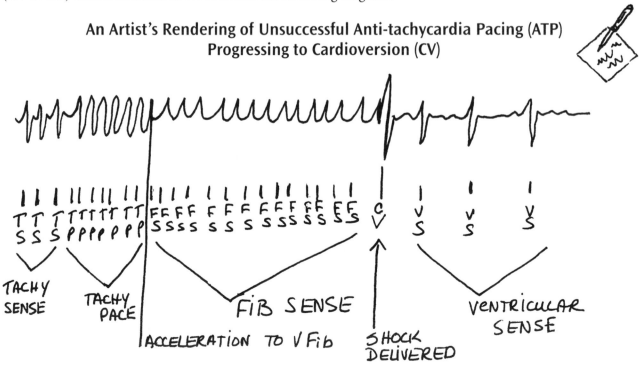

A Bit More About ICDs

The therapy delivered by an ICD is based on programmed criteria. For example, the treatment for monomorphic (originating in one site) ventricular tachycardia (VT) is often overdrive or anti-tachycardia pacing (ATP). If ATP is unsuccessful, cardioversion (CV) is initiated. If CV is unsuccessful, defibrillation (DF) is used. In other words, when the least aggressive therapy (ATP) is unsuccessful, the more aggressive therapy (CV or DF) will be initiated as evidenced in the following diagram.

Atrial and Ventricular Electrograms with AF

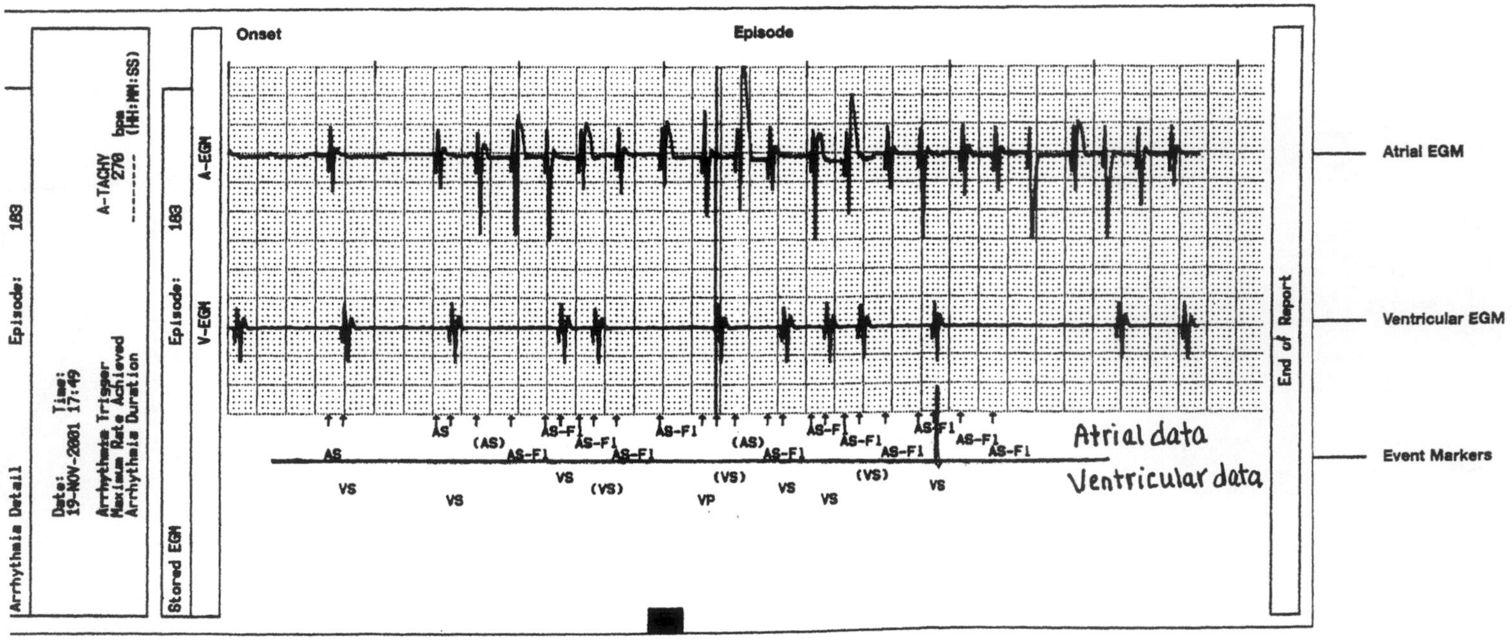

Atrial EGM

Ventricular EGM

Event Markers

The ICD device can discriminate between a supraventricular tachycardia (SVT) and ventricular tachycardia (VT) by comparing data from each lead and other discriminators as discussed below.

Supraventricular Discrimination Options

Supraventricular discriminator options assist the ICD device in *deciding* if the arrhythmia is atrial or ventricular in origin based on criteria other than rate and morphology. Discriminator options are *device specific* (differing by manufacturer) and are designed to prevent the patient from receiving unnecessary ventricular therapy for atrial arrhythmias. The supraventricular discriminators include the following comparative criteria.

THE DISCRIMINATORS

- *A to V comparison*—the number of atrial events compared to ventricular events.
- *Onset*—how fast the rate has changed. (Exercise may produce a high heart rate, but the increase in rate is gradual.)
- *Stability*—the measured intervals vary by < or > in a number of milliseconds. Atrial arrhythmias, such as atrial fibrillation, have inconsistent R-R (ventricular) intervals (owing to variable A-V conduction) compared to ventricular tachycardia.

> In the event that the ICD device cannot discriminate between an atrial and ventricular dysrhythmia, it treats the rhythm as ventricular, delivering the ventricular arrhythmia therapy.

An Example of Onset Enabled Discriminators

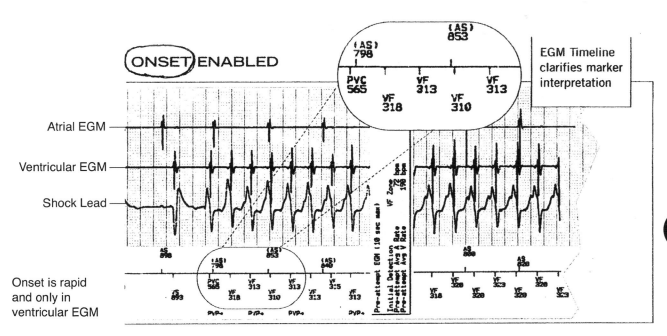

From *Guidant, Vitality 2 ICD Systems.* Copyright © 2004 by Guidant Corporation. Reprinted by permission.

Two discriminators are in effect:

1. Onset (VT onset is usually fast. If the atrial rate increases with exercise, the increase is gradual; thus, it is not VT).
2. Ventricular rate > Atrial rate (If the rhythm is atrial or sinus tachycardia, the A to V rate is equal.)

To complexify things just a bit 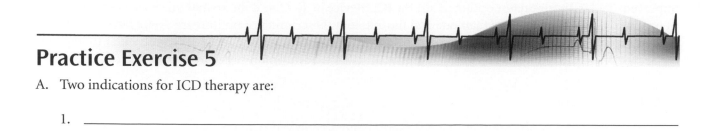, there are devices which treat rapid atrial dysrhythmias with atrial anti-tachycardia pacing (ATP) or suppression. Other clinically available devices treat atrial arrhythmias with cardioversion.

Practice Exercise 5

A. Two indications for ICD therapy are:

1. _____

2. _____

B. Two criteria necessary for initiating defibrillation therapy are:

1. _____

2. _____

For Feedback 5, refer to page 247.

input section   9.6   Bi-Ventricular Pacing

You have previously *learned* that AV or dual lead pacemakers are used to achieve synchronized atrial and ventricular functioning. As the name "bi-ventricular" implies, pacemakers can now stimulate both the right and left ventricle. Bi-ventricular pacing is the newest of pacing applications and, there is still *much* to learn about selecting treatment groups and evaluating (and increasing) efficacy.

Bi-ventricular pacing is becoming more popular due to attempts to avoid dyssynchrony caused or aggravented by right ventricular pacing. Currently, a bi-ventricular pacemaker is indicated for a patient with a prolonged QRS, >120 msec.

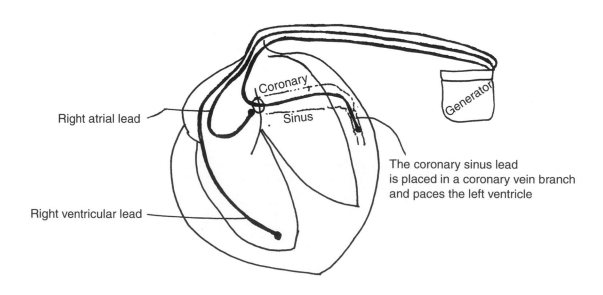

Right atrial lead

Coronary Sinus

Generator

The coronary sinus lead is placed in a coronary vein branch and paces the left ventricle

Right ventricular lead

As demonstrated in the previous diagram, the bi-ventricular pacemaker has three lead wires. The bi-ventricular (bi-V) pacemaker incorporates dual chamber AV pacing (a right atrial and a right ventricular lead) and (a third lead, positioned in a vein in the coronary sinus) (in the same device). These features are combined in a device with defibrillator capability, as well. A bi-ventricular pacemaker sends a stimulus to the atria, followed by a programmed AV delay. The stimulus is then simultaneously sent to both ventricles. The goal of bi-ventricular pacing is to control ventricular sychronous pacing as close to 100% of the time as possible.

A Bi-ventricular Programming Strip Demonstrating Programmed Parameters

Normal HF/Brady Parameters		
Individually programmable parameters for pacing	INITIAL VALUE	PRESENT VALUE
Basic Pacing		
Mode		DDD
A-Tachy Response		On
Lower Rate Limit		90 ppm
Max Tracking Rate		130 ppm
Max Sensor Rate		120 ppm
AV Delay (Paced)		120 ms
Pacing Chamber		BiV
Atrial ——— Atrial		
Pulse Width		0.4 ms
Amplitude		3.5 V
Right ——— Right Ventricular		
Ventricle Pulse Width		0.4ms
Amplitude		2.4 V
Left ——— Left Ventricular		
Ventricle Pulse Width		0.5 ms
Amplitude		3.5 V
Post-shock Delay		1.5 sec
Sensor		
Accelerometer		ATR Only
Activity Threshold		Med-Lo
Reaction Time		30 sec
Slope		11
Recovery		5 min

Next, it is helpful to think briefly about characteristic EKG patterns and cardiac muscle pathology. When a pacemaker is used in the right ventricle as in *AV* or *dual chamber* pacing, a conduction abnormality is created. On EKG, this abnormality resembles a left bundle branch block pattern. Pacemaker activation of the right ventricle causes the wave of ventricular depolarization to spread from right to left, outside the normal conduction pathway. This anomalous route of depolarization requires more time and delays left ventricular activation.

9

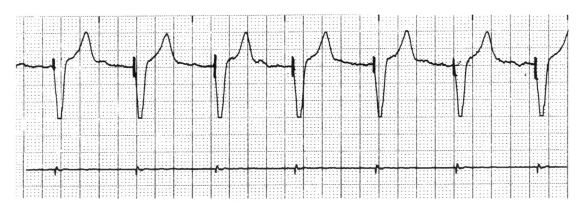

A characteristic LBBB pattern associated with right ventricular pacing

A left bundle branch pattern may also be observed in patients with muscle scarring associated with coronary artery disease, as demonstrated below. In both groups, the ventricles no longer work synchronously (together) as they would if normal conduction occurred from the SA to AV node and through the bundle branches and the His-Purkinje system.

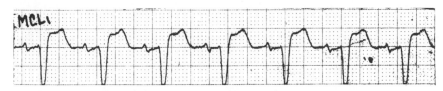

EKG demonstrating a LBBB conduction defect

Long-standing congestive heart failure often results in structural changes within the heart. The heart may become globally dilated (the entire heart takes the shape of a globe) as in a patient with dilated cardiomyopathy.

Large areas of cardiac muscle scarring may follow large scale myocardial infarction. In areas where infarction has occurred, the heart muscle becomes *dyskinetic* or *dysynchronous* (does not move together) as a result of scarring. *Re-synchronization therapy,* another name for bi-V pacing may be employed to achieve synchronized ventricular muscle functioning.

The following patient clinical conditions warrant consideration for bi-V pacing or re-synchronization therapy.

Eligibility for Bi-ventricular Pacing or Re-synchronization Therapy

WHO

- Patients with congestive heart failure continuing to experience moderate to severe symptoms despite maximum medical therapy
- Patients with delay in electrical conduction evident on the EKG (widened QRS)
- Patients with congestive heart failure, continuing to experience symptoms despite maximum medical therapy, and echocardiographic evidence of mitral regurgitation (backflow across the mitral valve when the left ventricle contracts)

WHAT

Bi-ventricular pacing affords an **improved** quality of life!

- *Functionally*, bi-V pacing improves exercise tolerance and decreases symptoms of shortness of breath and fatigue associated with activities of daily living.
- *Electrically*, bi-V pacing produces electrocardiographic (EKG) evidence of improved conduction (decreased QRS duration).

Quality of Life Changes

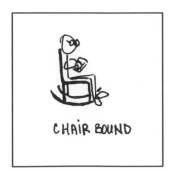

Versus

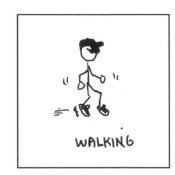

WHEN

The results associated with bi-ventricular pacing or re-synchronization therapy vary by patient.

- It *may* take months to see improvement in symptoms.
- Electrical (EKG) evidence may improve first.
- Improvement will vary among patients regardless of selection for device therapy.

WHERE AND HOW

As demonstrated in the next diagram, lead wires are positioned in the right atrium, the right ventricle, and in a branch of the coronary sinus (the large venous system of the coronary arterial system.)

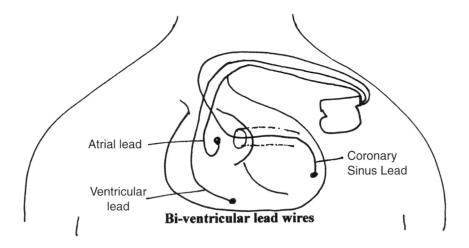

Bi-ventricular lead wires

Atrial pacing occurs if necessary, when the sinus rate falls below the programmed atrial rate. Pacing of the right and left ventricles occurs simultaneously. Remodeling or reshaping of the ventricles occurs over time, secondary to electrical (bi-V) re-synchronization. In other words, over time the improved electrical conduction is *expected* to produce a positive change in the mechanical functioning of the ventricles. The expected positive change includes improved septal and ventricular contractions and decreased mitral regurgitation.

Practice Exercise 6

A. Two differences between AV pacing and bi-V pacing are:

1. _____

2. _____

B. The third lead in a bi-V pacemaker is positioned in _____

_____

C. The goal of bi-ventricular pacing is _____

_____

D. Electrical improvement may precede _____

_____

_____

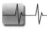 **For Feedback 6, refer to page 247.**

Now, a new generation of pacing has combined bi-ventricular pacing with anti-Tachy pacing and defibrillation! Therapies are now combined in many different ways. For example, bradycardic pacing therapies may be used alone or in combination with optional treatments for tachyarrhythmias. Combination therapies represent an *evolving* science and have likely changed since you began this Section! Stay tuned to the written and *virtual* resources available from all pacemaker manufacturers!

> **SPECIAL NOTE:** The left ventricular (or coronary sinus) lead is inserted transvenously through the right atrium and coronary sinus into a branch of the coronary vein. The coronary sinus lead is situated in a branch of the coronary vein rather than against the muscle wall of the heart. (You will recall that other leads rest on the muscle wall.) Owing to positioning, this lead behaves differently. If the position of the lead does not change, the impedance remains stable. The energy required to stimulate the heart muscle through a vein is often higher than direct muscle stimulation. As a result, the battery drain is greater (battery requirements and battery size may differ from a standard pacemaker).

Feedback 1

A. Two common indications for rate modulated pacing are:

1. Sinus bradycardia with chronotropic incompetence

2. Drug induced rate suppression

B. Electrograms (EGMs) are displays of internally recorded activity from the leads of implantable devices.

C. Intrinsic atrial and ventricular activity are represented as P and R on the EGM.

D. Atrial and ventricular pacing are represented as AP and VP on the EGM.

Feedback 2

A. Hysteresis is defined as a programmed option that allows the heart rate to lag behind the base pacemaker set rate.

B. Mode switch or ATR is recommended for the treatment of supraventricular tachycardia, atrial flutter and atrial fibrillation.

C. The #1 advantage for auto-capture is that it provides for increased energy output if a pacemaker stimulus fails to elicit a paced response. It corrects a failure to capture.

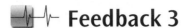 Feedback 3

A. Another name for rapid pacing is overdrive suppression.

B. Overdrive suppression is used to treat rapid atrial and ventricular arrhythmias.

Feedback 4

A. Two causes of PMT are:

1. P.V.C.s

2. Failure of atrial capture

Feedback 5

A. Indications for ICD therapy are

1. Documented episodes of sudden cardiac death

2. Documented inducible ventricular arrhythmias

3. High-risk conditions (ischemic heart disease, low ejection fractions)

4. Congenital cardiomyopathies or arrhythmogenic syndromes

B. Two criteria necessary for initiating defibrillation therapy are

1. Rate of onset (VT onset is usually fast)

2. Ventricular rate greater than the atrial rate

Feedback 6

A. Two differences between AV pacing and bi-V pacing are

1. An AV pacemaker (2 leads) paces the right atrium and right ventricle; a bi-V pacemaker (3 leads) paces the right atrium and the right and left ventricles

2. Bi-V pacing re-synchronizes ventricular functioning

B. The third lead in a bi-V pacemaker is positioned in the coronary sinus.

C. The goal of bi-ventricular pacing is synchronized ventricular muscle function.

D. Electrical improvement may precede improvement in symptoms.

9

Notes

Electrolyte Changes

Objectives

When you have completed Section 10, you will be able to describe or identify clinical conditions and EKG manifestations associated with

1. hypokalemia
2. hyperkalemia
3. hypocalcemia
4. hypercalcemia
5. hypomagnesemia
6. hypermagnesemia
7. prolonged QTc interval

input section 10.1 Ions, Electrolytes, and Potassium

Section 10 deals with certain electrolyte imbalances as reflected on the EKG. Even though that sounds less than intriguing, there are some unique and interesting things you should know. 😊 **Honest!**

The author is making the assumption that you have a reasonable understanding of electrolytes . . . but if you are uncertain, a *brief* overview follows.

Remember **ions**? They are the electrically charged particles contained in the various fluid compartments of the body—the intracellular fluid (ICF) compartment and the extracellular fluid (ECF) compartment. If your long-term memory is operative, you will recall that the ECF includes *both* the fluid in the blood vessels (intravascular fluid) and the fluid located between the cells (interstitial fluid).

Anions are negatively charged particles—like bicarbonate (HCO_3^-) and chloride (Cl^-).

Cations are positively charged particles—like potassium (K^+), sodium (Na^+), calcium (Ca^{++}), and magnesium (Mg^{++}).

Cat-ion

Electrolytes are combinations of anions and cations in solution.

It is interesting to consider what happens to all the ions or charges in the processes of heart contraction and relaxation and in the processes of cellular depolarization and repolarization.

All cells in the body, including the myocardial cells, have an electrical charge which is a result of all the ions (cations and anions) in the body. These ions are found both inside and outside of the cells—some in greater concentrations than others.

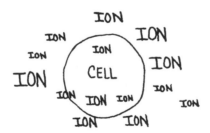

When a cell is at rest (polarized state), the inside of the cell has a net negative charge, while the cell membrane has a net positive charge. Sodium (Na^+) tends to be mainly outside the cell, and potassium (K^+) tends to be mainly inside the cell during this polarized state.

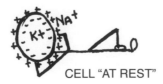

CELL "AT REST"

When a cell is electrically stimulated, sodium (Na^+) rushes into the cell, while potassium (K^+) moves out. Sodium and potassium basically change places for awhile.

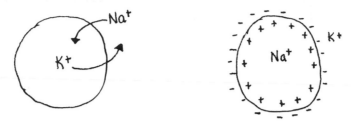

This movement of K^+ and Na^+ upsets the charge on the inside of the cell—giving it a net positive charge. This reversal of charges is **depolarization**. Depolarization causes calcium (Ca^{++}) to move into the cell. Calcium then causes the mechanical activity of **contraction**. Following depolarization, the ions move back to their "resting state" or repolarized positions in order to receive the next impulse.

It is important to recognize clinical conditions causing electrolyte imbalances and anticipate changes associated with depolarization, repolarization, and contractility of the myocardial cells.

Serum Potassium

We will begin by examining potassium (K^+), a major intracellular cation. A **normal serum potassium ranges between 3.6–5.2 mEq. per liter**. Potassium is the cation that influences myocardial cell **repolarization**.

HYPOKALEMIA

Hypokalemia is the term used to describe a **serum potassium (K^+) level below 3.6 mEq/liter**. Because the potassium ions play an important role in repolarization activities of myocardial cells, certain changes occur in the EKG pattern when the potassium level is unbalanced. Those changes may be subtle or pronounced.

For instance, *hypokalemia* may cause any or all of the following EKG changes.

A. *Depressed ST segment*

B. *Prominent U wave**

C. *Prolonged QT or QU interval*

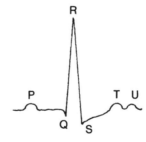

The QT interval (depicted on the following page) is measured from the beginning of the QRS complex to the end of the T wave. The QT interval simply represents the total time for ventricular depolarization and repolarization.

A U wave superimposed upon or near the T wave (more or less of a camel back presentation) gives the appearance of a prolonged QT interval. In effect, it is the U wave that makes the interval prolonged.

Just for the record, QT intervals vary with age, gender and heart rate, though, a normal QT interval should be no greater than half of the R-R interval. The QT interval is best measured in leads V_2 and V_3.

10

---

* The U wave is thought to represent the prolonged repolarization of the Purkinje fibers.

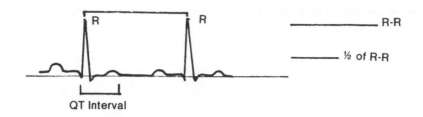

R-R

½ of R-R

QT Interval

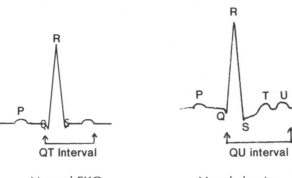

QT Interval

QU interval

Normal EKG   Hypokalemia

In a healthy state, the normal male QT interval averages 0.39 seconds; the normal female QT interval averages 0.41 seconds. Because the QT interval varies with heart rate, a formula (Bazet's formula) was derived to correct for heart rate variation.

$$\text{Bazet's formula} \qquad \mathbf{QTc} = \frac{\text{QT interval in seconds}}{\sqrt{\text{R} - \text{R interval in seconds}}}$$

QTc is the abbreviation utilized for a heart-rate corrected QT interval. Fortunately, QTc calculators are programmed into 12 lead EKG machines! See more detail on page 260.

Oftentimes it is difficult to visualize U waves or determine where a T wave stops and the U wave begins. It may help to view those leads where the T waves tend to be flat.

Here is a 12 lead EKG demonstrating hypokalemia (and demonstrating the difficulty of U wave identification!). V_6 provides the best view of the U wave.

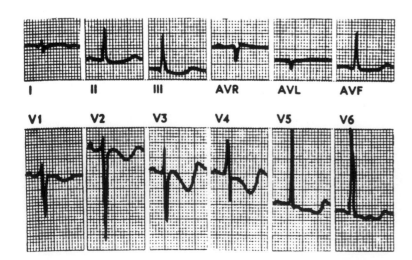

> **IMPORTANT NOTICE:** One can never diagnose hypokalemia from an EKG—it can only be suspected. Hypokalemia must be confirmed by a serum potassium level.

Hypokalemia may be associated with any of the following conditions or therapies.

- starvation
- vomiting
- diarrhea
- diuretic therapy

- intermittent gastric suction
- excessive digitalis therapy
- excessive use of steroids

Because hypokalemia *increases electrical instability*, the following dysrhythmias may be associated with low serum potassium levels.

- **P.V.C.s**
- **Atrial tachycardia**
- **Junctional tachycardia**

- **Ventricular tachycardia**
- **Ventricular fibrillation**

If this is *confusing, just remember that **potassium mainly affects the repolarization** period of cardiac activity. Since the T wave represents repolarization, **look for EKG changes near the T wave**. Probably the most common EKG feature associated with pronounced hypokalemia is the prominent *U wave*.

Here's a Poem for U . . .

Roses are Red
Violets are Blue
Potassiums that are *Low*
Will give you a U (wave)!

Hyperkalemia

Of course, there are EKG effects and electrical considerations associated with elevated potassium (K^+) levels, as well. **A serum potassium (K^+) level greater than 5.2 mEq. per liter** is termed **hyperkalemia**.

The most characteristic EKG features associated with **hyperkalemia** include

- Tall, peaked, narrow, tent-like T waves that are symmetrical in appearance.

- Diminished height or amplitude of the R wave.

- Small or low amplitude P waves.

- A widened QRS (intraventricular block) in severe hyperkalemia.

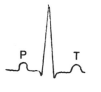

Normal

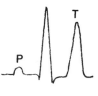

Hyperkalemia
(Mild)

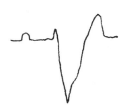

Hyperkalemia
(Severe)

10

Here is a rather impressive rhythm strip demonstrating a serum potassium level near 7.0 mEq. per liter.

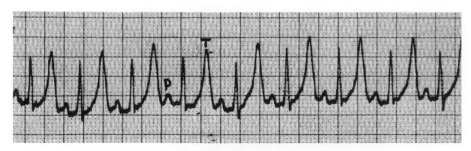

(It is difficult to miss the tall, peaked, tent-like T waves!)

> **IMPORTANT NOTICE:** One can never diagnose hyperkalemia from an EKG—it can only be suspected. Hyperkalemia must be confirmed by a serum potassium level.

Hyperkalemia *may* be associated with any of the following clinical conditions or therapies.

- excessive amounts of potassium replacement (**most common cause!**)
- burns
- crushing injuries
- adrenal insufficiency
- oliguria
- kidney disease

Hyperkalemia *depresses* **the normal electrical activity of the myocardial cells** and may result in any of the following dysrhythmias.

- **Sinus bradycardia**
- **Sinus arrhythmia**
- **First degree AV block**
- **Junctional rhythm**
- **Idioventricular rhythm**
- **Ventricular tachycardia**
- **Ventricular fibrillation**
- **Asystole** (the absence of rhythm)

Hint: Tall, peaked (tent-like), symmetrical T waves should lead one to suspect *hyperkalemia.*

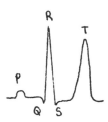

> ### Review Guide
>
> | Hypokalemia | Hyperkalemia |
> |---|---|
> | K^+ < 3.6 mEq./L. | K^+ > 5.2 mEq./L. |
> | Depressed ST segment | Tall peaked T waves |
> | Prominent U wave | Small P waves |
> | Prolonged (QU interval) | Widened QRS, when severe |

. . . I suppose we should try a bit of practice. . . . **right?**

Practice Exercise 1

A. Potassium plays an important role in the (circle one) repolarization / depolarization activity of the myocardial cells.

B. During a normal cardiac cycle, the _____ wave represents repolarization activity.

C. This one is easy!

Match the terms with the EKG complexes at the right.

Hypokalemia

Normal Conduction

Hyperkalemia

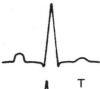
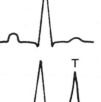
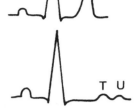

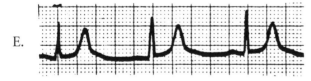

D. Briefly describe your observations and note any appropriate actions.

_____

_____

_____

_____

_____

E. Describe this rhythm strip and actions you might take.

_____

_____

_____

_____

_____

 For Feedback 1, refer to page 260.

10.2 Serum Calcium

That brings us to calcium. Remember calcium? Calcium is the cation (-ION) that moves into the cells following depolarization, causing mechanical activity or contraction. In other words, calcium (Ca^{++}) is a cardiac *stimulant* whose **main function is *contractility*.**

   Normal serum calcium levels range between 9–11 mg.%. EKG changes associated with hypocalcemia are seen in the ST segment of the cardiac cycle.

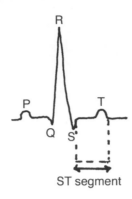

ST segment

Hypocalcemia

Hypocalcemia refers to a **serum calcium (Ca^{++}) level below 9 mg.%** and causes *decreased contractility of the heart*.

   On EKG, a low serum calcium presents as a *lengthening* or prolongation of the ST segment, without changing the appearance of the QRS or the T wave. There is no change in the QRS or T wave because calcium does its work between depolarization and repolarization.

> Always remember to observe for hypocalcemia when there is an upset in acid base balance and in the presence of hypoparathyroid disease.

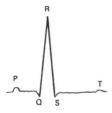

   In a hypocalcemic state, the ST segment appears flat (*isoelectric*) and *prolonged,* as illustrated in the above drawing. If you recall the earlier discussion of QT intervals, you will remember that the *QT interval is prolonged.* The other significant feature is the low amplitude T waves, squatty in appearance. (I'm not certain that *squatty* is a real word . . . but you get the idea!)

   Here are two EKG leads demonstrating hypocalcemia.

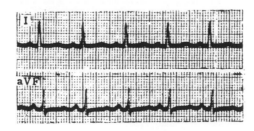

Hypercalcemia

Hypercalcemia, on the other hand, refers to a **serum calcium level greater than 11 mg.%.** A high serum calcium will cause *increased contractility of the heart*.

The EKG changes associated with hypercalcemia appear opposite to those of hypocalcemia (brilliant deduction, right 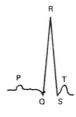?).

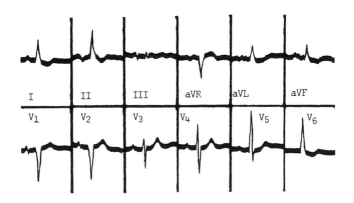

As seen in the above drawing, hypercalcemia causes a shortening of the ST segment (without changing the appearance of the QRS or T wave (because calcium does its work *between* depolarization and repolarization).

As a matter of fact, the ST segment is *commonly* absent! Often one observes an abruptly ascending T wave immediately following the QRS, as illustrated below.

Always remember to watch for hypercalcemia in the presence of acidosis.

Following is a 12 lead EKG demonstrating a high serum calcium level.

IMPORTANT NOTICE: One can never diagnose hypercalcemia from an EKG—it can only be suspected. Hypercalcemia must be confirmed by a serum calcium level!

Review Guide

Hypocalcemia	Hypercalcemia
$Ca^{++} < 9$ mg.%	$Ca^{++} > 11$ mg. %
↓ contractility	↑ contractility
prolonged ST segment	shortened ST segment

Practice Exercise 2

Surprise . . . it's practice time again!

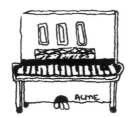

A. Calcium is a cardiac _____, so its main function is contractility.

B. Hypocalcemia refers to a serum calcium level (circle one) above / below 9 mg.%.

C. Hypocalcemia can be suspected when one sees a _____ ST segment.

D. Draw a cardiac cycle (PQRST) that demonstrates a low calcium effect.

E. Hypercalcemia refers to a serum calcium level above _____ mg.%.

F. Hypercalcemia can be suspected when one sees a _____ ST segment.

G. Draw a cardiac cycle (PQRST) that demonstrates a high calcium effect.

H. Hypocalcemia causes _____ cardiac contractility.

I. Hypercalcemia causes _____ cardiac contractility.

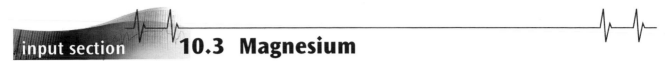 **For Feedback 2, refer to page 261.**

For Feedback 2, refer to page 261.

input section 10.3 Magnesium

Magnesium (Mg^{++}) is the second most frequently occurring intercellular cation. The normal serum magnesium level ranges between 1.8–3.0 mg/dL. However, serum magnesium levels are rarely diagnostic since 60% of magnesium resides in the bones, 40% resides in cells, and only 1% resides in the interstitial compartment and serum! Magnesium plays a number of important roles including mediating neural transmission and influencing the transport of ions regulating cardiac action potential.

Magnesium is particularly important in that a low magnesium level (hypomagnesemia . . . often suspected, rather than confirmed by lab values) causes an increase in the QTc interval. An abnormal QTc interval suggests that ventricular repolarization is delayed, and that delay poses a risk for dysrhythmias. **Quite frequently, hypomagnesemia occurs in tandem with hypokalemia and should be suspected when hypokalemia is present.** You will recall that a prolonged QT interval is associated with hypokalemia, as well.

When therapeutically administered, magnesium has both antidysrhythmic (similar to calcium channel blockers) and anti-platelet effects. It also has coronary vasodilator effects, reducing contractility. **Magnesium slows cardiac conduction and ventricular refractoriness.** Magnesium is often used to treat unresponsive lethal ventricular dysrhythmias (ventricular tachycardia, torsades de pointes) and may be given to acute myocardial infarct patients for its antiarrhythmic, anti-platelet and vasodilator effects. Clinical research is ongoing to determine the efficacy of magnesium in treating rapid, re-entry atrial dysrhythmias.

Hypomagnesemia may result from diarrhea, hypoparathyroid disease, pancreatitis, ulcerative colitis and alcoholism. Hypermagnesemia may be associated with chronic renal failure, dehydration, diabetic acidosis and oliguria.

Hypermagnesemia may be associated with chronic renal failure, dehydration, diabetic acidosis and oliguria.

There is no accompanying practice exercise! Instead, together we will evaluate a rhythm strip demonstrating a prolonged QT interval. Then, just for fun, we will calculate the QTc using Bazet's formula! You will recall (from Section 1), the QT interval is measured from the beginning of the QRS to the end of the T wave. Often times, the QT interval is most easily measured in leads V_2 and V_3.

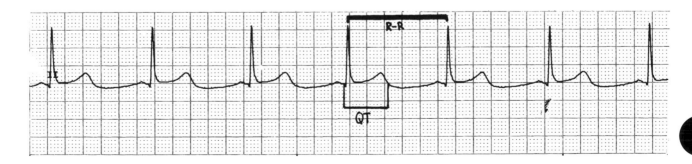

The above rhythm is a sinus bradycardia (approximate rate 55 beats per minute). The QRS is borderline, measuring just slightly less than 0.12 seconds. The QT interval measures 13 small squares or 0.52 seconds ($13 \times 0.04 = 0.52$). The R-R interval measures 27 small squares or 1.08 seconds ($27 \times 0.04 = 1.08$).

The QTc is a measure of the total time for depolarization and repolarization, corrected for heart rate. EKG machines automatically calculate the QTc rate, though a manual calculation can be performed using Bazet's formula.

$$\text{Bazet's formula} \qquad QTc = \frac{\text{QT interval in seconds}}{\sqrt{\text{R-R interval in seconds}}}$$

$$QTc = \frac{0.52 \ (\text{QT in seconds})}{\sqrt{1.08 \ (\text{R-R in seconds})}}$$

$$\sqrt{1.08} = 1.039$$

$$QTc = \frac{0.52}{1.039}$$

$$QTc = 0.50$$

The normal male QTc interval averages 0.39 seconds; the normal female QT interval averages 0.41 seconds. For both sexes, a normal QTc is less than 0.44 seconds. Thus, the above QTc interval is significantly prolonged at 0.50 seconds.

BREAK TIME! ☺

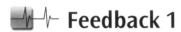 **Feedback 1**

How did you do? If your answers are similar to mine, you deserve a banana! (Bananas are packed full of potassium ⬭)

A.   Potassium plays an important role in the (repolarization)/depolarization activity of the myocardial cells.

B.   During a normal cardiac cycle, the <u>T</u> wave represents repolarization activity.

C.   If your matching does <u>not</u> match mine, the Great Banana suggests that you reread Input 9.1.

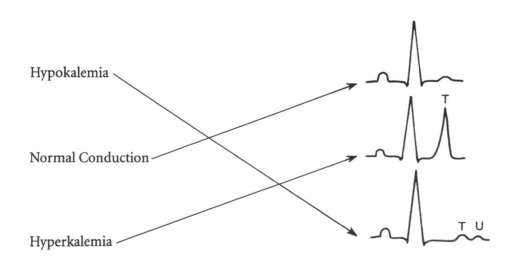

D. The rhythm appears to be a sinus bradycardia with a rate between 50–60 beats per minute. The ST segment is slightly depressed and there is a prominent U wave. I suspect hypokalemia, but would need to verify with a serum potassium level.

E. The rhythm is a borderline sinus bradycardia with a heart rate of 60. The P waves are small. The T waves are tall and peaked (tent-like). I suspect hyperkalemia, but would need to verify with a serum potassium level.

 ## Feedback 2

You're Doing Super . . .

. . . especially if you answered all the questions correctly!!

A. Calcium is a cardiac **stimulant**, so its main function is **contractility**.

B. Hypocalcemia refers to a serum calcium level (below) 9 mg.%.

C. Hypocalcemia can be suspected when one sees a <u>lengthened or prolonged</u> ST segment.

D.

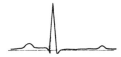

E. Hypercalcemia refers to a serum calcium level above <u>11</u> mg.%.

F. Hypercalcemia can be suspected when one sees a <u>shortened</u> ST segment.

G.

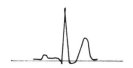

H. Hypocalcemia causes <u>decreased</u> cardiac contractility.

I. Hypercalcemia causes <u>increased</u> cardiac contractility.

A Final Refresher	
Hypokalemia	**Hyperkalemia**
K^+ < 3.6 mEq./L.	K^+ > 5.2 mEq./L.
Depressed ST segment	Tall peaked T waves
Prominent U wave	Small P waves
Prolonged (QU interval)	Widened QRS, when severe

10

Hypocalcemia	Hypercalcemia
$Ca^{++} < 9$ mg.%	$Ca^{++} > 11$ mg. %
↓ contractility	↑ contractility
prolonged ST segment	shortened ST segment

IMPORTANT NOTICE: Electrolyte effects on EKG are often subtle, and many times missed. When laboratory studies identify abnormal serum electrolyte levels, review a current 12 lead EKG to see if you can spot the subtle changes. ☺

Notes

10

Notes

The Identification of Ischemia, Injury, and Infarct

Objectives

When you have completed Section 11, you will be able to describe or identify

1. The classification scheme for myocardial infarction
2. The relationship between coronary blood supply and EKG patterns
3. the normal 12 lead EKG
4. the orientation of EKG leads to the left ventricular surfaces
5. EKG changes associated with ischemia
6. muscle layers in the heart
7. criteria for diagnosing or suspecting myocardial infarction
8. injury pattern in leads overlying an infarct
9. the hallmark of large scale myocardial infarction or necrosis
10. anteroseptal wall myocardial infarction
11. inferior wall myocardial infarction
12. criteria suggesting a posterior wall myocardial infarction
13. serum markers

Consider re-reading "LEADing into Section 1" before progressing!

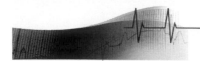

A Brief Introduction
by Stephanie L. Woods, Ph.D., R.N.

The Relationship between Coronary Blood Supply and the EKG

The conduction tissues generate electrical energy which is observable on the EKG as it travels through and activates cardiac muscle. Both the muscle and the conducting tissues require oxygen which is extracted from blood perfusing through the coronary arteries. When the blood supply is inadequate, both muscle and conducting tissues suffer secondary to the inadequate oxygenation. A diminished blood supply to the muscle typically results in pain (*angina*). The inadequate blood flow to conduction tissue results in characteristic changes on the EKG.

Decreased coronary blood flow sufficient to interfere with oxygen (O_2) and carbon dioxide (CO_2) exchange is referred to as *ischemia*. If the ischemia is transient or episodic in nature, there is usually no permanent damage, serving more as a warning. If ischemia persists, it can lead to varying degrees of cardiac muscle and conduction tissue damage. This damage, known as *injury,* may result in changes in both muscle and conduction tissue functioning. When marked ischemia persists over time, or with complete vessel occlusion, the muscle and conduction tissue will become injured and actually die, thus ceasing both electrical and mechanical activity. Muscle and conduction tissue cellular death is termed *myocardial infarction.* Once cardiac cells die, there is an immediate loss of muscle activity (*contraction*) and electrical activity (*conduction*) in the involved tissues.

ISCHEMIA HAS THE FOLLOWING CLASSICAL PRESENTATIONS

- Intermittent or sustained ischemia typically produces chest pain known as *angina pectoris*. Anginal pain may also radiate to the neck, jaw, arms, and back. Some patients will describe feelings of pressure, and may experience nausea, vomiting, and diaphoresis (sweating). Intermittent or *transient* ischemia produces characteristic T wave inversion and ST segment depression patterns on the EKG.

> **IMPORTANT NOTES:**
>
> 1. While most patients will experience anginal pain during ischemia, some will not. Smokers and patients with certain neurological disorders may be unable to sense pain in the chest wall. When coronary blood flow is diminished but unassociated with pain, this is referred to as *silent ischemia*. This is a risky situation because, without pain, the patient is unaware of danger and may not seek help.
>
> 2. Chest pain can be associated with various types of illnesses. One must be able to correctly determine the cause of pain in order to institute the appropriate treatment. To *rule out* ischemia (versus other causative factors of chest pain), one must correlate chest pain with changes in the EKG pattern and the presence of serum markers in the blood.

- Persistent ischemia causes cell injury. In the *injury phase,* cell membranes break down (lysis) causing leakage of the cell contents into the blood stream. This leakage contains proteins and biomarkers which can be measured by specific lab tests. During injury, some degree of dysfunction occurs. Conduction tissue injury may manifest as changes in heart rate, ectopic activity or life-threatening rhythms. Injury to muscle tissue may present as pump failure or congestive heart failure. The EKG demonstrates a classic ST elevation pattern during the injury phase. Ischemia is frequently associated with ventricular dysrhythmias.

- Continuous and prolonged ischemia produces cellular necrosis and death (*acute myocardial infarction*). Large scale myocardial infarction or complete vessel occlusion is evidenced on the EKG as a *pathologic Q wave.*

It is important to recognize that the classifications for myocardial insult are evolving as the intricacies of pathology are better understood. In past years, myocardial infarction was classified as *Q wave* or *non-Q wave* infarction, the Q-wave infarct representing more extensive myocardial muscle involvement or damage. That classification scheme focused more on the outcome of the myocardial event. **Today's classification scheme for myocardial insult is oriented toward *early recognition and intervention* rather than outcome.** The newest classification scheme is as follows and will be discussed in greater detail in Section 12.

ST-Elevation Myocardial Infarction (STEMI)

ST elevation > or equal to 1 mm in 2 or more contiguous leads

- Anterior leads
- Inferior leads
- Lateral leads
- Antero-lateral leads
- Posterior leads

New (or presumably new) LBBB

Non-ST-Elevation MI (NSTEMI): Includes high-risk or unstable angina

ST depression < or equal to 0.5 mm in two or more contiguous leads
Marked symmetrical T wave inversion in multiple precordial leads
ST-T wave changes with chest pain

Indeterminate/Low Risk Unstable Angina: Includes normal or non-diagnostic changes in ST segment or T waves

ST depression < 0.5 mm
T wave inversion or flattening in leads with dominant R waves
Normal EKG

Before advancing further, it is helpful to preview a normal 12 lead EKG and review the leads representing the various surfaces of the heart.

11

The Standard 12 Lead Electrocardiogram

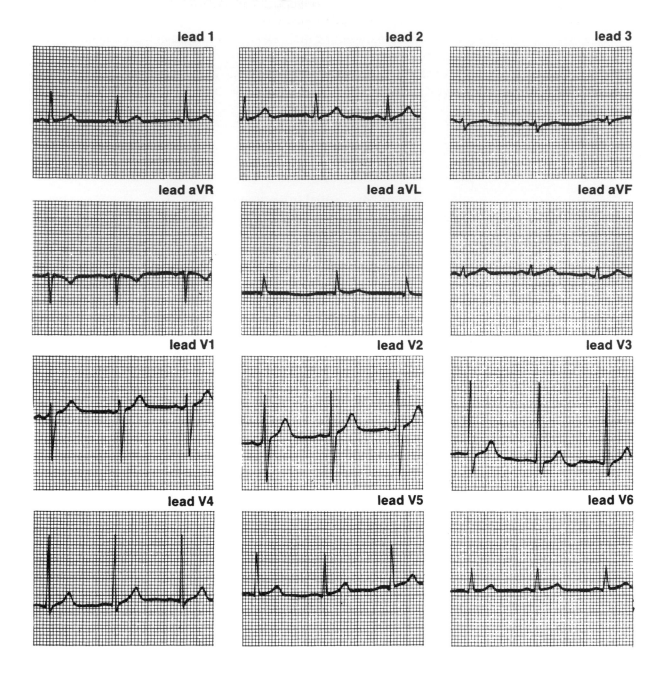

lead 1 lead 2 lead 3

lead aVR lead aVL lead aVF

lead V1 lead V2 lead V3

lead V4 lead V5 lead V6

   The standard 12 lead electrocardiogram allows one to view electrical activity on the surfaces of the heart—or, to look at the electrical activity from various angles or from various points of reference.
   The left ventricle is the most important chamber of the heart in that it functions as *the pump* or as the *driving force* for systemic circulation. Because the left ventricle is such an important structure, the 12 lead system is designed to view the various surfaces of the left ventricle!

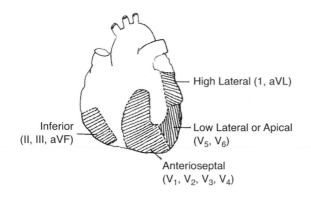

High Lateral (1, aVL)

Inferior
(II, III, aVF)

Low Lateral or Apical
(V₅, V₆)

Anterioseptal
(V₁, V₂, V₃, V₄)

Leads I and aVL look at the lateral surface of the left ventricle (high lateral).

Leads II, III, and aVF look at the inferior or diaphragmatic surface of the left ventricle.

Leads V₁, V₂, V₃, and V₄ look at the anteroseptal surface of the left ventricle.

Leads V₅ and V₆ look at the low lateral surface or apical surface of the left ventricle.

You will recall, there are no leads designated to look directly at the posterior surface of the left ventricle.

Up until now, this "lead business" may have seemed to be of little importance to you . . . but your thinking is about to be transformed!

Serious coronary artery events are typically reflected on the EKG as ischemic changes, patterns of injury, and/or areas of myocardial infarction or cellular death. That of course, is nothing new . . . but depending upon the extent of the cardiac embarrassment and the location of the insult, a patient's hospital course and prognosis can be anticipated. And you know what tells us the location of the insult? . . . **The leads!**

For both treatment and patient management purposes, one must also have an appreciation for myocardial blood supply.

Myocardial Blood Supply

The heart muscle is supplied by two main coronary arteries—the right coronary artery (RCA) and the left coronary artery (LCA). Both the RCA and the LCA arise from the base of the aorta, traveling on the outer surface of the heart muscle. Smaller branches of these major arteries penetrate into the deeper muscle layers, thus nourishing the inner muscle with an adequate blood supply. You will notice that the left coronary artery divides into the left anterior descending artery (LAD) and the left circumflex (Cx) artery. The table on the following page maps the supplying coronary artery branch with the various surfaces of the heart.

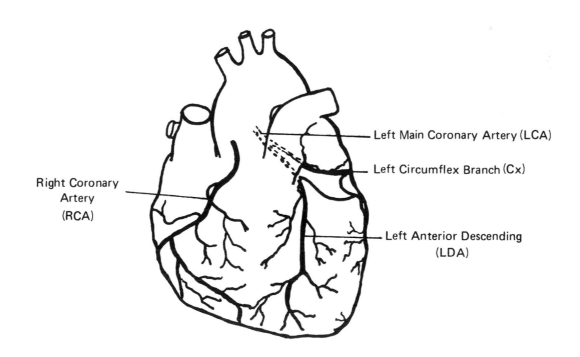

Right Coronary
Artery
(RCA)

Left Main Coronary Artery (LCA)

Left Circumflex Branch (Cx)

Left Anterior Descending
(LDA)

11

ARTERY	TISSUE SUPPLIED
Left Anterior Descending (LAD)	Anterior surface of the left ventricle Anterior surface of the septum The middle portion of the anterior surface of the right ventricle The lower portion of the posterior surface of the right ventricle
Right Coronary Artery (RCA)	The remainder of the right ventricle The upper portion of the posterior wall of the left ventricle (The SA node is supplied by the RCA in approximately 75% of the population, and the AV node is supplied by a branch of the RCA in about 90% of the population.)
Left Circumflex (Cx)	Lateral wall of the left ventricle Lower half of the posterior wall of the left ventricle

NOTE: This table, will be referenced throughout this Section.

By understanding which vessels commonly supply certain portions of the heart and by viewing EKG leads that reflect the electrical activity of the various surfaces, one can assess ischemia, tissue injury, and infarction changes in a noninvasive manner.

input section **11.1 Myocardial Ischemia**

Myocardial ischemia is sometimes referred to as angina or coronary insufficiency. As noted in the introduction to this section, *ischemia* is the change that results in the myocardial cells from a *temporary, insufficient* blood supply. Most usually, ischemia is due to atherosclerosis of the coronary arteries. Atherosclerosis is characterized by narrowing of the lumen (diameter) of the coronary arteries due to atheroma deposits, fibrosis, and calcification in the intima of the artery.

Following are schematics demonstrating first, the lumen of a healthy patent coronary artery and next,

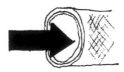

the lumen of a coronary artery compromised by severe atherosclerotic changes.

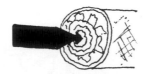

The dark arrows represent blood flow, normal and compromised.

A situational example demonstrating the temporary nature of myocardial ischemia begins with an elderly lady with known atherosclerotic disease.

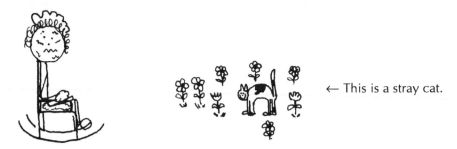

← This is a stray cat.

When rocking peacefully in her chair she experiences no symptoms because at rest, her myocardial cells receive an adequate blood supply. However, when she chases the stray cat from her garden, she experiences severe chest pain. Temporarily, the blood supply through her atherosclerotic coronary vessels is inadequate to meet tissue oxygenation needs. When she sits down to rest again, the pain subsides. This is *ischemia*. Typically, myocardial ischemia is precipitated by exertion and relieved by rest.

The oxygen requirements of the myocardium are approximately three times that of other body tissue. Normally, in a resting state, the myocardium extracts 70–75% of the oxygen from the blood flowing through the coronary arteries. When the oxygen demand increases with exertion, the myocardium cannot significantly increase its oxygen extraction rate. Rather, increased oxygen is realized through increased blood flow or perfusion. The heart rate increases and healthy coronary arteries dilate in response to increased myocardial oxygen demand. Healthy coronary arteries can increase perfusion five times that of normal. In the presence of coronary artery disease, the ability to increase blood perfusion is limited. **IMPORTANT NOTE: A coronary artery can be as much as 90% or greater obstructed before symptoms occur.**

EKG Wave Form Changes Associated with Myocardial Ischemia

Characteristic EKG patterns are commonly associated with ischemia episodes. Typically, myocardial ischemia presents on the EKG as ST segment and T wave changes in *leads looking at the ischemic surface*. Frequently, the T waves are inverted or upside down and tend to have a narrow appearance as demonstrated in the following strips.

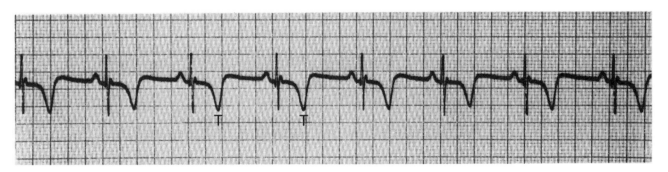

Again, notice the T waves are inverted in this strip.

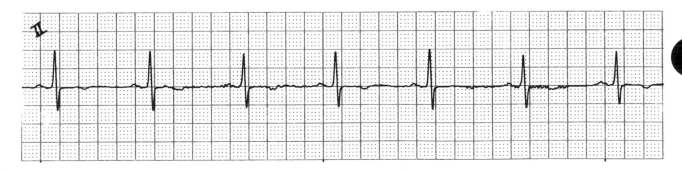

Coronary ischemia may also be reflected on EKG by ST segment changes. Note the following normal S-T segment. Note that the S-T segment is flat and at the same level as the segment that connects the P wave to the QRS. When the segments are flat they are said to be isoelectric. This means they are neither positive (elevated) or negative (depressed). The normal S-T segment is flat or isoelectric.

Normal

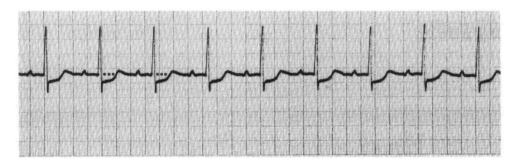

In ischemia, the ST segment will often be depressed.

Note the depression of the ST segment below the isoelectric (. . .) line.

If you think these ST-T wave changes resemble changes associated with certain electrolyte and drug effects, you are correct!! That is precisely why one never diagnoses any condition based solely on EKG findings!

. . . Okay, now back to the elderly lady chasing the stray cat out of her garden!

Following is the 12 lead EKG taken while she was experiencing chest pain. Notice the ST segment and T wave changes. For comparison, please refer to the example 12 lead EKG, page 268.

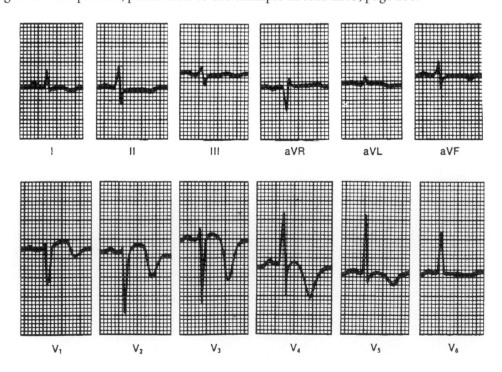

It is safe to say that our "rocking chair friend" has generalized ST-T wave changes throughout the 12 leads. Thus, it is likely that her myocardial blood flow is significantly compromised during exertion.

> **REMEMBER:**
>
> Leads I and aVL look at the high lateral surface of the left ventricle (LV);
>
> Leads II, III, and aVF look at the inferior surface of the LV;
>
> Leads V_1, V_2, V_3, and V_4 look at the anteroseptal surface of the LV;
>
> and
>
> Leads V_5 and V_6 look at the low lateral or apical surface of the LV.

> **IMPORTANT NOTE:** Coronary artery disease is a more dynamic process than once thought. Clots or thrombi may form, and then be broken down via the normal fibrinolysis process. The net effect of these two opposing processes is an unstable or changing clinical situation. Thus, symptoms of coronary artery disease may remain *steady state* or progress. Myocardial ischemia maybe temporary or *transient* in nature (less than 20 minutes) or sustained (*unstable*). When ischemia persists, myocardial injury begins and may result in infarction.

Practice Exercise 1

Are you ready for some practice?
Practice will be kept simple since this material has a tendency to be somewhat difficult!

A. The 12 lead EKG allows one to look at the electrical activity of the heart from various _____

_____

_____

_____

_____

B. The most important chamber of the heart is the left ventricle because _____

_____

_____

_____

_____

11

C. Match the leads with the correct surfaces of the left ventricle.

> Leads I and aVL   High lateral surface of the LV
>
> Leads II, III, and aVF   Low lateral surface of the LV
>
> Leads V_1, V_2, V_3, and V_4 Inferior surface of the LV
>
> Leads V_5 and V_6 Anteroseptal surface of the LV

D. By definition, *ischemia* is the myocardial change that results from _____ blood supply.

E. Myocardial ischemia presents on the EKG as _____ and _____ changes in leads looking at the ischemic surface.

F. Here is a 12 lead EKG. Describe the ST-T wave changes that you see.

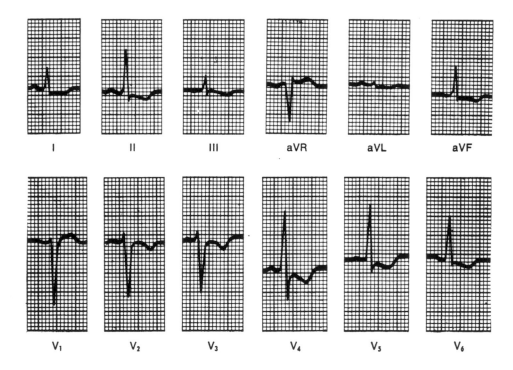

I   II   III   aVR   aVL   aVF

V_1 V_2 V_3 V_4 V_5 V_6

_____

_____

_____

_____

_____

_____

G. Describe the differences between an "ST-elevation myocardial infarction" (STEMI) and a "non-ST elevation myocardial infarction" (NSTEMI).

_____

_____

_____

 For Feedback 1, refer to page 300.

For Feedback 1, refer to page 300.

input section 11.2 Myocardial Injury and Infarction

Before delving into the subject of myocardial infarction, it is helpful to review the muscle layers of the heart.

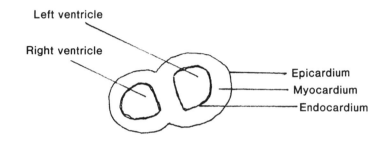

The *endocardium* is continuous with the endothelium that lines the veins and arteries. It lines the chambers of the heart. The *epicardium* is the outer muscle covering. The muscle layer between the endocardium and the epicardium is the *myocardium.*

Myocardial infarction is the term used to describe actual necrosis and death of a portion of heart muscle resulting from an insufficient blood supply. In other words, the heart muscle is deprived of an adequate blood supply over a period of time, thus causing *cellular destruction and death.* In most cases, a fatty arterial wall plaque ruptures, allowing red blood cells and platelets to aggregate, forming a clot which occludes (in part, or total) the lumen of a coronary artery.

A myocardial infarction may be limited to any one of the muscle layers, or may extend through all muscle layers. The extent of muscle damage is related to the duration or stability of the occlusion and the presence or absence of collateral circulation. Collateral circulation means that vessels other than the main coronary arteries begin to increase perfusion to the heart.

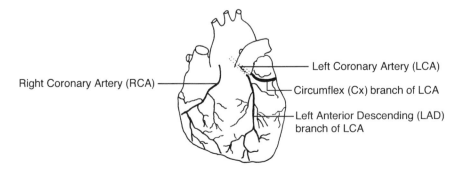

Because the two main coronary arteries, the right coronary artery (RCA) and the left coronary artery (LAD), and the circumflex (Cx) and descending (LAD) branches of the LCA supplying the heart muscle run along the epicardium, the inner muscle layers are more prone to injury in the face of coronary artery disease. The inner muscle layers receive their blood supply from smaller branches of the LCA and RCA that penetrate into the muscle. If these small branches are occluded, muscle destruction is inevitable. In fact, infarction may result from incomplete occlusion of a coronary artery if the blood supply is significantly limited to a portion of the heart muscle!

On the other hand, if coronary artery disease is slow progressing (over many years), sufficient collateral circulation may develop to supply the heart muscle with adequate blood and oxygen despite progressive occlusion of a supplying vessel. In this case, complete occlusion of a coronary artery branch *could* occur without significant muscle destruction. Complicated, right!

Before discussing the EKG findings associated with acute myocardial infarction, one must first memorize the following cautionary rule:

> **CAUTION:** The diagnosis of acute myocardial infarction is NEVER based solely on EKG findings.

The diagnosis of an acute myocardial infarction or acute coronary syndrome is based on:

- **Positive patient history** (chest pain, radiating pain, indigestion, jaw pain, elbow pain, sweating, nausea, vomiting, etc.)
- **Elevated serum markers** (indicating cellular membrane destruction . . . serum markers will be discussed on page 299).
- **Positive or suggestive EKG findings**

It should be noted that the EKG *may* remain normal in acute myocardial infarction . . . or show nonspecific changes that are not diagnostic. *Usually,* however, the following electrocardiographic findings are associated with ST-elevation myocardial infarction (STEMI).

Generally, the *first* electrocardiographic finding associated with acute myocardial infarction (STEMI) is *ST segment elevation* in two or more contiguous leads *overlying the area of injury.* The ST elevation measures 1 mm or greater in amplitude and represents current *injury.* ST elevation simply means that the ST segment rises above the isoelectric line. Usually, ST elevation is observable 30–40 minutes post vessel occlusion.

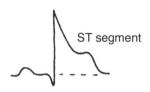

ST segment

ST segment elevation

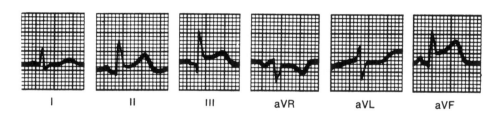

I   II   III   aVR   aVL   aVF

Observe the ST elevation evident in leads II, III and aVF above.

> **NOTE:** An injury pattern (ST elevation) cannot be determined in the presence of left bundle branch block! Look back to page 158. A LBBB pattern is often associated with ST changes that mimic injury pattern.

If monitoring is initiated at the very onset of acute myocardial infarction (STEMI), tall, peaked, "tent-like" T waves may be evident in leads overlying the infarct. It has been suggested that this is a result of intracellular potassium leaking from the damaged muscle cells into the extracellular space. Within several hours post infarct, however, the tall peaked T waves evolve. The ST elevation persists in leads overlying the infarct during the acute phase of the infarct.

What is meant by *leads overlying the infarct*?
Remember this chart?

> Leads I and aVL look at the lateral surface of the LV (high lateral).
>
> Leads II, III, and aVF look at the inferior surface of the LV.
>
> Leads V_1, V_2, V_3, V_4, look at the anteroseptal surface of the LV.
>
> Leads V_5 and V_6 look at the low lateral surface of the LV (apical).

If ST elevation is observed in leads I and aVL, one can assume there is current injury of the high lateral wall of the left ventricle . . . or, if ST elevation is seen in leads II, III, and aVF, one can assume there is injury of the inferior wall of the left ventricle, etc. (One can only *assume* there is injury because other conditions such as pulmonary embolus and pericarditis result in ST elevation!)

That's fairly easy, huh?

So, in STEMI, ST elevation will be observed in the leads overlying the injured myocardial surface. Additionally, *reciprocal ST segment depression* often occurs in the leads oriented toward the *uninjured* myocardial surfaces. Look at the illustration on the previous page. Notice the slight ST segment depression in leads I and aVL.

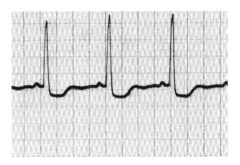

ST segment depression

The EKG *hallmark* of myocardial infarction is the presence of pathologic *Q waves*, observed in leads oriented toward the necrotic area. To qualify as abnormal, Q waves must be wide and deep in appearance, measuring at least **0.04 seconds in width** (one small EKG square) and measuring **deeper than ¼ of the R wave amplitude.**

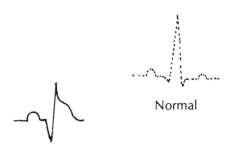

Normal

Pathologic Q Wave

The appearance of pathologic Q waves follows the appearance of the ST-T wave changes in many cases. The appearance of pathologic Q waves is an evolutionary phase of myocardial infarction and is usually evident several hours post occlusion. Additionally, there is a loss of the positive R wave (loss of R wave progression) found in leads oriented toward the necrotic area. Thus, the resulting wave pattern is a QS configuration.

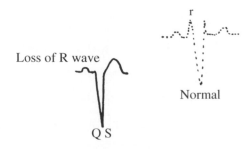

The loss of the R wave follows after the appearance of the ST-T wave changes. The loss of R waves is an evolutionary phase of an extensive acute myocardial infarct process.

Understanding pathologic Q waves or the loss of R waves requires first knowing a bit about normal or healthy ventricular depolarization. Depolarization of the ventricles begins in the left side of the intraventricular septum . . . and spreads to the right, through the septum.

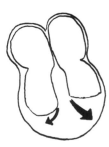

Next, ventricular depolarization spreads outward through the free walls of both the left and right ventricles.

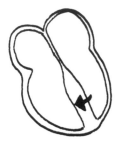

Because the left ventricle has greater muscle mass, the left ventricular depolarization forces are greater than the right ventricular forces. Thus, the net general direction of ventricular depolarization is leftward.

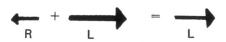

In summary, ventricular depolarization can be thought of as first ①, a left to right activation of the septum, followed by a large net force of activation moving from ② right to left through the free wall of the left ventricle.

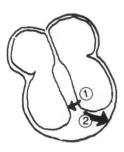

To lend clarity, let's explore the spread of ventricular depolarization, using the precordial leads V_6 and V_1 as examples. Remember, the V leads . . . $V_1, V_2, V_3, V_4, V_5,$ and V_6 . . . are all positive leads. (For a quick refresher on V leads, refer to page 7.)

This is the left ventricle . . .

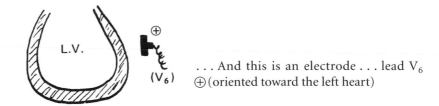

(V₆)

. . . And this is an electrode . . . lead V_6
⊕ (oriented toward the left heart)

The V_6 electrode will first see the left to right depolarization of the septum. Since the depolarization wave is moving away from the positive electrode, the first part of the QRS deflection will be negative.

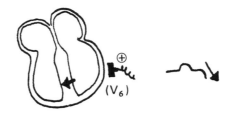

Next, the larger (net) force of depolarization moves from right to left through the free wall of the left ventricle toward the positive electrode. So, a large upward deflection is then seen on EKG. Note the positive R wave in the QRS below.

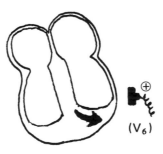

Thus, in a lead oriented toward the left ventricle (like V_6), the entire picture of ventricular depolarization will look like this.

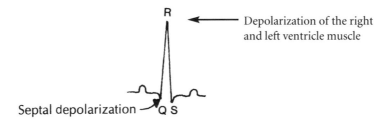

R ← Depolarization of the right and left ventricle muscle

Septal depolarization ⌐ Q S

Next, let's consider the ventricular depolarization process from a lead oriented toward the right ventricle (like V_1). Remember, all V leads are positive leads!

11

The first phase of ventricular depolarization is always septal activation, and you will remember that the interventricular septum is activated from left to right. That means that the initial depolarization force is moving toward the positive electrode.

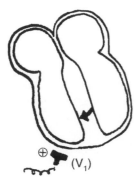

> When the depolarization force moves toward a positive electrode, the EKG deflection will be positive or upright.

Thus, the initial phase of the QRS deflection observed in this lead (V_1) is positive or upward.

Next, the wave (net force) of depolarization moves from right to left through the free wall of the left ventricle, away from the positive electrode.

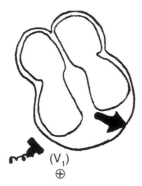

> When the depolarization force moves away from a positive electrode, the EKG deflection will be negative.

The entire picture of ventricular depolarization as seen from a right chest electrode looks like this (lead V_1 or V_2).

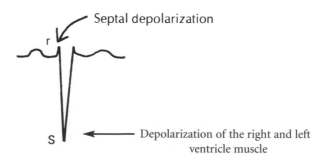

Septal depolarization

Depolarization of the right and left ventricle muscle

Here are leads V_1 through V_6 as recorded from a healthy individual.

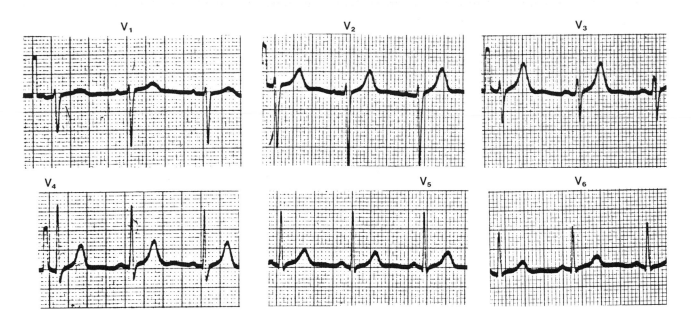

Knowing how the forces of depolarization move normally through the ventricular muscle, it's easy to understand why each of the V leads appear as they do!

In the previous strip notice how the R waves gets progressively larger in each lead until the complexes are upright in leads V_4, V_5, and V_6. This is known as *normal R wave progression*.

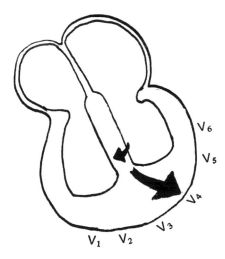

Leads V_1 and V_2 are oriented toward the right heart, while leads V_3 and V_4 are oriented toward the septum. Since the septal force of depolarization moves toward the right, these leads usually record a small initial R wave, a positive wave that progresses in size. Following septal depolarization, the net force (direction) of ventricular depolarization is leftward, moving away from the right V leads. Thus, the positive R wave is followed by a negative wave, a QS pattern.

Leads V_5 and V_6 are oriented toward the left heart. Since the septal force of depolarization moves away from these electrodes, a small negative Q wave is the first EKG deflection observed. The remainder of the QRS complex in these leads is positive, as the major ventricular wave of depolarization is moving toward the left chest electrodes.

Sounds relatively simple . . . right? ☺

11

Pathologic Q waves (in positive leads) and loss of R waves (in negative leads resulting in a QS pattern) represent *electrical death!* In other words, the area of muscle, represented by the leads demonstrating abnormal Q waves or loss of R waves, has lost its ability to transmit electrical impulses.

That is sometimes a difficult idea to grasp . . . so we will use a window analogy to add clarity. Tissue that is dead cannot repolarize or depolarize . . . it is electrically inactive. If all the muscle layers are involved in the infarct (transmural infarct), then electrically speaking, there is a "hole" or a "window" in the muscle.

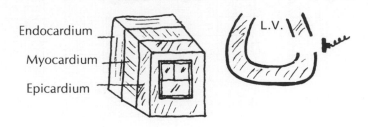

The Window Analogy Graphically Illustrated

Okay . . . this is you.

Suppose you are standing in a room looking at a wall . . . what will you see?

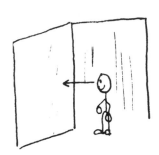

Naturally, you see the wall.

But, if instead of a solid wall, there is a window . . . what will you see?

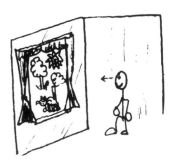

Naturally, you will see through the window, viewing the activity outside or beyond the window.

A similar phenomenon occurs in the case of an electrical "hole," or "window." If an electrode is placed over this window (over the electrically dead muscle tissue), the electrode will see the healthy electrical activity beyond the window!

Here are the precordial (chest leads) of a normal healthy individual. Note the normal progression of R waves, beginning small and progressing until the QRS is upright.

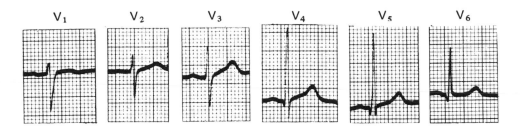

EXAMPLE

When a large scale infarct (STEMI) occurs in the anteroseptal wall of the left ventricle, the necrotic region becomes an "electrical" window. Since leads V_1–V_4 view the anteroseptal region of the left ventricle, they will look through the window at distant heart activity. Compare this example to the one directly above.

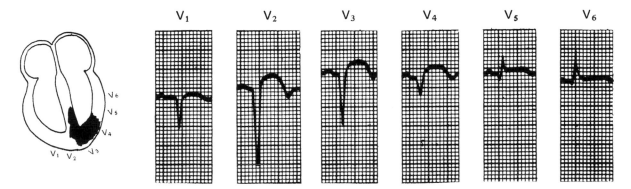

Anteroseptal Wall Infarction: Note the loss of R wave in leads V_1, V_2, V_3, and V_4 and the ST segment elevation in those same leads.

Remember, necrotic tissue has no ability to transmit electrical impulses! One would normally expect septal depolarization (the first phase of ventricular depolarization) to move toward the positive V_1–V_4 electrode producing a positive, upward stroke (R wave). In the presence of an anteroseptal infarct, the V_1–V_4 electrode captures only the second phase of ventricular depolarization, moving away from the electrode. Thus, there is no initial positive upstroke (loss of R wave). Rather, only a large negative wave (QS) is observed. The ST elevation signifies that the injury is current.

To review then, the positive R forces in these leads are completely lost. There are no initial positive R forces. The first deflection is a downward wave , a Q wave. When the deflection is negative (without an R wave), the complex is referred to as a QS—as opposed to a QRS.

11

IMPORTANT NOTE OF ELEVATED SIGNIFICANCE

ST segment changes are very important! Myocardial infarctions are now classified as ST elevation myocardial infarction (STEMI) or non-ST elevation myocardial infraction (NSTEMI). STEMI's are associated with a 1 mm or greater rise in ST amplitude in two or more contiguous leads. NSTEMI's are defined by a 0.5 mm or greater ST depression in two or more contiguous leads and marked symmetrical T wave inversion in multiple precordial leads.

Before progressing further, a brief summary is in order!

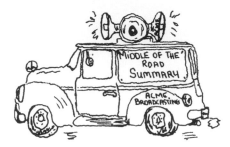

- The right and left coronary arteries and their branches supply the heart muscle with oxygen.
- If the blood supply to a portion of the heart muscle is only temporarily interrupted, EKG changes can be seen in those leads that look at the ischemic area.
- Ischemic changes include inverted or upside down T waves and ST depression, as noted in the strip below.

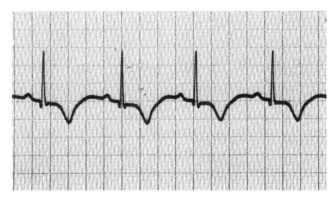

Inverted T waves

- When ischemia persists or when a coronary artery or a branch of an artery becomes occluded, myocardial tissue damage will rapidly ensue.
- Myocardial injury is generally seen on the EKG as ST segment elevation in the leads overlying the injured tissue.

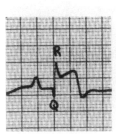

ST elevation in a positive QRS

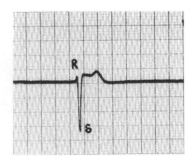

ST elevation in a negative QRS

- As myocardial cells die and the infarct evolves, abnormal (pathologic) Q waves may become evident (depending on the duration of the occlusion and the presence of collateral circulation) in leads overlying the infarct. Pathologic Q waves (measuring at least 0.04 seconds in width and deeper then ¼ of the R wave amplitude) in upright leads represent electrical death!

A Q wave = ¼ or greater adjacent R is a pathologic Q

- When a complete occlusion (Q wave infarct) occurs in areas of the heart reflected in the right precordial leads (V_1, V_2, V_3, and V_4), the initial R wave is lost, so that only a QS configuration is seen, as demonstrated in the drawing below.

Before looking at some actual electrocardiograms, there is another phase of myocardial infarct (STEMI) evolution to consider. As the infarct begins to resolve, the abnormal ST segments gradually return to the baseline. In this stage, the T waves will commonly be inverted, denoting *resolution*.

Evolutionary Phases of Myocardial Infarction

Injury	Cellular Neerosis	Resolution
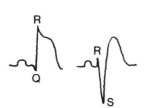	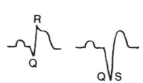	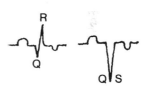
ST segment elevation	The appearance of the pathologic Q wave or the loss of R wave is almost always evident with complete occlusion.	T wave inversion

The only residual (long-term) EKG evidence of myocardial infarction (Q-wave infarct) will be the persistent Q waves or the absence of R waves. *Almost* all patients retain the Q waves or maintain the loss of R waves in the leads representing the affected muscle tissue.

. . . So when a patient comes back to see you—a hundred years from now . . . you can very intelligently ask him or her, "When was it you had your heart attack?" (You will know the infarct occurred because the pathologic Q waves or the absence of R waves will be evident on the EKG!)

On the next page, a **chart** is provided to assist you as you analyze upcoming 12 lead EKGs.

CHART DEPICTING CHANGES TYPICALLY ASSOCIATED WITH INFARCTION
(MUSCLE NECROSIS AND DEATH)

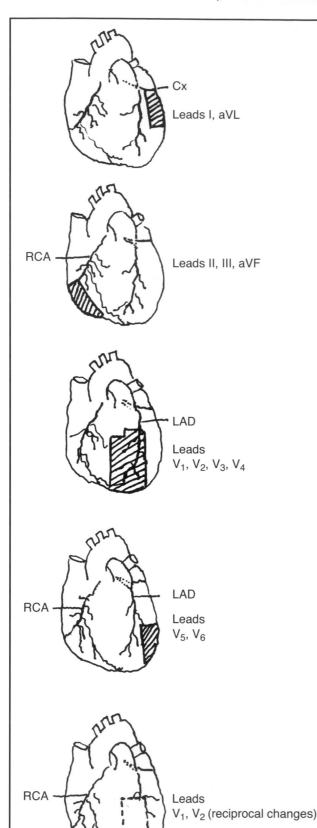

Cx
Leads I, aVL

RCA
Leads II, III, aVF

LAD
Leads V₁, V₂, V₃, V₄

LAD
RCA
Leads V₅, V₆

RCA
Leads V₁, V₂ (reciprocal changes)

Lateral wall infarction (**high lateral**) = pathologic Q waves in leads I and aVL [a lateral wall infarction is caused by an occlusion of the Circumflex Branch (Cx) of the Left Coronary Artery].

Inferior wall infarction = pathologic Q waves in leads II, III, and aVF (an inferior wall infraction is usually caused by occlusion of the Right Coronary Artery).

Anteroseptal wall infarction = loss of positive R waves (QS deflections only) in leads V_1, V_2, V_3, and V_4, (an anteroseptal wall infarction is caused by occlusion of the Anterior Descending branch of the Left Coronary Artery). The anterior wall is viewed by leads V_3 and V_4. The septal wall is viewed by leads V_1 and V_2.

Low lateral (apical) infarct = pathologic Q waves in leads V_5 and V_6 (a low lateral infarct may be caused by occlusion of the Anterior Descending Artery, the Posterior Descending Artery, or the marginal branch of the Right Coronary Artery).

Posterior wall infarction* = large R waves in leads V_1 and V_2, tall and wide symmetrical T waves in leads V_1 and V_2, possibly Q waves in lead V_6 (a posterior infarct is usually caused by an occlusion of the Right Coronary Artery or one of its branches).

* Posterior infarcts will be addressed on page 296.

There is only one more item to remember. *Ignore* lead aVR when looking for infarcts . . . Q waves appearing in this lead are *not* significant. Rather than being oriented to the left ventricular surface, lead aVR is oriented to the cavity of the left ventricle.

If you need to compare the following electrocardiograms to a normal EKG, reference page 268.

Okay! Following is a patient that has been experiencing severe chest pain for 24 hours. He has experienced nausea and vomiting since the onset of chest pain.

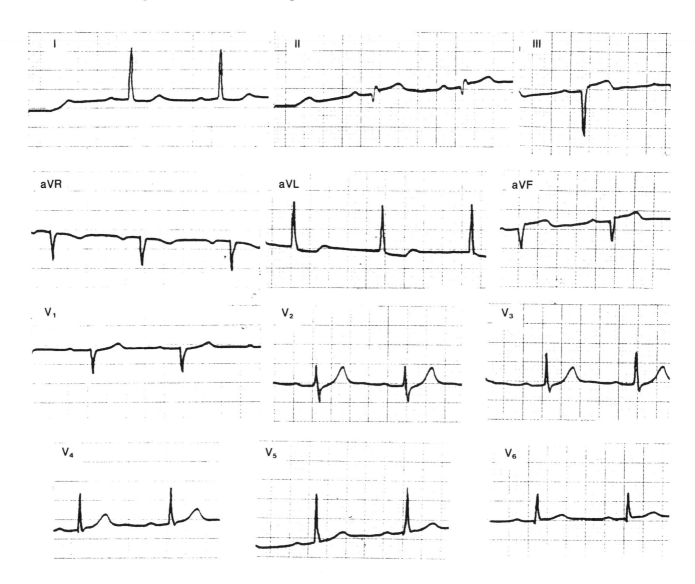

Observe each lead . . . look for evidence of current injury (ST elevation), and look for pathologic Q waves or loss of R waves (indicating cellular death or necrosis).

How about me helping you?

Lead I looks okay to me—there is a normal P, QRS, and T wave. The ST segment is "just a tad" below the isoelectric line.

Except . . . you know what . . . the P-R interval measures 6 small squares or 0.24 seconds! That is grounds for a first degree heart block! (First degree heart block can be reviewed on page 142.)

In *Lead II*, I see several abnormalities . . . there is a prominent Q wave and the ST segment is elevated above the isoelectric line.

Lead III also has a large Q wave and ST elevation. You will remember that *lead aVR* is the lead we are going to *ignore!*

11

Lead aVL shows slight ST segment depression—dipping below the isoelectric line.

Lead aVF also has a large Q wave and slight ST elevation.

All the V leads (V_1–V_6) look fairly normal.

So, in summary, there are pathologic Q waves and ST elevation in leads II, III, and aVF and slight ST depression in leads I and aVL.

What Does All of That Mean?

Well, review the summary chart on page 286. Elevated serum markers (see page 299) and pathologic Q waves in leads II, III, and aVF mean that there is an **Inferior Wall Myocardial Infarction**. The ST elevation implies current tissue injury. The slight ST depression noted in leads I and aVL is simply the reciprocal changes that appear in leads oriented toward the opposite uninjured myocardial surfaces.

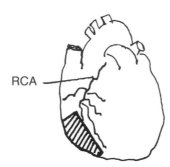

RCA

Anatomically, the inferior wall of the left ventricle borders the diaphragm. Thus, the patient with an inferior wall myocardial infarction may be troubled with persistent hiccoughs as well as nausea, and/or vomiting.

Typically, the Right Coronary Artery supplies the inferior wall of the left ventricle. In most individuals, the Right Coronary Artery feeds both the SA node and the AV node (refer back to page 269). Compromise of the RCA can precipate an array of dysrhythmias. As a matter of fact, that is no doubt why this patient has a first degree heart block! And you know what else—this patient later developed Wenckebach! Remember Wenckebach? If not, review page 145.

What do you think? Is looking for EKG evidence of infarcts tough business?

Let's try another one! The precordial (V) leads appear on the next page.

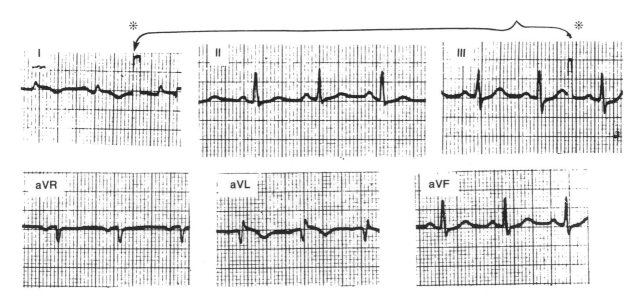

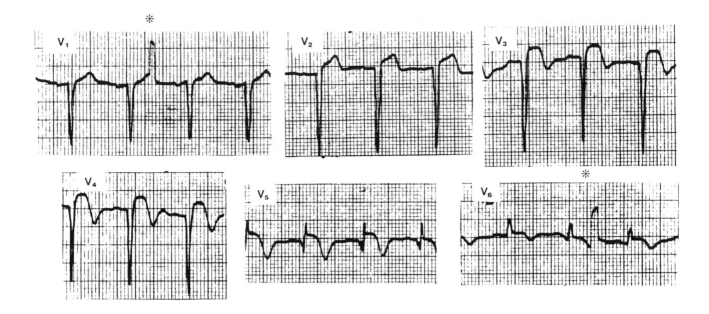

> **NOTE:** These are artifacts produced by the EKG machine, *not* waveforms. To make certain that the EKG machine is properly calibrated, a standardized 1 millivolt pulse (10 vertical boxes) is periodically introduced into the tracing.

Lead I looks rather "squatty" (low voltage) and the T waves are inverted. There is probably an initial Q wave, but it's difficult to tell for certain. There may also be slight ST elevation.

Leads II, III, and *aVF* appear normal, though there is slight ST sagging in leads *III* and *aVF.*

Lead aVL demonstrates very pronounced Q waves and inverted T waves. Further, there is slight ST elevation.

Leads V₁–V₄ show no R waves, only large negative QS deflections. In addition, there is pronounced ST elevation in leads V₂, V₃, and V₄.

Lead V₅ shows abnormal Q waves, ST elevation, and deeply inverted T waves. Also the R waves are greatly diminished in size.

Lead V₆ shows diminished R waves, a slightly elevated ST segment and inverted T waves.

This one is tough! 🤨 Look back to the chart (page 286) if you need assistance! Sometimes, if there are multiple waveform changes, I begin in reverse order. For instance, *leads II, III,* and *aVF* are fairly normal, so I presume that the inferior wall of the left ventricle is uninvolved.

You will remember that *leads I* and *aVL* represent the high lateral wall of the left ventricle. Pathologic Q waves in both of these leads suggest high lateral wall myocardial infarction. Because there is accompanying slight ST elevation, I am assuming there is current injury. The inverted T waves tell me there is ischemia of the lateral wall as well. So, the Q waves in leads I and aVL probably represent a high lateral wall infarction. Does that make sense? Hope so!

Injury and infarction (STEMI) typically presents as follows:

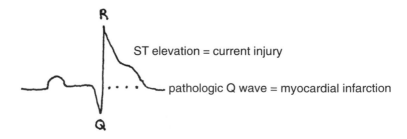

Moving on, leads V_1–V_4 show ST elevation and diminished or nonexistent R waves. Looking back at the chart on page 286, I see that leads V_1–V_4 reflect the electrical activity of the anteroseptal wall of the left ventricle. From the above changes in leads V_1–V_4, the patient's history of crushing chest pain and the elevated serum markers, I can assume the patient also has an anteroseptal infarction. That means there is probably occlusion of the Left Anterior Descending coronary artery (refer back to page 269).

Continuing on with analysis . . .

Lead V_5 demonstrates abnormal Q waves; leads V_5 and V_6 show ST elevation and inverted T waves. So, the Q waves represent necrosis, the ST elevation represents injury, and the inverted T waves represent ischemia. The following day, a prominent Q wave was evident in V_6, as well. Since leads V_5 and V_6 represent the low lateral or apical area of the left ventricle, it would appear that the patient suffered damage of the high and low lateral and anteroseptal walls of the left ventricle!

Ugh! Also, one should bear in mind that the more "lethal" types of dysrhythmias . . . Mobitz II and complete heart block . . . are associated with anterior wall myocardial infarction.

Identifying injury and Q-wave infarct patterns is a matter of looking at each lead *very carefully* to determine subtle or pronounced deviations from normal.

It should be emphasized that many factors distort and complicate EKG patterns, such as dysrhythmias, electrolyte imbalances, drug effects, and so forth. If only a portion of the heart muscle wall is involved, or an occlusion is intermittant, the EKG changes will be subtle. Thus, the diagnosis of myocardial infarction is *never* solely based on the EKG findings!

The patient suspected of having an acute myocardial infarction must be monitored closely and continuously. The cells in the injured area of the heart muscle are **electrically unstable**. You will recall from Section 4, ischemic tissue is thought to release a *substance* which is capable of increasing the automaticity of the Purkinje fibers, resulting in electrical instability. This electrical instability may predispose the patient to *lethal* ventricular dysrhythmias. When ventricular irritability is present, amiodarone is the antiarrhythmic drug therapy of choice.

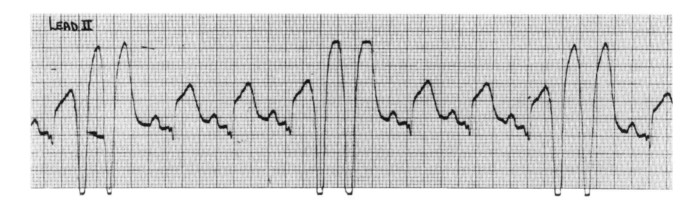

The above patient has a confirmed acute inferior wall myocardial infarction. Notice the extreme ST elevation and the prominent Q waves in lead II. This same pattern was evident in leads III and aVF, as well. P.V.C.s are falling on the downstroke of the vulnerable T waves and are occurring in couplets. This patient is at high risk for ventricular tachycardia or ventricular fibrillation. Amiodarone therapy is the usual treatment of choice.

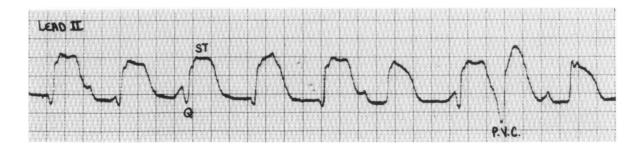

The rhythm strip on the bottom of page 290 was recorded following hospital admission for an acute inferior wall myocardial infarction. Note the extreme ST elevation and the pathologic Q waves. Near the end of the strip, a P.V.C. falls near the vulnerable T wave, warning of increasing ventricular irritability.

It is important to remember that decreased cardiac contractility occurs secondary to myocardial muscle injury. **Observe the acute myocardial infarct patient closely for signs of heart failure and shock-like symptoms.**

The treatment objectives and options for transient ischemia or persistent ischemia leading to acute myocardial infarction will be discussed in Section 12. **Principally, it is the degree of left ventricular muscle mass involvement, and secondarily, the occurrence of lethal dysrhythmias, that determine patient prognosis post infarct.**

At the outset of acute myocardial infarction, anti-platelet or thrombolytic drug therapy ("clot busters") may be used in an attempt to restore the patency of the blocked coronary artery.

Before moving on to the practice exercise, a few points regarding QT intervals are in order. (If you need a refresher on QT intervals, refer back to pages 123 and 252). Studies of QT intervals have reported a direct relationship between the duration of QT intervals and myocardial ischemia and injury. The duration of the QT interval and the QTd measurement appear to be markers of both the extension and severity of myocardial damage.

Ischemia and non-Q wave infarcts have shorter QT and QTd intervals; Q wave infarcts and sustained ischemia typically demonstrate QTd prolongation.

You will recall, the QTd interval (QT dispersion) is a measure of myocardial refractoriness. In this metric, the QT interval is measured on the same beat in all 12 EKG leads. The shortest QT interval measurement is then subtracted from the longest QT interval measurement. The resulting difference represents the degree of variation in refractoriness. (You may also remember, the greater the dispersion, the greater the presumed risk for ventricular tachycardia or ventricular fibrillation associated with proarrhythmic drug effects!)

Now, on to the Practice Range!

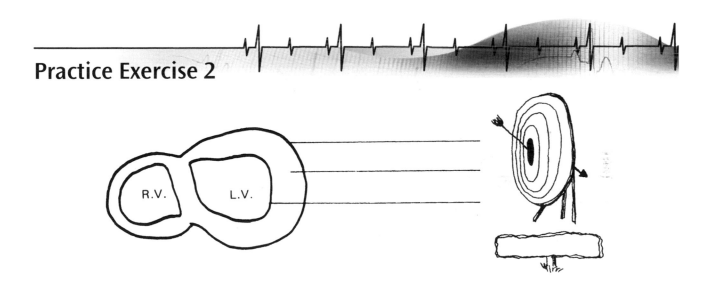

Practice Exercise 2

A. Above is a cross section view of the heart. Label the three muscle layers.

B. The diagnosis of large scale (Q-wave) myocardial infarction is based upon three criteria. List them!

1. _____

2. _____

3. _____

11

C. Draw a complex demonstrating a current injury pattern.

(Circle the correct word.)

D. Reciprocal ST (elevation / depression) will occur in the leads oriented toward the uninjured myocardial surfaces.

E. The hallmark of extensive myocardial infarction or necrosis is the _____ wave in positive leads and the _____ in negatively deflected leads.

F. To be pathologic, the abnormal Q waves must meet two criteria:

   1. The Q waves must measure at least _____ seconds in width or duration.

   2. The Q waves must be _____ the adjacent R wave.

G. Okay . . . here we go!

   This patient was admitted to the hospital with crushing chest pain radiating to his left elbow. Leads I, II, III, and aVL were essentially normal. Here are the precordial leads from his admission EKG. Study them closely, describe what you see, and make an interpretation using the chart on page 286.

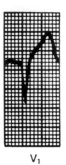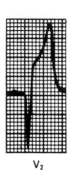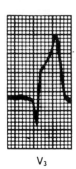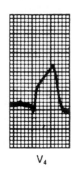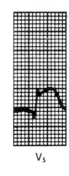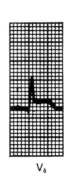

| V_1 | V_2 | V_3 | V_4 | V_5 | V_6 |

_____

_____

_____

_____

_____

_____

_____

_____

_____

H. The following patient presented with indigestion-type pain, nausea, vomiting, and elevated serum markers. Study the leads carefully, describe what you see, and make an interpretation using the chart on page 286.

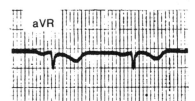
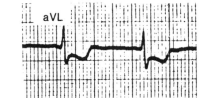
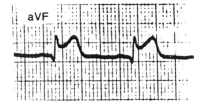
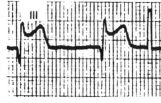
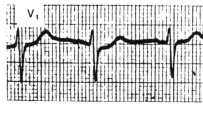
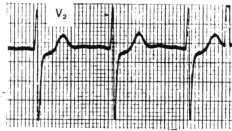
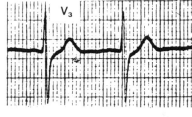
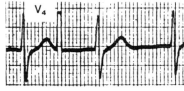
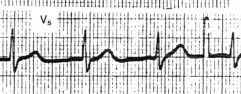
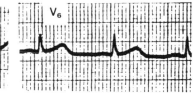

_____

_____

_____

_____

_____

_____

_____

_____

_____

_____

_____

11

I. Below are five examples of various EKG lead patterns. On the following page are five descriptions of EKG patterns. Study the EKG patterns closely! Then, write the number of the example EKG pattern next to the phrase that correctly identifies the strip. (See phrases on page 295).

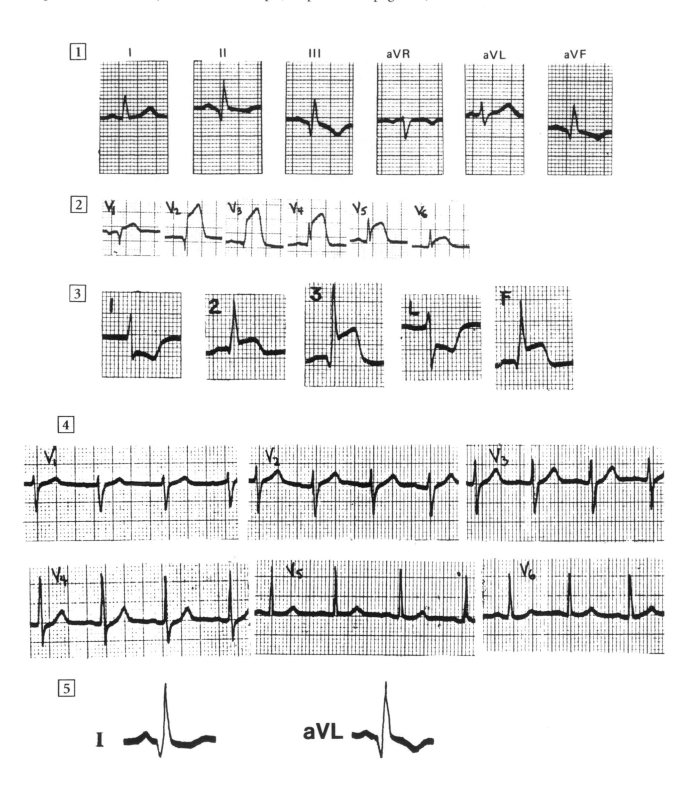

(number)

_____ Prominent Q waves in leads II, III, and aVF. Inverted T waves in leads II, III, and aVF. Probable old inferior wall infarction with ischemia of the inferior wall.

_____ Marked ST depression and T wave inversion in leads I and aVL. Prominent ST elevation in leads II, III, and aVF. Probable acute inferior wall myocardial infarction with reciprocal ST-T wave changes in the lateral leads.

_____ Pathologic Q wave in lead aVL. Inverted T waves in lead aVL. Probable old lateral wall infarction. The inverted T waves denote ischemia.

_____ Leads V_1–V_6 appear within normal limits. No pathology evident.

_____ Leads V_1–V_4 show abnormal QS deflections with marked ST elevation. Probable acute anteroseptal wall infarction with injury extending to the low lateral wall of the left ventricle.

J. Evaluate this rhythm strip. Describe the rhythm and your impressions.

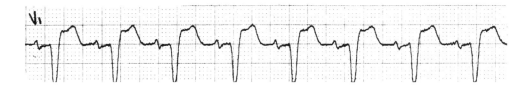

_____

_____

_____

_____

_____

_____

_____

_____

K. This next strip is a "Thinking Only" exercise. If perplexed, refer to Feedback 2.

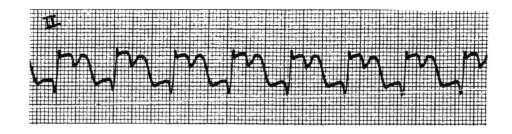

For Feedback 2, refer to page 301.

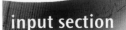

Seemingly, Section 11 has continued forever!

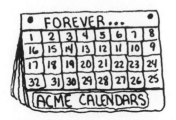

So, this final discussion on **posterior wall myocardial infarction** will be brief!

A posterior infarction is diagnosed by adding additional V leads. V_7, V_8, and V_9 can be used to evaluate the posterior (back) of the heart. V_7 is placed in the posterior fifth intercostal space in the posterior axillary line. V_8 is also in the fifth ICS at the scapular line. V_9 is placed in the fifth ICS on the spinal border. If the practitioner does not choose to use V_7, V_8, and V_9, another method can be used to diagnose a posterior infarct.

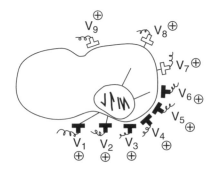

Leads V_1 and V_2 represent the anterior surface of the left ventricle and are *directly opposite* to the posterior left ventricular surface.

Posterior

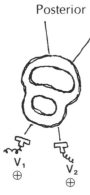

Anterior

In other words, leads V_1 and V_2 lie opposite to the posterior surface of the heart.

So when observing for a posterior wall infarction, one can view leads V_1 and V_2!

Electrocardiographic findings associated with posterior wall infarctions appear in leads V_1 and V_2 and present as *the opposite* of electrocardiographic findings associated with anterior wall infarctions. So, one must remember patterns associated with an anterior wall infarct!

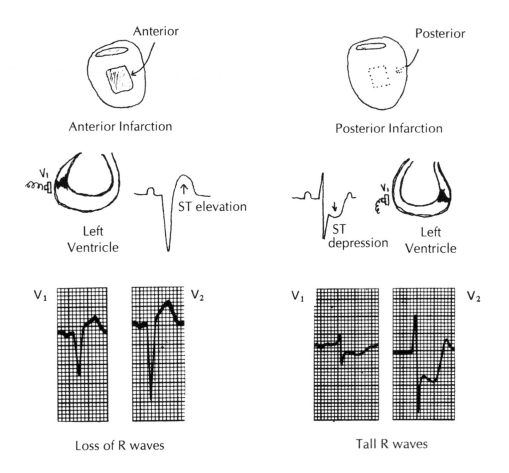

IMPORTANT: With an acute posterior wall myocardial infarction, one will see tall *R waves in leads V_1 and V_2* (instead of loss of R waves), *slight ST depression in leads V_1 and V_2* (rather than ST elevation), and tall, upright, symmetrical T waves.

The other factor to consider is that a posterior wall infarct is usually due to occlusion of the Right Coronary Artery, or one of its branches. It is not uncommon, then, for concurrent injury to occur in both the inferior and posterior walls of the left ventricle.

P.S. Watch out for dysrhythmias!

As you might suspect, the posterior wall infarct patient may present with back pain, and sometimes this pain is mistaken for "renal" or other pathology.

... Beware of the patient that presents with back pain ...
(A warning from the management.)

Since this exercise is **brief,** let's try some practice!

Practice Exercise 3

A. Leads _____ and _____ lie opposite the posterior surface of the left ventricle.

B. When looking at leads V_1 and V_2, the three EKG criteria arousing suspicion of a posterior wall infarction are:

1. _____

2. _____

3. _____

C. The following patient was admitted to the hospital with crushing chest pain radiating into his back. He was diaphoretic and nauseated. Look at each lead closely and describe what you see. Refer back to the chart on page 286 to help you with your interpretation.

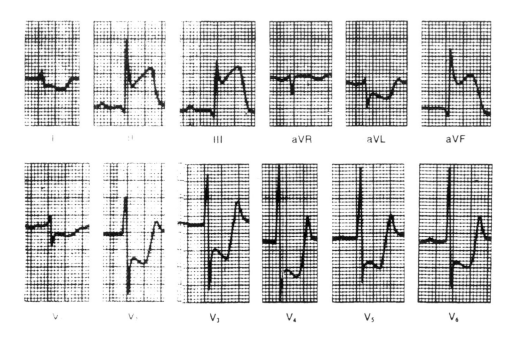

| i | :I | III | aVR | aVL | aVF |

| V | V, | V₃ | V₄ | V₅ | V₆ |

_____

_____

_____

_____

_____

_____

_____

_____

For Feedback 3, refer to page 303.

Important Notes about Serum Markers

As noted earlier in this Section, the *textbook* identification of acute myocardial infarction is based upon (1) a positive patient history; (2) the presence of serum markers; and (3) specific EKG changes. Unfortunately, not all patients resemble textbook cases! Progressive clinical research has demonstrated that a substantial percentage of patients with an acute myocardial infarction may not exhibit ST elevation (injury pattern) or a pathologic Q wave. In those cases, the diagnosis is based on patient presentation and serum marker elevations.

Serum markers are used to detect the presence of proteins released when myocardial cells are injured and dying. When myocardial cells die, the cell membrane reputures and releases myocardial proteins into the bloodstream.

It is worth emphasizing that earlier cardiac enzyme measures (CPK, LDH, SGOT) have been abandoned for serum markers (proteins) that demonstrate more site specificity and time sensitivity. Serum markers CK-MB, myoglobin and cardiac troponin (I and T), represent the current studies utilized to identify acute myocardial infarct. Biochemical researchers continue to search for even more precise markers to expedite the diagnosis and treatment of acute coronary syndromes. Specifically, research is ongoing to determine if future generations of assays for cardiac troponin may detect release of protein that occurs during reversible injury (ischemia without infarction).

CK-MB (Creatine Kinase-Myocardial Band)

CK-MB is dominantly a cardiac specific isoenzyme found in the serum of all acute myocardial infarct patients. (However, small concentrations (1–3%) are also found in skeletal muscles. Thus, severe trauma may cause a rise in CK-MB levels.) CK-MB begins to rise within 3–9 hours post infarct and is present for 48 hours. CK-MB is measured in ng/ml and reported as a % relative index. Levels of less than two percent are considered insignificant; levels of two to four percent are considered borderline; and, levels greater than four percent are considered positive. However, depending upon laboratory methods and instrumentation, percentage limits for both normal and abnormal values may vary slightly. Just for the record, occasionally CK-MB is referenced as CPK-MB.

Myoglobin

Myoglobin is a large molecule protein released secondary to muscle injury. This protein is non-specific to cardiac muscle and therefore, may be elevated with trauma and other muscle injury. Myoglobin normal values are less than 85 ng/ml. When associated with muscle damage, the myoglobin level begins to rise within the first one to two hours post injury and remains elevated during the first 24 hours. Though non-specific to cardiac muscle, myoglobin is considered an *early marker* and raises diagnostic suspicions when associated with classic cardiac physical symptoms.

Cardiac Troponins (T and I)

Cardiac troponins are the most specific markers for the definitive diagnosis of necrosis associated with cardiac muscle injury. The cardiac troponins begin to rise within four to nine hours following an ischemic event. Cardiac troponin I and T remain elevated for 10 to 14 days. Clinical research has demonstrated that elevated cardiac troponin I values associated with *non-Q wave* infarcts are associated with higher mortality rates. The accepted normal troponin I value is ≤ 0.4 ng/ml.

Of the three markers discussed above, myoglobin is considered an *early riser;* while CK-MB and the troponins are *late risers.* For the quick diagnosis of myocardial ischemic disorders, an early and late riser analysis are combined, often through serial blood draws.

The following graphic illustration demonstrates the timing of serum marker elevation.

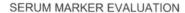

SERUM MARKER EVALUATION

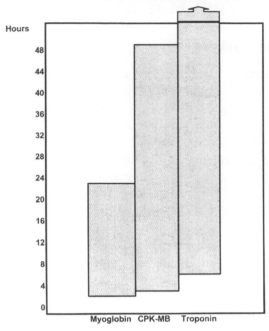

Hours

48
44
40
36
32
28
24
20
16
12
8
4
0

Myoglobin   CPK-MB   Troponin

Based on the previous discussion, it is clear that a single sampling of an isoenzyme or serum marker is inconclusive for the identification of an acute coronary syndrome.

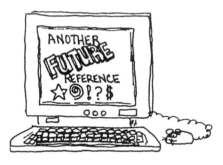

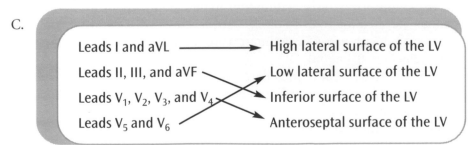

Feedback 1

How did you do? If all your answers are correct, you may advance to the head of the class!

A. The 12 lead EKG allows one to look at the electrical activity of the heart from various <u>angles or from various points of reference</u>.

B. The most important chamber of the heart is the left ventricle because it functions as "The Pump" or the driving force for systemic circulation.

C.

Leads I and aVL ⟶ High lateral surface of the LV

Leads II, III, and aVF ⟶ Low lateral surface of the LV

Leads V₁, V₂, V₃, and V₄ ⟶ Inferior surface of the LV

Leads V₅ and V₆ ⟶ Anteroseptal surface of the LV

For review, reference page 273.

D. By definition, *ischemia* is the myocardial change that results from a <u>temporary, insufficient</u> blood supply.

E. Myocardial ischemia presents on the EKG as <u>ST and T wave</u> changes in the leads looking at the ischemic surfaces.

F. Lead I shows a depressed and flat ST segment and a flattened T wave.

Leads II and III show slight ST depression and inverted T waves.

Lead aVL shows ST segment depression.

Lead aVF shows T wave inversion.

Lead V_1 shows ST elevation.

Leads V_2, V_3, V_4, V_5, and V_6 show ST depression and T wave inversion (generalized ischemic changes).

G. An STEMI presents on the EKG as ST elevation measuring 1 mm or greater in 2 or more contiguous leads. A LBBB pattern may be evident as well. In a NSTEMI, no ST elevation is present. Instead, ST depression measuring 0.5 mm or less is evident in 2 or more contiguous leads. There may also be marked symmetrical T wave inversion in multiple precordial leads.

 Feedback 2

Whew! 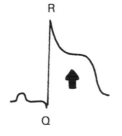 How did you do with this practice section? Sometimes, learning this material is a S-L-O-W process. It may help to read it through several times!

A.

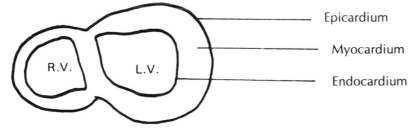

B. The diagnosis of myocardial infarction is based upon three criteria.

1. <u>Positive patient history</u>.

2. <u>Elevated serum markers</u>.

3. <u>Specific EKG changes</u>.

C. The first complex demonstrates a current injury pattern (ST elevation) in an upright complex. The second complex depicts a current injury pattern in a negative complex.

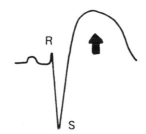

11

D. Reciprocal ST (elevation / (depression)) will occur in leads oriented toward the uninjured myocardial surfaces.

E. The hallmark of extensive myocardial infarction or necrosis is the **pathological Q** wave in positive leads and the **loss of R wave** (QS pattern) in negatively deflected leads.

F. To be pathologic, the abnormal Q waves must meet two criteria:

   1. The Q waves must measure at least <u>0.04</u> seconds in width or duration.

   2. The Q waves must be at least 25% (¼) the size of the adjacent R wave.

G. **Interpretation:**

There are abnormal QS patterns and marked ST elevation in leads V_1–V_4. Leads V_5 and V_6 demonstrate Q waves and ST elevation. These changes represent probable acute anteroseptal wall myocardial infarction, including infarction of the apical surface of the left ventricle.

H. **Interpretation:**

Lead I shows depression of the ST segment.

Leads II, III, and aVF demonstrate pronounced ST elevation and a pathological Q wave in Lead III.

Lead aVL shows ST depression and inverted T waves.

Leads V_1–V_6 appear normal.

This EKG represents probable acute inferior wall myocardial infarction.

I. <u>**1**</u> Prominent Q waves in leads II, III, and aVF. Inverted T waves in leads II, III, and aVF. Probable old inferior wall infarction with ischemia of the inferior wall.

<u>**3**</u> Marked ST depression and T wave inversion in leads I and aVL. Prominent Q waves and ST elevation in leads II, III, and aVF. Probable acute inferior wall myocardial infarction with reciprocal ST-T wave changes in the lateral leads.

<u>**5**</u> Pathologic Q waves in leads I and aVL. Inverted T waves in aVL. Probable old lateral wall infarction. The inverted T waves denote ischemia.

<u>**4**</u> Leads V_1–V_6 appear within normal limits. No pathology evident.

<u>**2**</u> Leads V_1–V_4 show abnormal QS deflections with marked ST elevation. There is marked ST elevation in leads V_5 and V_6. Probable acute anteroseptal wall infarction with injury extending to the low lateral wall of the left ventricle.

J. **Interpretation:**

Hope this rhythm strip did not fool you! This is a sinus rhythm (rate 94) with a left bundle branch block. (If you need a review of LBBB, turn back to page 158.) REMEMBER: IN LBBB, ST SEGMENT CHANGES OCCURS SECONDARY TO THE ABNORMAL ACTIVATION OF THE LEFT VENTRICLE. It is the delayed activation of the LV that causes abnormal ventricular repolarization (recovery). Thus, a current injury pattern cannot be determined in the presence of left bundle branch block!

K. Someone inadvertently labeled (II) this strip upside down! To correct, turn the book upside down and again view the strip. When a rhythm strip makes no sense whatsoever, consider human error!

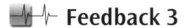 **Feedback 3**

If you answered all three questions correctly, you are entitled to the "official" EKG merit badge.

(Please cut along the dotted lines.)

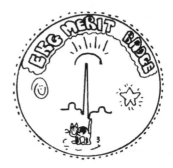

A. Leads V$_1$ and V$_2$ lie opposite the posterior surface of the left ventricle.

B. When looking at leads V$_1$ and V$_2$, the three EKG criteria arousing suspicion of a posterior wall infarction are:

1. Tall R wave

2. Slight ST depression

3. Tall, upright symmetrical T waves

P.S. Remember, the diagnosis of acute myocardial infarction is never solely based on the EKG findings.

C. **Interpretation:**

Leads I and aVL show significant ST depression.

Leads II, III, and aVF show marked ST elevation.

Lead V$_1$ demonstrates a small R wave and ST depression.

Lead V$_2$ shows a tall R wave, ST depression, and a tall, upright T wave.

Leads V$_3$–V$_6$ show a fairly normal progression of R waves and severely depressed ST segments.

The T waves remain upright.

The pathologic Q waves and ST elevation in leads II, III, and aVF suggest an acute inferior wall myocardial infarction. The ST depression noted in leads I and aVL is simply the reciprocal change occurring in leads oriented toward the uninjured myocardial surface.

Though by itself, V$_1$ is only suspicious of a posterior wall myocardial infarction, V$_2$ confirms any doubts. The ST depression noted in V$_3$–V$_6$ is no doubt reciprocal in nature.

. . . So, there appears to be acute injury and necrosis of both the inferior and posterior surfaces of the left ventricle! **Ugh!**

A *Summary of Coronary Artery Compromise* is included on page 304 for future reference!

SUMMARY OF CORONARY ARTERY COMPROMISE

Stages of Compromise	Patient Symptoms	Cellular	Electrical	Mechanical	Wave Forms	Serum Markers
Transient ischemia (< 20 minutes)	Intermittant chest pain; diaphoresis; nausea and vomiting	Intermittant disruption of O_2 and CO_2 exchange	Ectopic activity associated with irritability may be present	No disruption	Inverted T waves; flattened T waves; modest ST depression	No serum marker release
Persistent ischemia (> 20 minutes)	Persistent chest pain; pain may radiate to arms, neck or jaw: diaphoresis: nausea and vomiting	O_2 and CO_2 exchange disrupted; cells rupture, leaking enzymes into the blood stream	Ectopic activity associated with irritability may be present	Disruption related to any significant ectopic activity	ST segment depression pronounced (NON-STEMI)	No serum marker release
Current injury (30–40 minutes)	Persistent chest pain; may be crushing in nature and/or may radiate; diaphoresis; nausea and vomiting	O_2 and CO_2 exchange severely compromised; cells rupture expelling total contents into the blood stream	Ventricular irritability (P.V.C.s) often present	May be compromised depending upon the extent of injury	ST elevation in leads overlying the injury; reciprocal ST segment depression (STEMI)	No serum marker release
Tissue necrosis and death (begins 1–2 hours post occlusion)	Crushing chest pain, pain may radiate; diaphoresis; nausea and vomiting; shock-like symptoms often present (hypotension, altered mental status, pulmonary edema)	O_2 and CO_2 exchange disrupted. Cells necrose and die	Ventricular irritability usually observed; depending on the affected vessel(s), various forms of heart block may be observed.	Compromised secondary to loss of muscle contractility associated with cellular death {ventricular failure}; may be further compromised secondary to dysrhythmias	When associated with extensive damage, pathologic Q waves (or loss or R waves) develop in leads overlying the areas of damage	Early markers begin to rise 1–2 hours post occlusion
4–9 hours post occlusion						Definitive diagnosis based on rise of cardiac specific serum markers

Notes

11

Notes

_____

_____

_____

_____

_____

_____

_____

_____

_____

_____

_____

_____

_____

_____

_____

_____

_____

_____

The Diagnosis and Treatment of Acute Coronary Syndromes

Objectives

When you have completed Section 12, you will be able to describe or identify

1. the general diagnostic approaches for coronary artery disease (CAD)
2. the general treatment options for coronary artery disease
3. differences in treatment options for non-emergent vs. acute coronary syndromes

It is imperative that practitioners be able to assess and diagnose Acute Coronary Syndrome (ACS). When a patient presents the signs and symptoms suggesting ACS, time is of the utmost importance.

This section will focus on the EKG changes that correspond to Non-ST Segment Elevation Myocardial Infarction (NSTEMI) and ST Segment Myocardial Infarction (STEMI).

input section 12.1 Coronary Artery Disease and Progression to Acute Coronary Syndrome

Diet, a sedentary lifestyle and genetics predispose individuals to atherosclerosis. Metabolic syndrome is a precursor to atherosclerosis, coronary artery disease and acute coronary syndrome. Metabolic syndrome includes:

- Dyslipidemia (increased fat in the bloodstream)

- Glucose intolerance (increased blood sugar)

- Increased blood pressure

- Central obesity (carrying more weight in the abdomen, sometimes called having an "apple shape")

Atherosclerosis is the process whereby lipids (fats) are deposited within the walls of arteries. This process results in decreased blood flow to vital organs including the heart, brain and kidneys. For the purposes of this discussion, atherosclerosis will be related to the coronary arteries and the resulting decreased blood flow to the heart.

Coronary artery disease (CAD) begins with early plaque formation in the coronary arteries. Plaques are made up of lipids (fats) that are deposited along the wall of the artery. As this lipid-laden plaque builds up in the vessel wall, blood flow turbulence and inflammatory changes predispose the plaque to rupture. When the plaque ruptures, the fatty contents of the plaque protrude toward the center of the artery. As blood flows past the ruptured plaque, platelets are snagged and begin to stick to one another (agglutination) and clump (aggregation). A thrombus (blood clot) begins to form when clotting factors such as fibrinogen and thrombin are generated. Micro-emboli (small blood clots) can also break off of the original thrombus, sending small clots to occlude the smaller branches of the coronary arteries.

The thrombus may partially occlude, intermittently occlude or completely occlude arteries, blocking blood flow to the heart.

- Partial occlusions can produce symptoms associated with ischemia (decreased blood flow): angina (chest pain), shortness of breath (SOB), diaphoresis (sweating) and fatigue

- Intermittent occlusion may cause the symptoms associated with ischemia and progression to myocardial necrosis (death of heart muscle) producing a NSTEMI.

- Occlusion for a prolonged time usually produces a STEMI.

  See page 310 for a table relating ACS to EKG changes.

input section 12.2 Diagnosis and Treatment of Coronary Artery Disease

It is definitely preferable to diagnose and treat coronary artery disease before symptoms. Most typically, CAD is initially considered as patients seek routine medical advice and as their caregivers identify a high risk profile. Depending upon the presence of suspicious symptoms or high risk factors, diagnosis will occur using minimally invasive versus invasive diagnostic tests. Based upon diagnostic test results, treatment options are chosen.

Minimally Invasive Diagnostic Tests

Minimally invasive means that nothing more invasive than a small needle is used (phlebotomy, injection of a radioisotope). *Invasive* diagnostic tests require percutaneous approaches (through the skin) using large bore needles, threading of catheters, infusion of radiopaque dyes, infusion of drugs, and use of electrical energy (pacemaking, ablation).

The minimally invasive diagnostic tests cluster under three major headings: electrocardiography, medical imaging, and laboratory.

- **Electrocardiography**—You know the importance of obtaining a 12-lead EKG in the diagnosis of ischemia, injury, and infarction (Section 11). And, throughout this study of dysrhythmias, you have seen the value of rhythm strips. However, both the 12 lead EKG and rhythm strips are transient, representing a snapshot in time. The Holter monitor is a device capable of recording a 24 hour rhythm. There are also more sophisticated monitors which can record and store information for up to 30 days. If, while wearing the device, a patient feels he is experiencing a dysrhythmia, most of these have telephonic capability, allowing the patient's rhythm to be transmitted over the phone to a diagnostic center.

- **Medical Imaging**—The echocardiogram is a sonogram of the heart, produced by the soundwaves generated with systole. Echocardiograms allow one to estimate chamber size and cardiac output, evaluate valve function and look for presence of blood clots in the atria (often associated with atrial fibrillation).

  Stress tests are used to diagnose ischemia while the heart responds to exercise ($\uparrow$HR, $\uparrow$contractility). Scanning is accomplished with an imaging camera while radioisotopes are injected into the patient's vein. As the patient exercises, the radioisotope flows through the coronary arteries "lighting up" the well-perfused areas of the heart. Under-perfused areas show up as "cold spots" (ischemic areas). **MRI and Single Photon Emission Computed Tomography (SPECT)** are sophisticated non-invasive scans that allow for imaging of the heart. Again radioisotopes are injected and the patient is scanned to evaluate both the coronary arteries and myocardial perfusion.

- **Laboratory**—Cardiac serum markers are drawn to determine if actual damage is occurring to the myocardium.

Invasive Diagnostic Tests

- **Coronary Angiography** is often referred to as cardiac catheterization or in clinical lingo a "cardiac cath." **A cardiac cath is considered the "gold standard" for evaluating the coronary arteries and is undertaken before surgery or other interventions are considered**. A patient is taken to the catheterization laboratory and placed on an xray table. A surgical cutdown is performed on both an artery and a vein (usually femoral). An arterial catheter is advanced antegrade (against the flow), up through the abdominal aorta, up to the aortic arch and then through the coronary sinus to the coronary arteries. Radiopaque dye is injected to "light up" the coronary arteries. Stenotic (narrowed) areas as well as areas of blockage will show up. A venous catheter is advanced with venous flow through the vena cava up to the superior vena cava into the right atrium and ultimately, the right ventricle. Again, radiopaque dye can be used to evaluate chamber size and blood flow across the valves. Pressures in the right atrium, ventricle and pulmonary artery can also be directly measured (to be discussed in Section 13!) A precise measure can also be made of cardiac output.

- **Chemical Stress Tests**—For patients who are physically unable to tolerate a standard treadmill test, a chemical stress test is done. The patient is given a drug that increases heart rate and contractility (mimicking the effects of exercise) and a scan is done to identify the "cold spots" as discussed above.

- **Electrophysiology studies** (EPS) were briefly discussed in Section 2. These studies, accomplished in specialized catheterization labs, are used to both diagnose and treat patients with various dysrhythmias, particularly tachydysrhythmias. Special catheters are used to identify the areas from which the dysrhythmias originate. Then, treatment options are pursued that best resolve the dysrhythmia. Primarily radiofrequency ablation (RFA), specialized implantable pacemakers and defibrillators, and various drug therapies are used as treatments.

12

Elective Treatment Options

Elective treatment options are medical management, interventional procedures, and surgical procedures.

- **Medical Management Options** include the use of drugs to control or diminish the patient's symptoms. Most patients with CAD require some form of medical treatment. It is noteworthy that there is a large population of patients who are *poor risks* for interventional or surgical options. Therefore, those patients have only a medical management option. **Vasodilators** increase the diameter of the coronary arteries allowing better blood flow to the myocardium. **Anti-Platelet (platelet inhibitors) and Lipid-Lowering Drugs** change the properties of the blood itself. Lipid-lowering drugs decrease the amount of circulating lipids (fat, cholesterol) in the blood stream. Therefore, less lipids can be deposited as fatty plaque (atheromas) in the walls of the coronary arteries. Additionally, when circulating lipids are reduced, the viscosity (thickness) of the blood is decreased, allowing better blood flow through narrowed arteries. Anti-platelet drugs make the blood less likely to form clots in the narrowed coronary arteries.

ACUTE CORONARY SYNDROMES (ACS)

Signs and Symptoms:
Chest pain, fullness, pressure
Radiation of pain to neck, jaw, shoulder
Lightheaded, fainting
Sweating
Nausea, vomiting
Shortness of breath

Pathophysiology:

Lipid plaque is unstable, inflamed, and ruptures, activating the coagulation system. ⟶ **EKG Changes:** May be normal or non-diagnostic

Partial occlusion of artery resulting in ischemia and possibly intermittent occlusion, which can cause a NSTEMI. ⟶ ST depression or T-wave inversion

As thrombus continues to grow larger, small clots may break off (microemboli) and occlude smaller coronary vessels.

When the vessel becomes occluded for an extended time a STEMI may occur. ⟶ ST elevation

---

- **Interventional Options** actually increase the diameter of diseased coronary arteries. This is accomplished through the use of balloons, roto-rooters, or springs!! These percutaneous coronary interventions (PCI) are done in concert with a cardiac catherization and are performed in the cardiac catheterization lab by an interventional cardiologist. **Percutaneous transluminal coronary angioplasty (PTCA)** uses an inflatable *balloon tipped catheter,* threaded across the narrowed area (stenosis) in the coronary artery. The balloon is inflated to compress and fracture the fatty plaque. When the balloon is deflated, the anticipated result is a larger diameter vessel, with less fatty plaque blocking blood flow. **Athrectomy** is accomplished using a catheter with a very small whirling blade or diamond tipped drill. Athrectomy works *roto-rooter style* to pulverize fatty plaque in the coronary artery. The resulting fragments are so small they are of little danger in the circulation. **Stents** are *slinky-like* springs that are loaded onto a catheter that is threaded across the narrowed area in the coronary artery (stenosis). Once the catheter is positioned at the stenosis, a balloon is inflated, expanding the spring. The spring actually holds open the coronary artery by compressing the fatty plaque against the vessel wall.

- **Surgical Options** are used when interventional options are not possible. **Coronary Artery Bypass Grafting (CABG)** uses vein grafts (the patient's own or those of a cadaver) that are sewn into the patient's aorta and distal to (below) the area of stenosis. This creates a "bypass" around the stenotic area, thus creating a source of oxygenated blood. **Valve replacement** is done when either valvular stenosis (narrowing of the opening) or valvular regurgitation (backward flow of blood) is leading to a decrease in cardiac output. Valvular stenosis in either the tricuspid or mitral valves decreases ventricular filling, therefore compromising stroke volume. Pulmonic and aortic stenosis obstructs ejection of blood from the ventricles. When blood flow is obstructed across the valve, the ventricles must work harder to pump out blood. This chronic overwork leads to ventricular hypertrophy (enlargement) and ultimately, to failure. A hypertrophied ventricle requires a greater blood supply. In the patient with CAD, this increased demand cannot be met and ischemia results. Valvular regurgitation in the mitral and tricuspid valves allows for backward flow of blood into the atria during ventricular systole. Since part of the blood does not leave the heart as cardiac output, blood flow to the lungs and/or the body is compromised. Replacement valves are either mechanical or porcine (pig).

input section 12.3 Diagnosis and Treatment of Acute Coronary Syndrome (ACS)

> Diagnosis and Treatment are based upon the following:
> *Time Since Symptoms Started + EKG Evidence*

The algorithm on page 314 summarizes the diagnosis and treatment of acute coronary syndrome.

Acute coronary syndrome (ACS) describes a cluster of signs and symptoms in patients presenting with ischemic chest pain and one of the following diagnoses:

- unstable angina
- ST elevation myocardial infarction (STEMI), or
- Non-ST elevation myocardial infarction (NSTEMI)

These three diagnoses are related, in that all are a part of a progressive continuum of coronary artery disease. An assessment of symptoms, cardiac serum markers, and 12-lead electrocardiograms **over time**, determine where a patient is on this continuum.

12

Ask–Assess–Treat

One of the greatest challenges in caring for the patient with acute coronary syndrome is that one must be able to ask questions, assess, and treat all at the same time! When a patient enters the emergency department with chest pain, you must focus your "asking and assessing" while treating the chest pain as ischemia. This is challenging for the inexperienced practitioner, but after some experience, quite doable. The goal is to classify the type of acute coronary syndrome the patient is experiencing within **10** minutes of arrival!

ASK Targeted Questions: You are most interested in knowing **"when did the symptoms start?"** Every minute of ischemia counts when it comes to saving heart muscle. A patient with chest pain should be triaged quickly and evaluated within ten minutes of arrival. **Twelve hours or less** since symptom development is the cut-off time for use of fibrinolysis (clot-busting) drugs. Since thrombolytic drugs break down blood clots, it is imperative to ask **"have you had a recent stroke?"** Clot-busting drugs are usually contraindicated for patients with a recent stroke history. Additionally, you want to know **"are you taking any blood thinners or herbal medicines?"** Many herbal medications can cause bleeding when combined with traditional medications. Finally, you want to ask, **"do you have a family or personal history of cardiovascular or pulmonary disease, or diabetes?"** since these all relate to coronary artery disease (CAD).

Conduct a Targeted ASSESSMENT: Vital signs may or may not be definitive; however, look for **signs of shock (low blood pressure, cool and clammy skin, scant urinary output)**. Then, of course, listen to breath sounds and carefully assess for **rales** (a sign of cardiogenic shock) and evaluate the **pulse oximetry reading**. The 12-lead EKG must be observed for **waveforms indicating ischemia, injury, or infarct** (discussed in Section 11) as well as for dysrhythmias. Now as you are doing this, make certain that a chest x-ray is taken and that **serum markers**, coagulation and electrolyte studies are being drawn!

INTERVENE AS IF THIS IS ISCHEMIC PAIN: During the history and assessment phase (and while firing off orders for the various tests), start a large bore IV and oxygen at 4L/min with your free hand! Oh, and don't forget to give the patient 160–325 mg of aspirin and possibly a nitroglycerine tab under his tongue. (Are YOU having chest pain yet??)

CLASSIFYING PATIENTS ACCORDING TO 12-LEAD EKG EVIDENCE

ST Elevation MI (STEMI)

- ST elevation > or equal to 1mm in 2 or more contiguous leads
  - * Anterior leads
  - * Inferior leads
  - * Lateral leads
  - * Antero-lateral leads
  - * Posterior leads
- New (or presumably new) LBBB

Non-ST-Elevation MI (NSTEMI) (Includes High-Risk or Unstable Angina)

- ST depression < or equal to 0.5 mm in two or more contiguous leads
- Marked symmetrical T-wave inversion in multiple precordial leads
- ST-T wave changes with chest pain

- ST depression < 0.5 mm
- T wave inversion or flattening in leads with dominant R waves
- Normal EKG

Treatment Plans

Once the patient is classified according to 12-lead EKG evidence, serum marker results have been received and time since symptom onset is established, a treatment plan begins.

- Adjunctive treatments are supportive in nature and have been shown to improve outcomes. In ACS, STEMIs and non-STEMIs receive adjunctive treatments. Additionally, patients without significant EKG changes who are unstable, are new onset of angina, or who are troponin positive will receive these treatments.

- Time since onset of symptoms and resources available also affect the treatment plan. As has been stated, the critical time frame for myocardial tissue is 12 hours. Access to a catheterization laboratory, cardiologists capable of performing percutaneous coronary interventions (and who have done high volumes of such procedures), and ability to do cardiac surgery, if necessary, all impact choices of treatment.

  If fibrinolysis is a treatment option, the goal is to infuse these drugs within thirty minutes of the patient's arrival in the emergency department (door to drug).

  If percutaneous coronary interventions (PCI) are an option, the goal is to have the patient in the catheterization lab and begin intervention within 90 minutes from the time of patient's arrival in the emergency department (door to balloon).

  In summary, early identification of high risk patients is the goal. This is best done non-emergently. However, when patients present, **time is critical**. By following research-based guidelines, care can be standardized and outcomes improved.

Practice Exercise

Critical Thinking Questions

1. When considering the following treatment options, match them to a commonly understood plumbing concept!

   _____ Thrombolysis

   _____ Athrectomy

   A. *Roto-Rooter-like* clearing out of a sewer line

   B. Dissolution of a clog in a drain

   C. Using a plunger to unstop a sink drain

12

THE DIAGNOSIS AND TREATMENT OF ACUTE CORONARY SYNDROME (ACS)

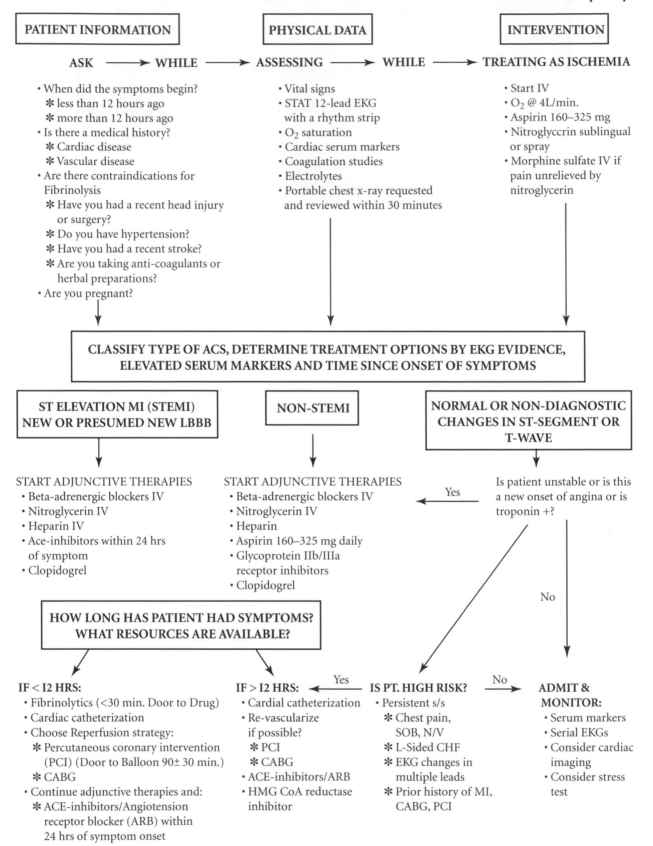

PATIENT INFORMATION	PHYSICAL DATA	INTERVENTION

ASK ⟶ WHILE ⟶ ASSESSING ⟶ WHILE ⟶ TREATING AS ISCHEMIA

- When did the symptoms begin?
  - ✱ less than 12 hours ago
  - ✱ more than 12 hours ago
- Is there a medical history?
  - ✱ Cardiac disease
  - ✱ Vascular disease
- Are there contraindications for Fibrinolysis
  - ✱ Have you had a recent head injury or surgery?
  - ✱ Do you have hypertension?
  - ✱ Have you had a recent stroke?
  - ✱ Are you taking anti-coagulants or herbal preparations?
- Are you pregnant?

- Vital signs
- STAT 12-lead EKG with a rhythm strip
- O_2 saturation
- Cardiac serum markers
- Coagulation studies
- Electrolytes
- Portable chest x-ray requested and reviewed within 30 minutes

- Start IV
- O_2 @ 4L/min.
- Aspirin 160–325 mg
- Nitroglyccrin sublingual or spray
- Morphine sulfate IV if pain unrelieved by nitroglycerin

CLASSIFY TYPE OF ACS, DETERMINE TREATMENT OPTIONS BY EKG EVIDENCE, ELEVATED SERUM MARKERS AND TIME SINCE ONSET OF SYMPTOMS

ST ELEVATION MI (STEMI) NEW OR PRESUMED NEW LBBB	NON-STEMI	NORMAL OR NON-DIAGNOSTIC CHANGES IN ST-SEGMENT OR T-WAVE

START ADJUNCTIVE THERAPIES
- Beta-adrenergic blockers IV
- Nitroglycerin IV
- Heparin IV
- Ace-inhibitors within 24 hrs of symptom
- Clopidogrel

START ADJUNCTIVE THERAPIES
- Beta-adrenergic blockers IV
- Nitroglycerin IV
- Heparin
- Aspirin 160–325 mg daily
- Glycoprotein IIb/IIIa receptor inhibitors
- Clopidogrel

Is patient unstable or is this a new onset of angina or is troponin +?

Yes ⟶

No ⟶

HOW LONG HAS PATIENT HAD SYMPTOMS? WHAT RESOURCES ARE AVAILABLE?

IF < I2 HRS:
- Fibrinolytics (<30 min. Door to Drug)
- Cardiac catheterization
- Choose Reperfusion strategy:
  - ✱ Percutaneous coronary intervention (PCI) (Door to Balloon 90± 30 min.)
  - ✱ CABG
- Continue adjunctive therapies and:
  - ✱ ACE-inhibitors/Angiotension receptor blocker (ARB) within 24 hrs of symptom onset

IF > I2 HRS: ⟵ Yes
- Cardial catheterization
- Re-vascularize if possible?
  - ✱ PCI
  - ✱ CABG
- ACE-inhibitors/ARB
- HMG CoA reductase inhibitor

IS PT. HIGH RISK? ⟶ No
- Persistent s/s
  - ✱ Chest pain, SOB, N/V
  - ✱ L-Sided CHF
  - ✱ EKG changes in multiple leads
  - ✱ Prior history of MI, CABG, PCI

ADMIT & MONITOR:
- Serum markers
- Serial EKGs
- Consider cardiac imaging
- Consider stress test

Based in part on the ischemic chest pain algorithm & the acute coronary syndrome algorithm, ACLS guidelines, American Heart Association, 2003.

2. A stent is a spring or mesh-like device placed in a coronary artery to hold open the narrowed vessel. Given this device is a foreign object, what sort of complications might compromise the stent and/or the patency (flow through) the artery?

_____

_____

_____

_____

3. Which of the following is not a characteristic of metabolic syndrome?

    a. Dyslipidemia

    b. Glucose intolerance

    c. B/P >140/90

    d. Central obesity

    e. Elevated troponin

4. You are asked to speculate on the cost-effectiveness of:

    PCI vs. CABG

    Provide a brief answer with your rationale.

_____

_____

_____

_____

_____

5. Describe the differences between minimally invasive and invasive testing.

_____

_____

_____

_____

_____

12

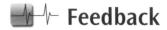 **Feedback**

CRITICAL THINKING QUESTIONS

1. When considering the following treatment options, match them to a commonly understood plumbing concept!

   (B) Thrombolysis

   (A) Athrectomy

   A. *Roto-Rooter-like* clearing out of a sewer line

   B. Dissolution of a clog in a drain

   C. Using a plunger to unstop a sink drain

2. A stent is a spring or mesh-like device placed in a coronary artery to hold open the narrowed vessel. Given this device is a foreign object, what sort of complications might compromise the stent and/or the patency (flow through) the artery?

   <u>Coating and closing off of the stent due to platelet adhesion and aggregation. Closure of the vessel secondary to scar tissue</u>. Vasoconstriction due to SPASM after stent insertion.

3. Troponin is a cardiac marker and does not relate to metabolic syndrome.

4. You were asked to speculate on the cost-effectiveness of:

   PCI vs. CABG

   The average length of hospital stay for a patient who is having a PCI (stent, athrectomy or angioplasty) procedure is 2 days. However, the average length of stay for a patient having a CABG is 5 days. Therefore, PCI procedures are usually more cost-effective.

5. The difference between minimally invasive and invasive testing is that with minimally invasive testing, nothing more than a small needle is used. Invasive testing may require percutaneous approaches, use of large bore needles and threading of catheters, injection of dyes and isotopes, and/or the use of electrical energy.

Notes

12

Notes

_____

_____

_____

_____

_____

_____

_____

_____

_____

_____

_____

_____

_____

_____

_____

_____

_____

_____

_____

_____

The Fundamentals of Hemodynamic Monitoring

Objectives

When you have completed Section 13, you will be able to describe or identify

1. blood flow through the heart identifying chambers, valves, and major vessels
2. normal right atrial, right ventricular, pulmonary artery, and pulmonary capillary wedge pressures
3. typical pressure waveforms associated with right heart chambers and the pulmonary artery
4. relationships among pulmonary artery diastolic pressure, pulmonary capillary wedge pressure, and left ventricular end-diastolic pressure
5. causes for abnormal pressures
6. this section as a future reference!!

13.1 Hemodynamic Monitoring and Cardiac Output

Hemodynamics is defined as the *flow of blood*. Hemodynamic monitoring is the study of blood flow to, and oxygenation status of, the body tissues. Blood flow is accomplished via the heart and vasculature, and oxygenation occurs in the lungs. Specific hemodynamic measures and techniques allow a practitioner to monitor the ability of the heart, lungs and vasculature to deliver oxygen to the body tissues. While the EKG allows the practitioner to assess the electrical functioning of the heart, hemodynamic monitoring allows the assessment of the heart's mechanical action (pumping).

Hemodynamic parameters can be monitored both non-invasively and invasively. **Non-invasive** monitoring does not require puncturing the skin or the insertion of catheters. Topical applications of technology allow for the monitoring of blood pressure, pulse rate, respiration rate and oxygen saturation. **Invasive** hemodynamic monitoring, requiring both the puncture of the skin and insertion of catheters, is reserved for critically ill and unstable patients. Invasive hemodynamic monitoring requires the insertion of a pulmonary artery (PA) catheter, also known as the Swan-Ganz catheter. A PA catheter can be inserted at the bedside. Appropriate patient populations include, but are not limited to, myocardial infarction, congestive heart failure, pulmonary hypertension, and septic shock.

Invasive monitoring provides specific clinical data to guide precise therapeutic intervention. Invasive hemodynamic monitoring allows differentiation between cardiac and pulmonary disease, and provides data regarding the extent of pathology. Hemodynamic monitoring can be done continuously or intermittently. For example, a patient with congestive heart failure (CHF), may have a PAC inserted, pressures obtained, and the catheter removed. The obtained pressures, guide treatment. In other patients, the catheter may be left in for several days.

Blood Flow through the Heart

It is important to remember that the primary functions of the cardiovascular system are to deliver oxygen and nutrients to the cells and to remove wastes.

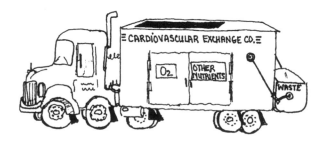

In order to perform this nutrient/waste exchange, the left heart circulates oxygenated blood from the pulmonary vasculature throughout the system to the cells via arteries. The oxygen/waste exchange occurs at the cellular level. Deoxygenated blood and waste is then returned via the veins to the right heart.

As can be seen in the following diagram, deoxygenated blood enters the right atrium (RA) via the inferior and superior vena cava. From the right atrium (RA), the blood crosses the tricuspid valve into the right ventricle (RV). The right ventricle (RV) pumps deoxygenated blood across the pulmonic valve into the pulmonary artery (PA). The blood then flows through the pulmonary vascular beds, a passive activity owing to the absence of contracting vessels and valves. Carbon dioxide (CO_2) is exchanged for oxygen (O_2) as the blood flows through the pulmonary vasculature.

The oxygenated blood then returns to the left atrium (LA) via the pulmonary veins. After passing across the mitral valve, the blood begins to fill the left ventricle (LV). The left ventricle has both the largest and strongest muscle mass of any of the four heart chambers. This muscle mass allows the left ventricle (LV) to generate a pressure of sufficient magnitude to eject the blood past the aortic valve into the aorta, and out to the vascular beds (systemic circulation).

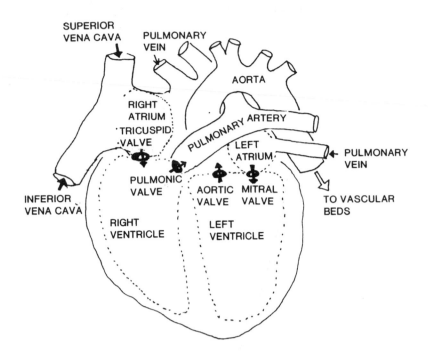

The blood flow cycle can be broken down into two major phases: (1) *systole,* or the contraction/ejection phase; and (2) *diastole,* the relaxation/filling phase. During each phase, the pressure and blood volume in each chamber differs. It is this pressure difference that permits the cardiac valves to open and close appropriately. The valves (tricuspid, pulmonic, mitral, and aortic) perform gatekeeper functions, keeping the blood flowing in a forward direction (antegrade) and preventing backward flow (retrograde).

Filling of the chambers occurs during diastole. As blood flows into the right and left atria, atrial chamber pressures increase. These increasing pressures force the tricuspid and mitral valves open, allowing the right and left ventricles to fill. The increased pressure in the atrial chambers and electrical activation (depolarization) stimulates the atria to contract. The P wave seen on the EKG monitor corresponds with ventricular diastole or filling. You will remember that the P wave represents atrial depolarization.

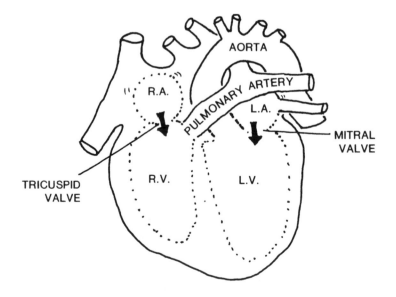

Ventricular filling. Increasing atrial pressures force open the Tricuspid and Mitral valves.

Ejection of blood occurs during systole. Ventricular systole occurs when the pressure and volume in the right and left ventricles exceed atrial pressures. The rising ventricular pressures force the mitral and tricuspid valves closed. The aortic and pulmonic valves are then forced open, allowing blood to flow out of the ventricles. Blood is ejected from the right ventricle into the pulmonary artery where it is taken to the right and left lungs for oxygenation.

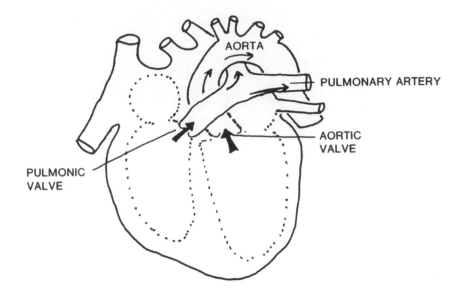

Blood returns to the left atrium via the pulmonary veins. This oxygenated blood will be ejected against the high resistance in the arterial system. The more muscular wall of the left ventricle contracts (systole) with great force, opening the aortic valve and allowing flow to the system.

Ventricular muscle contraction immediately follows electrical activation (depolarization) of the ventricles. Electrical depolarization produces the QRS seen on the EKG monitor!

This systole and diastole business is sometimes confusing! It may be helpful to remember . . .

Diastole = relaxation and filling
Systole = contraction and ejection

The diagram on the next page depicts the relationships between the EKG waveforms, diastole and systole, pressure changes and valve openings and closures.

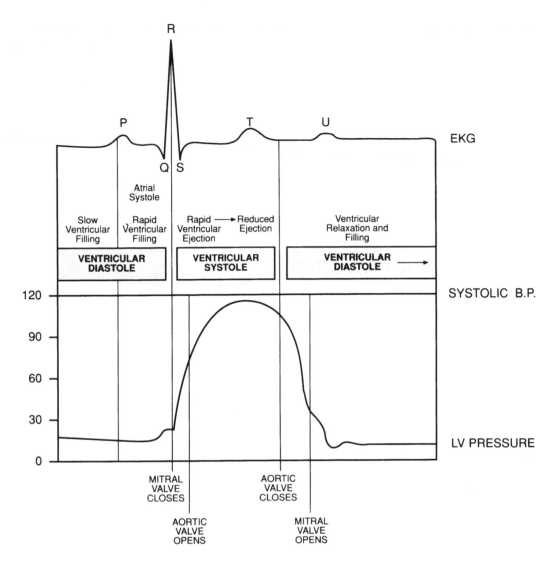

Cardiac cycle demonstrating EKG relationship to ventricular diastole, systole and valve function.

The Effects of Pressure, Vessel Characteristics, Viscosity, Resistance and Volume

Hemodynamies, or blood flow, is affected by pressure, vessel characteristics, viscosity, resistance, and volume.

PRESSURE

· Blood tends to flow from areas of **high pressure to low pressure (pressure gradient)**. The greater the pressure difference between flow into and out of a blood vessel, the greater the pressure gradient. If there is *no* pressure difference, then there is no flow. For instance, the pressure in the left ventricle must be higher than the pressure in the aorta, for blood to be ejected during systole.

VESSEL CHARACTERISTICS

· The longer the **length of a vessel**, the lesser the flow. A practical example of this can be observed in the backyard. If a gardener desires to water flowers far out by the back fence, he may need to attach multiple water hoses. The more water hose extensions he attaches, creating a longer hose, the less water flow will occur at hose end! Likewise in the body, the further the distance blood must travel, the lesser the flow at the end point.

- The larger the **diameter of a vessel**, the greater the flow (*vasodilation*). The smaller the diameter the vessel, the lesser the flow (*vasoconstriction*). When a person is under stress, the stress hormone norepinephrine causes vasoconstriction. As a result, flow is compromised to the periphery of the body. When under stress, the feet and hands often become cold. This is a sign of reduced blood flow, due to reduced diameter (vasoconstriction) of the blood vessels in the feet and hands. The disease process of atherosclerosis also affects the diameter of arterial vessels. As fatty deposits called atheromas build up within the vessel wall, flow is diminished.

- The greater the **viscosity of blood**, the lesser the flow. Viscosity is the thickness of blood. In states of dehydration or increased cell counts, blood becomes thicker. Thicker blood flows less well than thinner blood. Simply speaking, iced tea pours (flows) more rapidly into a glass than does a milkshake.

- **Resistance** is that factor that impedes blood flow. When blood vessels are constricted, resistance is increased. When vessels are dilated, resistance is decreased.

- **Volume** is related to pressure. When volume is increased within a vessel, pressure is increased. When pressure within vessels increases, the diameter of the vessel also increases. In response to the increased diameter, resistance decreases. This ability to respond to changes in pressure is called *distensibility*. Veins are much more distensible than arteries. A very personal example of distensibility *may* be found in your closet. There are two vintage pairs of favorite jeans:

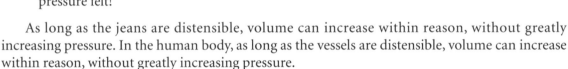

  ✳ One pair of jeans has a fixed waist band and button closure, thus limiting distensibility. Despite some acquired distensibility from hundreds of washings, a few extra pounds (increased volume) may create extreme pressure when buttoning those jeans!

  ✳ The second pair of jeans has an elastic waist band and possibly a Velcro closure! The elastic in the waist band allows greater distensibility following a big meal, thus reducing the pressure felt!

As long as the jeans are distensible, volume can increase within reason, without greatly increasing pressure. In the human body, as long as the vessels are distensible, volume can increase within reason, without greatly increasing pressure.

Understanding Cardiac Output

Cardiac output is affected by all the previously discussed concepts: pressure, vessel characteristics, viscosity, resistance, and volume. **Cardiac output (CO) is defined as the amount of blood ejected from the left ventricle in one minute**. The normal cardiac output is **4–8 L/minute**. This normal however, is a gross measure. To determine if a cardiac output is adequate for an individual, the cardiac output should be indexed to the individual's height and weight. This is calculated by dividing the cardiac output by the body surface area (derived from a height and weight nomogram.)

The equation for calculating CO is **heart rate times stroke volume**. From a practical standpoint, stroke volume cannot be calculated at the bedside. Therefore more practical measures of cardiac output are needed.

THE FOUR COMPONENTS OF CARDIAC OUTPUT

There are four components of cardiac output: preload, contractility, heart rate and afterload.

Preload

Maximum muscle contractility is achieved when the myocardial muscle fiber is stretched from 2.0–2.2 microns. The sarcomeres (bundles of muscle fibers) of the ventricles are stretched with blood volume received from the atria. The optimal stretch of a sarcomere requires a normal to slightly higher blood volume. This volume is called **preload**.

Preload is the blood volume from the veins that returns to the right side of the heart. Theoretically, whatever returns to the right side of the heart also returns to the left side. Since the left heart is the major pump of the heart, we are most interested in the left ventricular volume at the end of diastole. This volume generates a pressure known as the left *ventricular end diastolic pressure,* or (**LVEDP**). LVEDP or preload is measured as a *pulmonary capillary wedge pressure* (**PCWP**).

13

$$PRELOAD \ = \ PCWP \ = \ LVEDP$$

When blood volume is increased, preload is increased. When blood volume is decreased, preload is decreased. One must have a normal or slightly higher volume to achieve a maximum cardiac output. In a volume overload situation (preload), the sarcomeres are overstretched and produce a lesser cardiac output.

The relationship between optimal volume (preload) and optimal sarcomere stretch is explained as Starling's Law.

Starling's Law (Scientifically Speaking)

The force of contraction is proportional to the muscle fiber length up to a critical length. When the critical length is exceeded, myocardial contractile force decreases.

Starling's Law (Simply Speaking)

When the normal, or slightly above normal amount of blood volume flows from the atria into ventricles, the ventricular muscle fibers are stretched to an optimal length. Optimal stretch leads to a strong contraction that moves blood forward to the lungs and body leaving very little blood left in the ventricles.

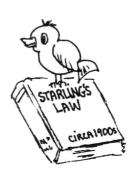

Starling's Law is often compared to a rubber band stretching. The rubber band length can be compared to myocardial fiber length. If the rubber band (muscle fiber) is stretched (diastole) a SHORT distance, contraction (systole) is *weak.* If, however, the rubber band is **fully** stretched (diastole) to its optional length, contraction (systole) is *forceful* and *efficient!* If a rubber band is repeatedly **overstretched** (diastole), it becomes *weakened* and its contractile force (systole) is *diminished.* And so goes the Starling Theory of rubber bands!

Contractility

As discussed above, contractility and preload are intimately related. In addition to the effect of preload, contractility is affected by the integrity of muscle fibers, sympathetic nervous system effects, and calcium.

Myofibrils are the muscle fibers in the heart which allow for contractility. Made up of actin (thin) and myosin (thick) filaments, these filaments interweave to form bands. When these filaments interact, contraction occurs. The adequate pumping of blood requires intact, functional myofibrils. Conditions that impair integrity of the myofibrils include ischemia, injury, infarction, and inflammation. Sarcomeres are groups of myofibrils. They encompass fluid and mitochondria which supply energy to the heart.

The sympathetic nervous system (SNS) affects the heart via beta adrenergic affects. *Beta-1* effects are increased heart rate (*chronotropy*), increased speed of impulse conduction (*dromotropy*) and increased strength of contractility (*inotropy*).

Calcium interacts with "active" sites on the actin filament leading to contraction. Influx of calcium into the cardiac cell also affects the *cardiac action potential* (impulse formation).

CALCIUM = CONTRACTILITY

Heart Rate

Heart rate is also an important dimension of cardiac output.

Within a given target range, as heart rate increases, so does cardiac output. It often becomes necessary to control heart rate in order to maximize cardiac output.

Afterload

Finally to further optimize cardiac output, the vasculature must be able to accept blood ejected from the left ventricle. With vascular vasoconstriction, there is greater resistance; with vascular vasodilation, there is lesser resistance. This resistance is called *afterload*. There are specific mathematical equations for calculating afterload. Afterload for the right ventricle is referred to as *pulmonary vascular resistance* (PVR). Afterload for the left ventricle is referred to as *systemic vascular resistance* (SVR). Afterload is measured in resistance units known as dynes/second. Changes in afterload affects cardiac output. When afterload is high, cardiac output falls. When afterload is low, cardiac output is high.

AFTERLOAD for the Left Heart = SVR

Systemic Vascular Resistance (SVR) = Resistance the left ventricle must overcome to eject blood into the systemic circulation. It is calculated:

$$SVR = \frac{\text{Mean Arterial Pressure} - \text{Right Artrial Pressure}}{\text{Cardiac Output}} \times 80$$

(Normal SVR = 900–1400 dynes/sec)

AFTERLOAD for the Right Heart = PVR

Pulmonary Vascular Resistance (PVR) = Resistance the right ventricle must overcome to eject blood into the pulmonary vascular beds. It is calculated:

$$PVR = \frac{(\textit{Mean Pulmonary Artery Pressure - PCWP})}{\text{Cardiac Output}} \times 80$$

(Normal PVR = 150–250 dynes/sec)

In summary, the four components of cardiac output are contractility, preload, heart rate and afterload.

How Does A Pulmonary Artery Catheter Work?

The development of the pulmonary artery (PA) catheter, also known as the Swan-Ganz catheter, permitted indirect invasive measurement of cardiac output. Though the pulmonary artery catheter is placed in the right side of the heart, this right-sided catheter allows the practitioner to monitor the left-sided pressures of the heart.

The PA catheter is usually inserted via the subclavian vein through the superior vena cava, into the right atrium. A small balloon on the tip of the PA catheter is inflated to assist the catheter flow across the tricuspid valve into the right ventricle (RV). From the RV, it floats across the pulmonic valve out into the pulmonary artery (PA). It then wedges into one of the small diameter pulmonary capillaries.

There are no valves in the pulmonary vessels. When the mitral valve is open during diastole, left ventricular pressure can be measured. If one thinks of the cardiac circulatory system being laid "end to end," it is easier to understand how a right heart catheter can measure pressures in the left ventricle. (It is much like being able to view the back room from the front room of a *shotgun house,* if all the interior room doors are open!)

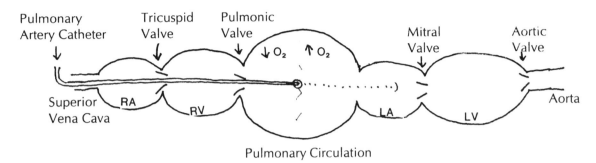

How a right-sided catheter is used to measure left-sided pressures

Practice Exercise 1

A. Invasive hemodynamic monitoring is accomplished via a _____ catheter.

B. The size (mass) and strength of the left ventricle allows oxygenated blood to be ejected past the

_____ valve into the _____, and out to systemic circulation.

C. Correctly label the four cardiac valves

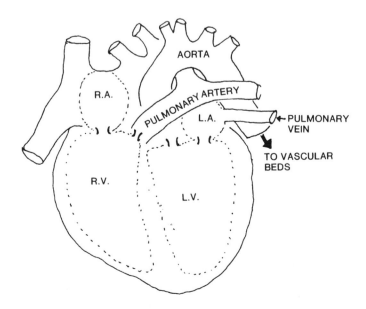

D. The contraction/ejection phase of the blood flow cycle is termed _____ ;

the relaxation/filling phase of the blood flow cycle is known as _____ .

E. If a muscle fiber is stretched (diastole) a short distance, contraction (systole) is _____ .

If a muscle fiber is fully stretched to its optimal length, contraction is _____ . If

a muscle fiber is repeatedly overstretched, contractile force is _____ .

F. Starling was a

☐ bird

☐ plane

☐ law man

(sense of humor poll conducted by the management ☺)

G. List the four components of cardiac output:

1. _____

2. _____

3. _____

4. _____

For Feedback 1, refer to page 344.

input section **13.2 The Pulmonary Artery Catheter (Swan-Ganz)**

The pulmonary artery catheter (PA) is a hollow latex tube with three internal lumen (channels). In addition, a thermistor runs through the length of the catheter. A thermistor measures blood temperature. If one were to cut the catheter in half, it would look like the following diagram.

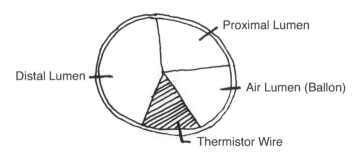

Cross Section: Pulmonary Artery Catheter

Proximal Lumen—This lumen opens into the right atrium. Right atrial pressure (**RAP**) is measured via this lumen. RAP is also called the central venous pressure (**CVP**). This lumen can be used for fluid administration as well as for monitoring pressure.

Distal Lumen—This lumen runs the entire length of the catheter and opens into the pulmonary artery.

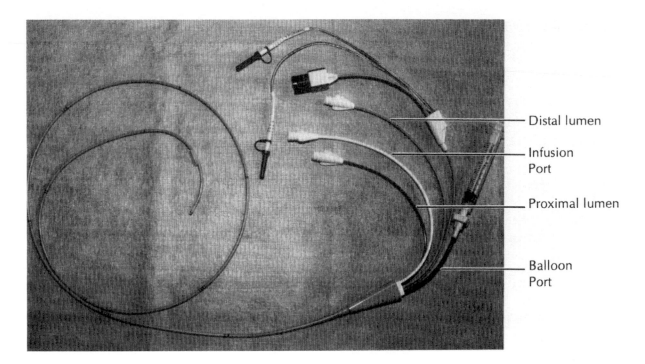

- Distal lumen
- Infusion Port
- Proximal lumen
- Balloon Port

Infusion Port—Some PA catheters have an extra lumen used for fluid and medication infusion.

Thermistor—This lumen is used to measure the patient's core temperature and to measure cardiac output (when connected to a cardiac output computer).

Balloon Port—This port allows inflation of a small balloon located near the end of the catheter. The balloon is inflated during catheter insertion and for obtaining the pulmonary capillary wedge pressure.

Cardiac Output (CO) can be measured in a number of ways. The PA catheter measures cardiac output using the thermodilution method. A known volume of fluid (10cc) at a known temperature (room temperature) is injected into the right heart via the proximal lumen of the pulmonary artery catheter. As the fluid mixes with the blood and passes by the thermistor, an attached external computer calculates the cardiac output. **Normal cardiac output ranges between 4–8 liters/minute**.

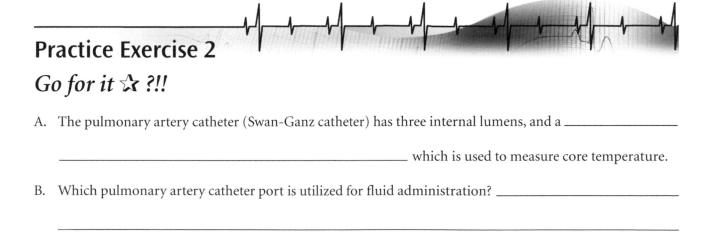

Practice Exercise 2

Go for it ☆ *?!!*

A. The pulmonary artery catheter (Swan-Ganz catheter) has three internal lumens, and a _____

_____ which is used to measure core temperature.

B. Which pulmonary artery catheter port is utilized for fluid administration? _____

_____

C. _____ atrial pressure is monitored at the proximal lumen opening.

D. An inflated pulmonary artery catheter balloon causes the catheter to _____ into a small pulmonary vessel.

E. Normal cardiac output (CO) ranges between _____ and _____ liters per minute.

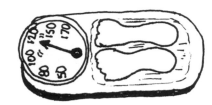 **For Feedback 2, refer to page 345.**

input section 13.3 Pressures and Waveforms

Hemodynamic monitoring requires an understanding of normal pressures and waveforms originating from the cardiac structures. Beyond the placement of a pulmonary artery catheter (PAC), hemodynamic monitoring requires both a bedside monitor and, transducer to measure pressures and display waveforms.

A *transducer* system is utilized to convert the mechanical pumping action into an electrical waveform displayed on a monitor. A transducer is much like a bathroom scale! When weight or pressure is applied to a bathroom scale, the gauge on the scale moves.

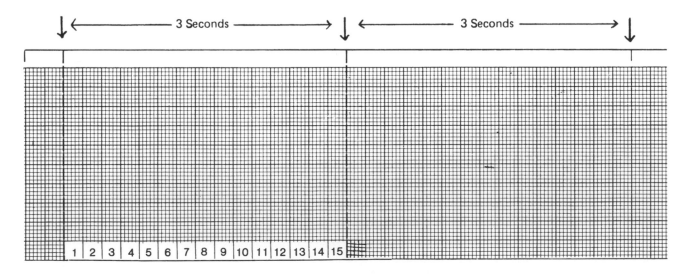

When pressure is applied to a transducer, the resulting waveform rises on the monitor and then falls as pressure is removed. Easy so far, right? As you progress through this section, you will learn that each cardiac chamber presents unique pressures and waveform characteristics!

You will recall from Section I, page 24, that monitor paper has both a time and amplitude dimension. Moving horizontally monitor paper measures **TIME**.

Moving *vertically* measures **AMPLITUDE**. Each small square horizontally represents 1mm amplitude, and each large square represents 5mm amplitude. As we move forward in the section, waveforms and the pressure they represent will be measured in amplitude dimension. Waveforms with great pressure differences are read as sytole over diastole. Lower pressure waveforms are read as mean or average measures.

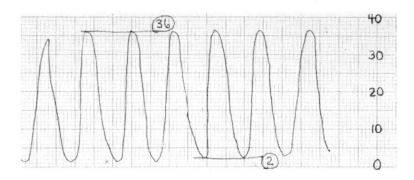

Right Atrium

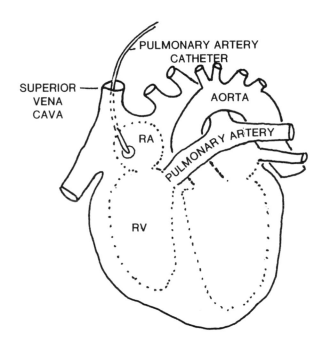

The pulmonary artery catheter is situated in the right atrium.

The above diagram demonstrates the placement of pulmonary artery catheter in the right atrium. You will recall that blood enters the right atrium (RA) passively. Intrathoracic pressure changes occurring secondary to respiration assist blood return to the right heart. Owing to its small muscle mass, the normal right atrial pressure is low. The low pressure produces a low amplitude, oscillating waveform demonstrated in the following diagrams. Because there is only a minimal difference between right atrial systolic and diastolic pressures, a mean or averaged RA pressure is utilized.

Right Atrial (RA) Pressure Waveform

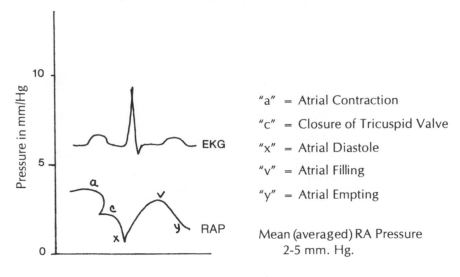

"a" = Atrial Contraction

"c" = Closure of Tricuspid Valve

"x" = Atrial Diastole

"v" = Atrial Filling

"y" = Atrial Empting

Mean (averaged) RA Pressure
2-5 mm. Hg.

Right Atrial (RA) Pressure

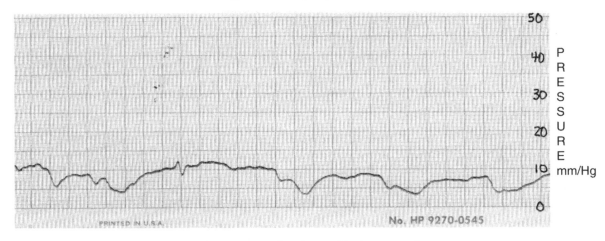

Note the low amplitude, oscillating waveform

Normal mean (averaged) right atrial pressure = 2–5mm Hg.

Low RA pressure may indicate hypovolemia or vasodilation. Elevated pressures may indicate fluid overload, RV failure, tricuspid insufficiency, chronic left heart failure or pulmonary disease.

Right Ventricle

Before you move forward, a bit of review is in order! Earlier in this section, the cardiac valves and their gatekeeper function were discussed. The cardiac valves serve to keep blood flowing in a forward direction. The tricuspid valve is located between the right atrium and the right ventricle. When the tricuspid valve opens, the blood volume in the right atrium (RA) flows into the right ventricle (RV). You will recall that filling pressure is the same as diastolic pressure. So, the right ventricular diastolic pressure is equal to the mean right atrial filling pressure of 2–5mm Hg.

> **Right ventricular (RV) diastolic pressure = 2–5mm Hg.**

As ventricular systole begins, pressure increases. The systolic or emptying pressure of the right ventricle ranges between 20–30mm Hg. This pressure is low in comparison to the systolic pressure of the left ventricle. This is due to the marked difference between the small muscle mass of the right ventricle and the large muscle mass of the left ventricle. Under normal conditions, pulmonary vascular resistance is low. Therefore, it only requires a small muscle mass to pump blood to the lungs.

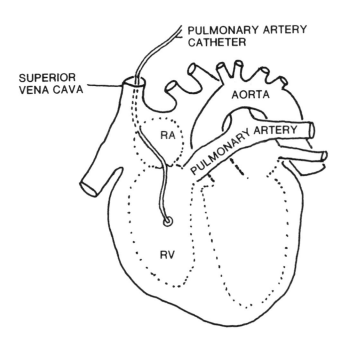

The above diagram demonstrates the placement of a pulmonary artery catheter in the right ventricle.

> $$\text{Normal right ventricular (RV) pressure} = \frac{20\text{–}30\text{mm Hg. (systolic)}}{2\text{–}5\text{mm Hg. (diastolic)}}$$

The following diagrams demonstrate normal right ventricular (RV) waveforms.

Right Ventricular (RV) Pressure Waveform

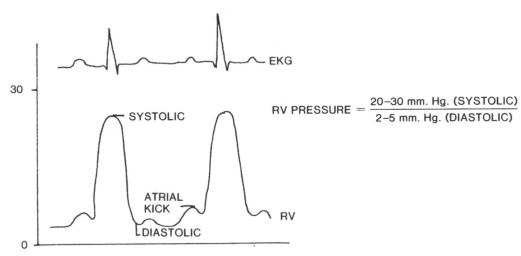

$$RV\ PRESSURE = \frac{20\text{--}30\ mm.\ Hg.\ (SYSTOLIC)}{2\text{--}5\ mm.\ Hg.\ (DIASTOLIC)}$$

NOTE: The RV waveform and pressure can *only* be recorded during catheter insertion. There is no catheter port that opens into the right ventricular chamber. As the catheter is inserted, pressure in the right ventricle is noted, and then the catheter is floated out into the pulmonary artery.

Right Ventricular (RV) Pressure

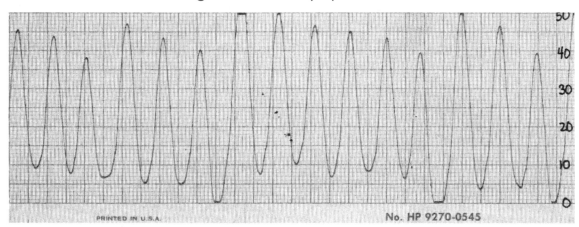

RV pressure is affected by the volume of blood in the ventricle (preload), the pumping ability of the muscle (contractility), and the resistance to ejection found in the pulmonary artery and the lungs (after load). When preload, contractility or afterload changes, so does RV pressure.

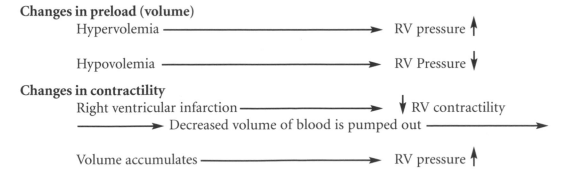

Changes in preload (volume)

Hypervolemia —————————————→ RV pressure ↑

Hypovolemia —————————————→ RV Pressure ↓

Changes in contractility

Right ventricular infarction —————————→ ↓ RV contractility

—————→ Decreased volume of blood is pumped out —————————→

Volume accumulates —————————→ RV pressure ↑

Changes in afterload (resistance)

Pulmonary hypertension (↑ resistance in pulmonary artery) → ↓ blood is pumped out ⟶

Volume accumulates ⟶ RV pressure ↑

*Chronic obstructive lung disease (COPD) is a common cause of pulmonary hypertension that increases RV pressure. Over time, the right ventricle fails as a pump and right-sided CHF results.

How are you doing thus far! At best, the hemodynamic monitoring concepts should create a stretch in your thinking!

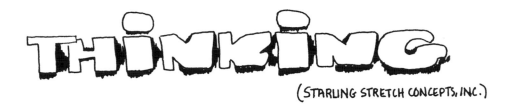

(STARLING STRETCH CONCEPTS, INC.)

Pulmonary Artery

When the pulmonic valve opens secondary to increasing right ventricular pressure, blood and the pulmonary artery catheter moves out of the right ventricle into the pulmonary artery (PA). Though the pulmonary artery has no contractile properties, both systolic and diastolic pressures can be measured.

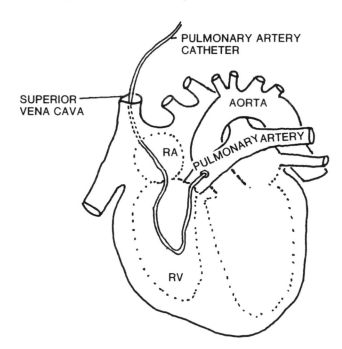

The above diagram demonstrates the pulmonary artery catheter placed in the pulmonary artery. Pulmonary artery filling occurs with right ventricular contraction and emptying. The pressure generated (systolic pressure) by the right ventricle is the same as the pulmonary artery (PA) systolic pressure!

RV Systolic Pressure = PA Systolic Pressure
20–30mm Hg.   20–30mm Hg.

Let's backtrack a minute. You will remember that right atrial (RA) pressure measures 2–5mm Hg. Right atrial (RA) pressure drives the filling of the right ventricle (RV). As the RV fills, the right ventricular muscle stretches, forcing the pulmonic valve open. This stretch stimulates the RV muscle to contract. As the muscle contracts, it generates a higher pressure, thus allowing complete emptying of the RV chamber. In the healthy heart, emptying pressure measures 20–30mm Hg. When the pulmonic valve opens, the RV volume is ejected into the pulmonary artery. So the highest or systolic pressure in the pulmonary artery is also 20–30mm Hg.!

Pressure Points Summary

	Right Atrium (RA)	Right Ventricle (RV)	Pulmonary Artery (PA)
Systolic		20–30mm Hg.	20–30mm Hg.
Mean	2–5mm Hg.		
Diastolic		2–5mm Hg.	

Makes sense, right!

Following pulmonary artery filling, the pulmonic valve closes to prevent blood from flowing backwards. Valve closure creates a back flow of blood against the valve, producing a distinctive notching in the waveform. This notching is referred to as the *dicrotic notch.* Please see the following diagram.

Pulmonary Artery (PA) Pressure Waveform

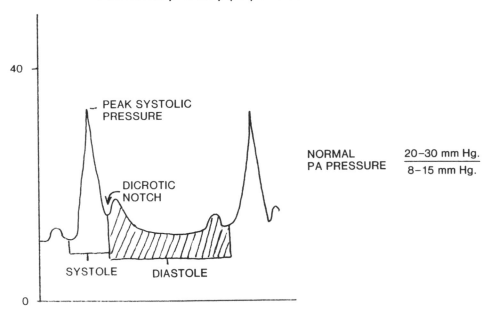

NORMAL PA PRESSURE $\dfrac{20-30 \text{ mm Hg.}}{8-15 \text{ mm Hg.}}$

The dicrotic notch is produced by closure of the pulmonic valve.

Low systolic pulmonary artery (PA) pressures would signify hypovolemia or vasodilation. Elevated pressures may be associated with a number of causes including pulmonary emboli, mitral insufficiency, left ventricular failure, cardiac tamponade, mechanical ventilation or COPD.

From the pulmonary artery, blood then flows passively through the pulmonary vasculature. Remember, there are no valves or "other blood flow controlling devices" in the pulmonary beds. Oxygenation occurs as the blood flows through the pulmonary system. As the blood disperses across the pulmonary vascular beds, the pressure drops to a resting or diastolic level. The pulmonary artery (PA) diastolic pressure ranges between 8–15mm Hg.

In summary, a normal pulmonary artery pressure (PAP) will reflect the following norms:

$$\frac{\text{Pulmonary Artery}}{\text{Pressure (PAP)}} = \frac{\text{20–30mm Hg. (systolic)}}{\text{8–15mm Hg. (diastolic)}}$$

Left Atrium

Earlier discussion indicated that there are no valves present in the pulmonary vascular system. Thus, blood flows passively from the pulmonary artery under low pressure to left atrium (LA). Since the PA catheter stops in the PA, there is no waveform or direct pressure reading from the LA. Indirectly, the PA diastolic correlates with the LA pressure.

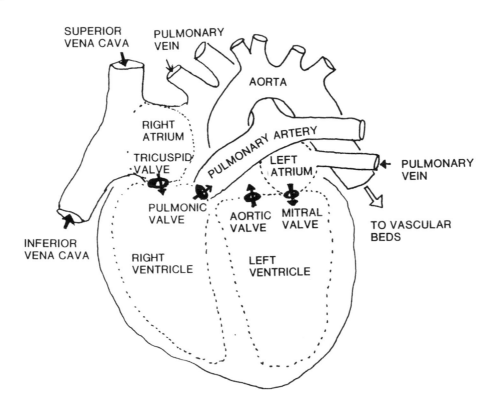

The following table maps pressure relationships from the right atrium to the left atrium.

	Pressure Points (continued)			
	Right Atrium (RA) Pressure	Right Ventricle (RV) Pressure	Pulmonary Artery (PA) Pressure	Left Atrial (LA) Pressure
Systolic		20–30-mm Hg.	20–30-mm Hg.	
Mean	2–5-mm Hg.			8–15mm Hg.
Diastolic		2–5-mm Hg.	8–15mm Hg.	

Clear as a foggy day, right! Bear in mind that no one masters hemodynamic concepts on the first pass. Mastery is gained through repetition and practice. /ᓚᕊᗩ

Important Detail

Before going further, it is important to point out that the pulmonary artery catheter cannot be passed beyond the pulmonary artery! Therefore, left atrial and left ventricular pressure measurements cannot be made directly using the pulmonary artery catheter. Read on for clarification . . .

Pulmonary Capillary Wedge Pressure (PCWP) vs. Left Atrial Pressure

The notion that a catheter inserted into the right heart can measure left heart functioning is confusing. The secret is the 1.5cc latex balloon at the tip of the pulmonary artery catheter. When inflated with a syringe, the balloon occludes or wedges into a small branch of the pulmonary artery and blocks any information coming *from the right heart.* At the tip of the catheter, distal to the balloon, there is a pressure reading device. When the balloon is inflated, the device reads pressure in the left atrium at the end of diastole. Remember, this is filling pressure or preload!

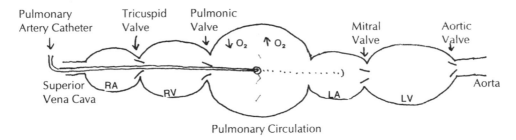

A right-sided catheter used to measure left side pressures.

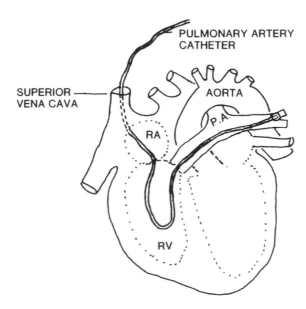

The inflated balloon on the pulmonary catheter is wedged into a small branch of the pulmonary artery.

Both the pulmonary capillary wedge pressure (PCWP) and the left atrial pressure (LA), should be 8–15mm.Hg. (mean values) under normal circumstances.

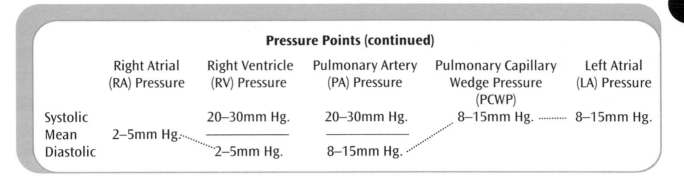

13

Pressure Points (continued)

	Right Atrial (RA) Pressure	Right Ventricle (RV) Pressure	Pulmonary Artery (PA) Pressure	Pulmonary Capillary Wedge Pressure (PCWP)	Left Atrial (LA) Pressure
Systolic		20–30mm Hg.	20–30mm Hg.	8–15mm Hg.	8–15mm Hg.
Mean	2–5mm Hg.				
Diastolic		2–5mm Hg.	8–15mm Hg.		

The pulmonary capillary wedge pressure (PCWP) waveformation is presented in the next two diagrams.

Pulmonary Capillary Wedge Pressure (PCWP)

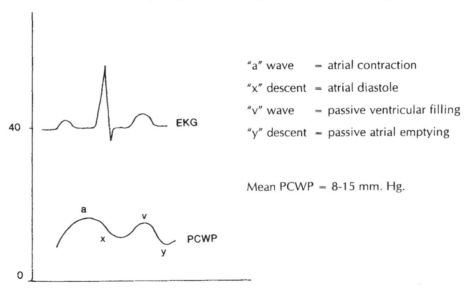

"a" wave = atrial contraction

"x" descent = atrial diastole

"v" wave = passive ventricular filling

"y" descent = passive atrial emptying

Mean PCWP = 8-15 mm. Hg.

The PA waveform "flattens out" as the pulmonary artery catheter balloon is inflated and subsequently wedges in the pulmonary artery. The resulting waveform has little systolic-diastolic pressure change. Thus, as with the RAP, the PCWP is reported as a mean pressure.

The following diagram demonstrates a pulmonary artery catheter moving from the right ventricle into the pulmonary artery. Note that both the RV and PA pressures are elevated.

Right Ventricular (RV) Pressure ⟶   Pulmonary Artery (PA) Pressure

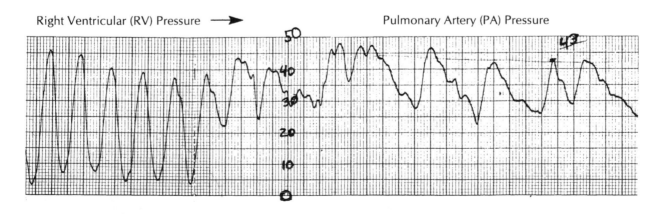

Pulmonary Capillary Wedge Pressure (PCWP)

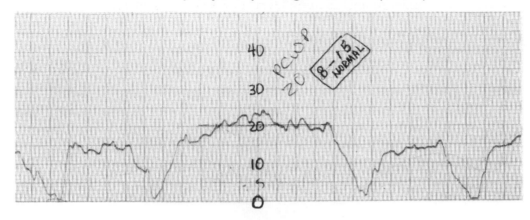

Note the elevated pulmonary capillary wedge pressure (PCWP).

Pulmonary Capillary Wedge Pressure (PCWP) vs. Left Ventricular End Diastolic Pressure (LVEDP)

Finally, the last topic in the hemodynamic monitoring process is to relate previously discussed pressures to left ventricular (LV) function. The left ventricle is the major pump of the heart! The left ventricle (LV) has the greatest muscle mass of the four cardiac chambers.

Earlier we presented the concept that the right ventricular (RV) diastolic or filling pressure is equivalent to the mean right atrial (RA) pressure. These pressures are equivalent owing to the *passive* flow of blood from the right atrium to the right ventricle. **Voila!** The same phenomenon occurs in the left side of the heart!

The left ventricular filling or diastolic pressure should equal the left atrial mean pressure because blood flows passively from the left atrium into the left ventricle. Makes sense, right? Thus, at the conclusion of the left ventricular filling phase, the *left ventricular end diastolic pressure* (LVEDP) equals the mean left atrial pressure. Whew!

Now, have a look at the entirety of pressure relationships.

Pressure Points

	(RA) Pressure	(RV) Pressure	(PA) Pressure	(PCWP)	(LA) Pressure	(LV) LVEDP
Systolic		20–30mm Hg.	20–30mm Hg.			
Mean*	2–5mm Hg.			8–15mm Hg.	8–15mm Hg.	
Diastolic		2–5mm Hg.	8–15mm Hg.			8–15mm Hg.

*means pressures are reported for the right and left atria and PCWP because minimal differences exist between systolic and diastolic pressures in those chambers/vessels.

Key:
RA = Right Atrium
RV = Right Ventricle
PA = Pulmonary Artery
PCWP = Pulmonary Capillary Wedge Pressure
LA = Left Atrium
LVEDP = Left Ventricular End Diastolic Pressure

So, in reviewing the pressure points, the PA diastolic, PCWP, LA, and LVEDP should be equal pressures. Thus, a catheter placed in the right heart *can* assess left heart function!!

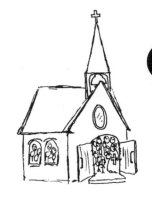

The left ventricular end diastolic pressure (LVEDP) is a critical measure of left ventricular function. If the LVEDP rises, it is an indication that left ventricular emptying is incomplete. Incomplete left ventricular emptying may occur secondary to pump failure (left ventricular failure) caused by acute myocardial infarction (muscle injury and necrosis). Incomplete LV emptying may also result from *aortic stenosis.* In aortic stenosis, the aortic valve fails to open completely, thus restricting the free flow of blood out of the left ventricular chamber.

HINT: Aortic stenosis reminds me of a Sunday morning church service finale, where 200 people attempt to exit a single door obstructed by a bastion of hand shakers! The hand shakers create congestion and crowd backup. This "obstructed emptying" causes tension (pressure) to rise!

A decrease in the pulmonary capillary wedge pressure (PCWP)/left ventricular end diastolic pressure (LVEDP) results from a reduced preload. A reduced preload is often due to hypovolemia, dehydration, or extreme vasodilation of the venous system.

Cardiac Output Can Be Assessed Without Invasive Hemodynamic Monitoring

There are times when invasive hemodynamic monitoring may not be indicated. However, the measurement of cardiac output is still important. One can assess some information regarding cardiac output indirectly. While the information is not specific, it may guide treatment decisions.

- Increases and decreases in **preload** may be reflected, in part, by changes in
  * Volume status – Intake and output, daily weights
  * Edema
  * Changes in serum sodium or hematocrit (due to dilution or concentration)

- Increases and decreases in **contractility** may be reflected, in part, by changes in
  * Skin temperature
  * Pulse strength
  * Neurological status
  * Urine output

- Fast, slow or irregular **heart rates** can affect cardiac output.

- Increases and decreases in **afterload** may be reflected, in part, by changes in
  * Skin temperature. Warm, flushed skin reflects vasodilation and therefore, decreased afterload.
  * Skin temperature. Cold skin reflects vasoconstriction and therefore, increased afterload.

Practice Exercise 3

Note: Difficulty Ahead . . . Be Prepared to Stop for Review

A. Owing to its (circle one) small/large muscle mass, the normal right atrial pressure is low/high.

B. Minimal differences between systolic and diastolic pressures are reported as _____ pressures.

C. Mean right atrial pressure normally ranges between _____ and _____ mm Hg.

D. Correctly match right atrial pressure abnormalities with probable pathologies by placing the letter L or H in the spaces provided.

L = Low right atrial pressure

H = High right atrial pressure

_____ Right ventricular failure

_____ Fluid overload

_____ Vasodilation

_____ Tricuspid valve insufficiency

_____ Chronic left heart failure

_____ Hypovolemia

E. Explain why the right ventricular diastolic pressure equals the mean right atrial pressure (to cheat, turn to page 333).

_____

_____

_____

_____

F. Normal right ventricular (RV) pressure is (circle one).

2–5mm Hg.   20–30mm Hg. $\dfrac{20\text{–}30\text{mm Hg.}}{2\text{–}5\text{mm Hg.}}$

G. The dicrotic notch in the pulmonary artery waveform is produced by

_____

_____

_____

❑ Check if you are alive and well . . .

❑ Check if you are uncertain!

H. Correctly match systolic pulmonary artery pressure abnormalities with suspect pathologies by placing the letter L or H in the spaces provided.

L = Low systolic PA pressures

H = High systolic PA pressures

_____ Pulmonary emboli

_____ Hypovolemia

_____ Mechanical ventilation

_____ Left ventricular failure

_____ Vasodilation

I. Normal pulmonary artery pressure (PAP) is _____ mm Hg.

8–15mm Hg.

J. The pulmonary artery (PA) resting or diastolic pressure equals the mean left atrial (LA) pressure

because there are no _____ in the pulmonary vascular system or left atrial junction.

The absence of _____ allows the pressures to equalize.

K. If the diastolic PA pressure is 10mm.Hg., the mean LA pressure will be _____ mm Hg.

L. The pulmonary artery catheter cannot be passed beyond the _____!

BREAK TIME ...
Please return in 15mm Hg. 🙂

❏ I returned on time

❏ I was tardy

M. Left ventricular filling or end diastolic pressure equals the left atrial mean pressure because _____

_____

_____

N. Correctly match left ventricular end diastolic pressure (LVEDP) abnormalities with associated pathologies by placing the letter H (high) or L (low) in the spaces provided.

H = elevated LVEDP (> 15mm Hg.)   _____ Hypovolemia

L = low LVEDP (< 8mm Hg.)   _____ Aortic stenosis

_____ Incomplete LV emptying

_____ Left Ventricular failure

_____ Dehydration

O. In the spaces provided, write the words represented by the following abbreviations. *Then*, note normal pressures for the various hemodynamic measures!

Pressures

RA = _____

RV = _____

PA = _____

PCWP = _____

LA = _____

LVEDP = _____

P.

There are four components of cardiac output: Preload, Heart Rate, Contractility and Afterload				

Please review the following list of drugs, factors, and interventions. Evaluate how each of these would increase or decrease the patient's preload, heart rate, contractility and/or afterload. Some of the drugs, factors, and interventions will impact one of the four components, others may impact two or more of the components. Use an arrow up for increase and an arrow down for decrease. See Digoxin as an example.

Drugs, Factors and Interventions	Preload	Heart Rate	Contractility	Afterload
Digoxin				
Anxiety				
Lasix				
Nitroglycerin				
Blood Transfusion				
Fever				
Bolus of IV fluids				
Atropine				
Caffeine				
Hypoxia				
Thyroid Hormone				
Calcium				
Hemodialysis				
Elevate Head of Bed				
Cooling Blanket				
Pacemaker Insertion				
Nicotine				

Bravo

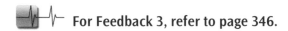 For Feedback 3, refer to page 346.

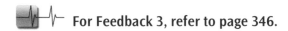 Feedback 1

Great Job!

A. Invasive hemodynamic monitoring is accomplished via a <u>pulmonary artery</u> catheter.

B. The size (mass) and strength of the left ventricle allows oxygenated blood to be ejected past the <u>aortic</u> valve into the <u>aorta</u> and out to systemic circulation.

C.

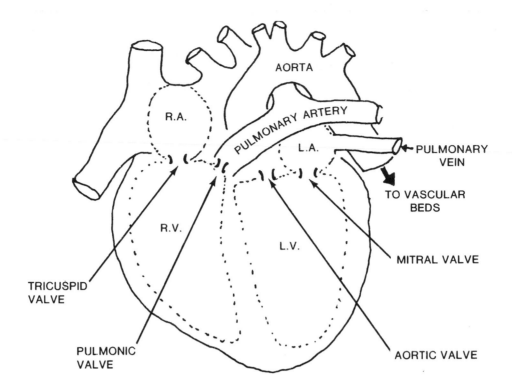

D. The contraction/ejection phase of the blood flow cycle is termed <u>systole</u>; the relaxation/filling phase of the blood flow cycle is known as <u>diastole</u>.

E. If a muscle fiber is stretched (diastole) a short distance, contraction (systole) is <u>weak</u>. If a muscle fiber is fully stretched to its optimal length, contraction is forceful. If a muscle fiber is repeatedly overstretched, contractile force is <u>diminished</u>.

F. Starling was a   ☐ Bird

                    ☐ Plane

                    ☒ Law man

G. The four components of cardiac output:
1. Contractivity
2. Heart rate
3. Pre-load
4. Afterload

 ## Feedback 2

A. The pulmonary artery catheter (Swan-Ganz catheter) has three internal lumens, and a <u>thermistor</u> which is used to measure core temperature.

B. The <u>proximal</u> pulmonary artery catheter port is utilized for fluid administration.

C. <u>Right</u> atrial pressure is monitored at the proximal lumen opening.

D. An inflated pulmonary artery catheter balloon causes the catheter to "<u>wedge</u>" into a small pulmonary vessel.

E. Normal cardiac output (CO) ranges between <u>4</u> and <u>8</u> liters per minute.

⊸⋀⋏⊸ Feedback 3

A. Owing to its small muscle mass, the normal right atrial pressure is low.

B. Minimal differences between systolic and diastolic pressures are reported as averaged or mean pressures.

C. Mean right atrial pressure normally ranges between <u>2</u> and <u>5</u>mm Hg.

D. L = Low right atrial pressure   __H__   Right ventricular failure

    H = High right atrial pressure   __H__   Fluid overload

                          __L__   Vasodilation

                          __H__   Tricuspid valve insufficiency

                          __H__   Chronic left heart failure

                          __L__   Hypovolemia

E. When the tricuspid valve opens, the blood volume in the RA flows passively into the RV. It is the mean right atrial pressure that forces the valve open. That pressure is maintained in the systolic stage of right atrial ejection and the diastolic stage of RV filling via the open tricuspid valve.   Whew!

F. Normal right ventricular (RV) pressure is $\dfrac{20\text{--}30\text{mm Hg.}}{2\text{--}5\text{mm Hg.}}$

G. The dicrotic notch in the pulmonary artery waveform is produced by <u>the back flow of blood against the closed pulmonic valve. The pulmonic valve closes following pulmonary artery filling</u>.

H. L = Low systolic PA pressures   __H__   Pulmonary emboli

    H = High systolic PA pressures   __L__   Hypovolemia

                          __H__   Mechanical ventilation

                          __H__   Left ventricular failure

                          __L__   Vasodilation

I. Normal pulmonary artery pressure (PAP) is $\dfrac{20\text{--}30\text{mm Hg.}}{8\text{--}15\text{mm Hg.}}$

J. The pulmonary artery (PA) resting or diastolic pressure equals the mean left atrial (LA) pressure because there are no <u>valves</u> in the pulmonary vascular system or left atrial junction. The absence of <u>valves</u> allows the pressures to equalize.

K. If the diastolic PA pressure is 10mm Hg., the mean LA pressure will be <u>10</u>mm Hg.

L. The pulmonary artery catheter cannot be passed beyond the <u>pulmonary artery</u>!

M. Left ventricular filling or end diastolic pressure equals the left atrial mean pressure because <u>the blood</u> <u>flows passively from the left atrium into the left ventricle via the open mitral valve.</u>

N. Correctly match left ventricular end diastolic pressure (LVEDP) abnormalities with associated pathologies by placing the letter H (high) or L (low) in the spaces provided.

H = elevated LVEDP (> 15mm Hg.)   __L__   Hypovolemia

L = low LVEDP (< 8mm Hg.)   __H__   Aortic stenosis

                                              __H__   Incomplete LV emptying

                                              __H__   Left ventricular failure

                                              __L__   Dehydration

O. In the spaces provided, write the words represented by the following abbreviations. <u>Then</u> note NORMAL pressures for the various hemodynamic measures!

	Pressures
RA = right atrium	2–5mm Hg.
RV = right ventricle	20–30mm Hg.
	2–5mm Hg.
PA = pulmonary artery	20–30mm Hg.
	8–15mm Hg.
PCWP = pulmonary capillary wedge pressure	8–15mm Hg.
LA = left atrium	8–15mm Hg.
LVEDP = left ventricular end diastolic pressure	8–15mm Hg.

P. Answers to question P on next page.

There are four components of cardiac output: Preload, Heart Rate, Contractility and Afterload

Please review the following list of drugs, factors, and interventions. Evaluate how each of these would increase or decrease the patient's preload, heart rate, contractility and/or afterload. Some of the drugs, factors, and interventions will impact one of the four components, others may impact two or more of the components. Use arrow up for increase and an arrow down for decrease. See Digoxin as an example.

Drugs, Factors and Interventions	Preload	Heart Rate	Contractility	Afterload
Digoxin		↓	≠	
Anxiety	≠	≠	≠	≠
Lasix	↓			↓
Nitroglycerin	↓			↓
Blood Transfusion	≠			
Fever		≠	≠	↓
Bolus of IV fluids	≠			
Atropine		↓		
Caffeine	↓	≠	≠	≠
Hypoxia		≠	≠	
Thyroid Hormone		≠	≠	
Calcium			≠	
Hemodialysis	↓			
Elevate Head of Bed	↓			
Cooling Blanket	≠			≠
Pacemaker Insertion		≠		
Nicotine		≠	≠	≠

☆ *Stellar performance!*

Notes

_____

_____

_____

_____

_____

_____

_____

_____

_____

_____

_____

_____

_____

_____

_____

_____

_____

_____

Kidstuff

Objectives

When you have completed Section 14, you will be able to describe or identify

1. cardiac variants in children
2. normal heart rates for children
3. normal duration of P, P-R, QRS, and QT intervals
4. recognition of the following cardiac dysrhythmias in kids:

- sinus arrhythmia
- sinus bradycardia
- sinus tachycardia
- sinus arrest/sinus block
- sick sinus syndrome
- atrial tachycardia
- P.A.C.s
- atrial flutter
- atrial fibrillation
- wandering atrial pacemaker
- junctional escape rhythms
- premature junctional beats
- junctional tachycardia

- S.V.T.
- P.V.C.s
- ventricular tachycardia
- ventricular flutter
- ventricular fibrillation
- P.E.A.
- long QT syndrome
- first degree heart block
- second degree heart block
- third degree heart block
- bundle branch blocks

5. drug and electrolyte manifestations

Contributions by:
Karen Corlett, R.N., M.S.N., A.P.N.
Jane D. Werth, M.S., R.N.

Back in the days of Michelangelo, painters frequently painted children as little adults—same body shape, same body proportions, and the same skin tone. It didn't work then and it doesn't work now. . . .

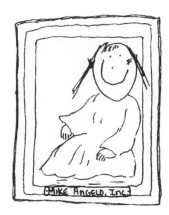

. . . children are not just adults in miniature. They have different health care problems and different body function norms . . . so follows the reason for this section. It is important to understand both the similarities and differences between adult and pediatric electrocardiography.

Birth through 18 years of age covers a wide time span! However, for the sake of simplicity we will use the term *pediatrics* to cover this age span in most references. The term *newborn* applies to babies 0–1 month of age, and the term *infant* applies to infants 1 month–one year.

So bearing that in mind, let's start! . . . Just one more thing. . . .

. . . you may find it helpful to read the corresponding "adult" version as you ponder pediatric dysrhythmias . . . that's why the rest of this book is attached!

The stable EKG pattern seen in the normal adult does not completely develop in the child until around the age of ten. Most changes that do occur in pediatric EKGs are due to a shift from right ventricular dominance (seen in the newborn) to left ventricular dominance (seen in the adult).

At birth, the right ventricle is thicker than the left side counterpart. During the first month of life, there is a dramatic decrease in right ventricular pressure and a subsequent decrease in right ventricular wall thickness. It is also probably important to note that the size of the infant heart is large in comparison to the size of the thoracic cavity.

In many instances, dysrhythmias in children differ in *cause* and *frequency* from adults. For instance, ventricular dysrhythmias are seen less frequently in children owing to the absence of atherosclerotic heart disease. More commonly seen in children are the EKG dysrhythmias and abnormalities which occur secondary to structural problems in the heart. Now, just take a minute and remember atrial septal defects . . . tetralogy of Fallot . . . and patent ductus arteriosus (you may have studied those in Anatomy 101). Basically, many congenital heart defects, like those named above, create artificial openings in heart chambers that can greatly increase chamber pressure gradients. These pressure increases can cause chamber **hypertrophy**. Since congenital heart defects occur in approximately eight to ten of every 1,000 newborns, hypertrophy induced EKG changes are very common.

Let's look at *atrial hypertrophy* for a moment. As you will recall, the P wave represents atrial depolarization. The P wave then reflects depolarization of both the right and left atria. In reality, the P wave can be divided into two components.

Right Atrial Component ↘   P   ↙ Left Atrial Component

(Remember, leads II, III, and aVF display the most prominent P waves.) In the presence of atrial hypertrophy, one observes an increase in the *amplitude* or the *duration* of the P wave.

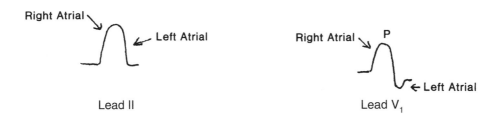

Amplitude   Duration

Looking at atrial depolarization in lead II, right atrial hypertrophy is reflected as a prominent (often pointed) P with increased amplitude (greater than 3 mm). Lead V_1 is included here for comparison purposes.

Lead II   Lead V_1

Left atrial hypertrophy presents as a prolonged P wave and may be notched.

Lead II   Lead V_1

When both right and left atrial hypertrophy are present, the P wave may reflect a combination of the above patterns.

Lead II   Lead V_1

Leading Statements

You will recall that leads view electrical activity from different perspectives or angles. Since ventricular dysrhythmias are less common in children, usually "kids" are monitored on leads which best reflect atrial activity. Commonly then, children will be monitored on leads II, III, and aVF. Generally speaking, the differences observed in normal or healthy adult and pediatric EKG tracings have to do with variations in rate, ventricular wall thickness, and the position and orientation of the heart, itself.

input section ## 14.1 General Rules and Concepts

There are a few general rules and concepts that aide the understanding and identification of pediatric EKGs and rhythm anomalies. As one would suspect, the age of the infant is a critical factor in any rhythm analysis.

Heart rate norms vary in children from year to year (and sometimes month to month). Though the norms presented on page 354 are approximations, most authorities generally agree with these parameters.

Pediatric Heart Rate Norms

Age	Range	Average Rate
0–1 month	90–200	160
2–3 months	90–200	150
4–12 months	100–180	140
1–3 yrs.	80–180	130
4–5 yrs.	70–150	100
6–8 yrs.	68–140	100
9–11 yrs.	60–120	88
12–16 yrs.	60–125	80
> 16 yrs.	60–90	75

As demonstrated above, there is a tremendous variation in the age-related norms. However, as a general rule . . .

> **RULE #1**   As age ↑ heart rate ↓

In the absence of a rate guide, a *field* estimate of an age-specific heart rate is often determined by the following formula:

> HEART RATE = 150 minus (5 × age in years)

In any case, *heart rate must be evaluated in relation to the age of the child and the underlying clinical condition.* Heart rate increases may be related to crying, agitation, fear, pain, fever, etc. In fact, the heart rate may increase eight to ten beats per minute for each Fahrenheit degree increase in temperature. (*Remember that?*) Decreases in heart rate may be related to sleep, increased vagal tone, abdominal distention, increased intracranial pressure, apnea, and a variety of *other* factors.

Another general rule that can be applied to pediatrics is . . .

> **RULE #2**   As age ↑, the duration of the P-R and QRS
> intervals ↑ and the duration of the QT interval ↓.

So . . . let's explore each of those intervals separately. In fact, let's explore all the wave forms!

The P Wave

You will recall that the P wave represents atrial excitation spreading from the SA node through the right and left atria. Normally the duration of the P wave is 0.06 ± 0.02 seconds in children.

Remember each small EKG paper square represents 0.04 seconds!

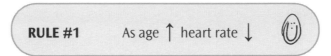

.06 ± .02

The maximum P wave duration is 0.10 seconds in children and 0.08 seconds in infants. A prolonged P wave may be due to atrial hypertrophy as was discussed on page 353.

The P-R Interval

You will remember that atrial activation and atrial repolarization are represented on the EKG as a P wave followed by a straight line, the P-R interval. The P-R interval is measured from the beginning of the P wave to the start of the QRS complex. The P-R interval represents atrial depolarization (P wave) and the delaying or holding of the impulse on the AV node (straight line).

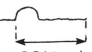
P-R interval

The P-R interval further represents the time for the impulse to pass from the SA node through the AV junction, through the ventricles to the Purkinje fibers. Like the duration of the P wave, the duration of the P-R interval varies with age and heart rate.

Pediatric P-R Intervals

Age	Duration of P-R Interval
0–4 months	0.09–0.12 seconds
4–12 months	0.09–0.14 seconds
1–3 years	0.1–0.14 seconds
3–8 years	0.12–0.17 seconds
9–16 years	0.15–0.18 seconds
> 16 years	0.15–0.20 seconds

A prolonged P-R interval represents increased conduction time and may be seen in conditions such as first degree heart block, myocarditis, digitalis toxicity, hyperkalemia, or atrial septal defect. A shortened P-R interval may be seen in rhythms with accelerated conduction such as Wolff-Parkinson-White (W.P.W.) Syndrome.

QRS Duration

Remember, the duration of the QRS indicates the time elapsed during ventricular activation or depolarization. Normal pediatric QRS durations appear below.

Kid's QRSs

Age	QRS Duration
Premie	0.04 seconds
0–3 years	0.04–0.08 seconds
4–16 years	0.05–0.09 seconds
> 16 years	0.05–0.10 seconds

When the QRS is greater than the prescribed upper limit, i.e., 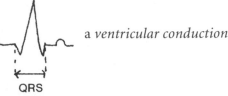 a *ventricular conduction*

delay exists. This conduction delay may be caused by a number of factors including

- severe hyperkalemia
- quinidine toxicity
- procainamide toxicity

- bundle branch block
- ventricular pacemaker device

QT Interval

The QT interval represents the time for both ventricular depolarization and repolarization to occur. It is measured from the beginning of the Q wave to the end of the T wave. Just like the adult, the QT interval varies with heart rate and a variety of other factors. In the infant, however, the *QT interval principally varies with age!* In infants (less than 6 months), the maximum QT interval is 0.45 seconds. In children, the maximum QT interval is 0.44 seconds. As a comparison, the maximum QT interval for adults and adolescents is 0.425 seconds. When measuring the QT interval you must correct for heart rate (QTc) by looking at a table or calculating using Bazet's formula:

$$\text{Bazet's formula} \qquad \mathbf{QTc} = \frac{\text{QT interval in seconds}}{\sqrt{\text{R} - \text{R interval in seconds}}}$$

Though QT intervals may not be routinely measured, it is worthwhile noting that QT interval *prolongation* is associated with hypokalemia, hypocalcemia, myocarditis, and the administration of various antiarrhythmic drugs. The QT interval is also prolonged in long QT syndrome (LQTS), discussed on page 420. A *shortened* QT interval may be seen with hypercalcemia and digitalis effect.

The ST Segment

The ST segment occurs after ventricular depolarization and before ventricular repolarization (T wave). Similar to grown-ups, ST segment elevation may be associated with acute pericarditis (inflammation of membranes surrounding the heart) or acute myocardial infarct (rare in children), hyperkalemia, hypokalemia and digitalis effect.

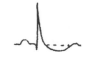

ST segment elevation   ST segment depression

ST segment elevation ST segment depression

As with adults, it is important to remember that EKGs are not diagnostic, only suggestive!

The T Wave

The T wave is the recovery phase (repolarization) following ventricular depolarization. Tall, peaked T waves may be seen in hyperkalemia and ventricular hypertrophy. Flat, low T waves may be seen in newborn infants as a normal phenomenon or associated with hypothyroidism, hypokalemia, pericarditis, myocarditis, or digitalis effect.

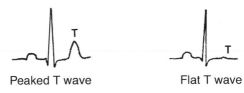

Peaked T wave   Flat T wave

All these components come together for the *normal EKG lineup:*

- Rate—varies with age and clinical condition
- Rhythm—regular
- P waves—each QRS will be preceded by a P wave. All P waves will appear uniform
- QRS—all QRS complexes will appear uniform in configuration
- Conduction—each P will be followed by normal QRS
- T wave—may be flipped (inverted) from birth to adolescence in the right precordial leads V_1, V_2
- P-R interval and QRS duration normal for age

It is important to recognize that multiple subtle EKG pattern changes occur as an infant develops. Some of the major, early observed changes are now discussed.

> **RULE #3**   Expect *subtle* EKG pattern changes.

PREMIE EKG (BIRTH BEFORE 37 WEEKS GESTATION)

- Lower voltage QRS and T wave in limb leads (I, II, III).
- Shorter P-R, QRS, QT intervals.

NORMAL NEWBORN EKG

- Normal duration QRS in limb leads (this time you tell me . . . leads ____, ____, and ____).
- T wave in V_1 usually becomes flipped (inverted or negative) by third day and remains flipped until the age of five (this phenomenon occurs because of the changing nature of the developing heart)!

Before examining rhythm anomalies, let's review the steps you learned previously for analyzing EKGs—these steps are as appropriate for pediatric rhythms as they are for adult rhythms!

- Determine the heart rate using methods discussed on page 29
- Determine whether the rhythm is basically regular or irregular. Are there unexpected premature beats, pauses or dropped beats?
- Look at atrial activity (P waves). Is atrial depolarization occurring at an expected rate with a regular rhythm? Are the P waves so rapid that there are more atrial impulses than there are QRS complexes? Is it difficult to distinguish atrial activity?
- Observe ventricular activity. Are the QRSs of normal duration? Does a QRS following each P wave? Are the QRSs occurring regularly (consistent R-R interval)?
- Determine the relationship between atrial activity and ventricular activity. Is each P wave producing a QRS? Is the P-R constant?

Remember—*What's in a name?* A dysrhythmia by the *wrong* name may spell defeat! *It is more important to accurately describe what you observe than to apply a label.* (Unfortunately, people disagree over labels . . . actually, without labels, this is all very logical!)

Practice Exercise 1

A. The heart rate, the duration of P-R, QRS, and QT intervals all vary with _____.

Circle the correct answer in the following statements (B–E).

B. The heart rate increases / decreases with increasing age.

C. The P-R interval lengthens / shortens with increasing age.

D. The duration of the QRS is greater / lesser with increasing age.

E. The duration of the QT interval increases / decreases with increasing age.

F. Evaluate and describe this cardiac complex.

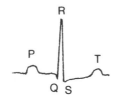

_____

_____

_____

 For Feedback 1, refer to page 391.

For Feedback 1, refer to page 391.

input section 14.2 Sinus Dysrhythmias

Sinus rhythms are so called because they originate in the sinoatrial node. The SA node is the normal pacemaker of the heart because it has the fastest pacemaking capability or the *highest automaticity.* As with everything in pediatrics, the inherent rate of SA node discharge (thus the rate of conduction or heart rate in a normal heart) varies with age . . . so much for precision! Need a quick rate review? Please turn back to page 354.

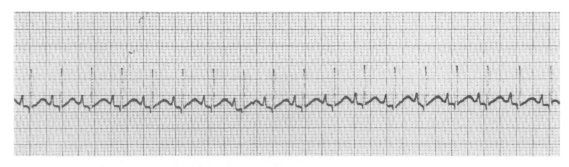

Normal sinus rhythm in a normal newborn. The heart rate is 166 because the baby is crying!

Sinus Arrhythmia

The first dysrhythmia to be considered is *sinus arrhythmia*. Sinus arrhythmia is a slightly irregular rhythm that is initiated by the SA node. Usually the irregularity of the rhythm is related to respiration. The heart rate tends to increase with inspiration and decrease with expiration. Sinus arrhythmia is more pronounced in adolescence than in childhood.

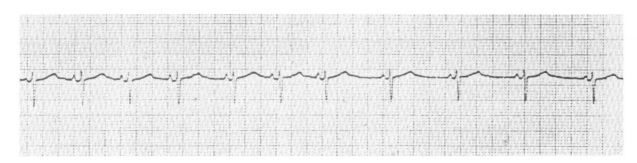

A nonpathologic sinus arrhythmia. Note the irregular P-P interval.

Sinus arrhythmia is a variation of normal and can be differentiated from a truly abnormal arrhythmia by having the child hold his or her breath. In sinus arrhythmia, brief cessation of breathing will cause the heart rate to remain steady.

Let's look at sinus arrhythmia in detail.

- Rate—variable with age.
- Rhythm—irregular, but may be patterned when related to respiration.
- P waves
  —uniform in appearance
  —irregular P-P interval
  —precede each QRS complex
- P-R interval nonvarying.
- QRSs are all of normal configuration, but the R-R intervals are irregular.

Sinus arrhythmia is a common dysrhythmia that is usually a *variation of normal.* Though no treatment is required, one should be aware that it exists. Just for fun, measure the varying P-P and R-R intervals in this rhythm strip.

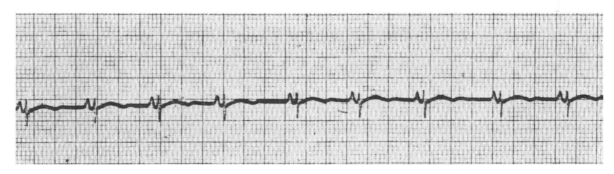

Normal newborn with sinus bradycardia and sinus arrhythmia secondary to maternal Inderal treatment for P.A.T.

Sinus Bradycardia

Bradycardia has a few drawbacks . . . remember bradycardia is a term used to describe a rate slower than the expected norm. Of course, the definition of bradycardia varies with age in pediatrics (and you're saying, "*What doesn't?"*). Generally speaking, sinus bradycardia is defined as a rate of less than 100 beats/minute in newborns and less than 70 beats/minute in children.

Getting back to the shortcomings of bradycardia . . . if sinus bradycardia develops gradually, compensatory cardiac changes (such as increased stroke volume and chamber dilation) may prevent a fall in cardiac output (*stable sinus bradycardia*). That's good! Unfortunately, if the bradycardia comes on more suddenly, the heart is less likely to compensate and cardiac output will be compromised (*unstable sinus bradycardia*).

$$\text{cardiac output} = \text{heart rate} \times \text{stroke volume}$$

> Remember that infants and young children are less able to increase stroke volume so bradycardia may significantly impact their cardiac output.

So, keeping that in mind, let's look at *sinus bradycardia* in greater detail.

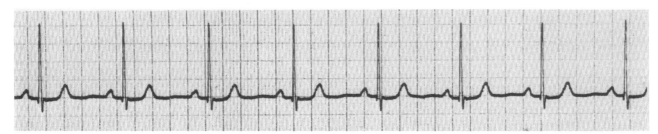

Sinus bradycardia with a heart rate of 62 per minute. This rhythm strip belongs to an eight year old girl. Notice that the P-R interval approaches the upper limit of normal.

Criteria for *sinus bradycardia:*

- Rate—less than 100 in newborns; less than 70 in children.
- Rhythm—regular.
- P waves precede each QRS; the P-R interval is constant; the P-P interval is regular.
- QRSs are all of normal configuration; the R-R interval is regular.

Some of the more common causes of sinus bradycardia include:

- hypoxia
- apnea in the healthy premature infant
- increased vagal tone (due to increased intracranial pressure, hypertension, abdominal distention, cough, stooling, etc.)
- adolescent athletes (normal rhythm of *pint-size champions*) ☺
- hypoglycemia

Most commonly, sinus bradycardia is a **secondary event** resulting from hypoxia. **Hypoxia suppresses the automaticity of the sinus node,** thus decreasing the rate of sinus impulse formation. If untreated, the hypoxia may result in hypotension and acidosis which, in turn, decreases cardiac contractility. A negative spiraling then ensues with the decrease in cardiac contractility causing further hypotension, hypoxia and bradycardia. Correcting the hypoxia and acidosis is critical. Epinephrine 0.01 mg/kg (1:10,000 solution) is the drug of choice for augmenting both the heart rate and myocardial contractility owing to its alpha- and beta-receptor stimulation.

Atropine (0.02 mg/kg) can be used for vagally mediated sinus bradycardia.

Transcutaneous pacing may be used to treat symptomatic bradycardias unresponsive (refractory) to drug therapy.

Most defibrillators have the capability for transcutaneous pacing. Make sure you know how to use this feature for this rare but life-threatening indication.

In summary, *sinus bradycardia* is treated when there is evidence of decreased cardiac output (decreased responsiveness, lethargy, loss of consciousness, cyanosis). The underlying cause, however, should always be investigated and treated as necessary.

It is important to consider that an exaggerated slow heart rate may allow escape beats or escape rhythms to be initiated from a lower, more distal pacemaker. Commonly, one would see the escape beats originating from the AV junction. When escape beats originate in the AV junctional tissue, there is no P wave, but they are conducted normally through the ventricular conduction system. Thus, the QRS is within normal limits. An escape beat originating from the ventricle would be even slower with a wider QRS complex.

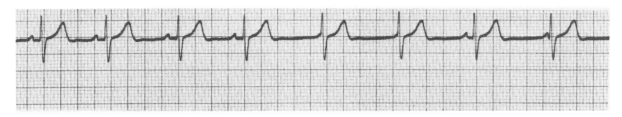

Notice that the heart rate gradually slows. An AV junctional pacemaker assumes intermittent command following beat 4.

Sinus Tachycardia

Tachycardia is a term used to describe a heart rate of greater than 140 in children and greater than 160 in infants. *Sinus tachy* (as those of us who are close call it) is a regular sinus rhythm with an *increased* rate. Usually *sinus tachycardia* will not exceed a rate of 180 in children and 200 in infants. Whew!

***Sinus tachycardia* has the following characteristics:**

- Rate—140–180 in children, 160–200 in infants.
- Rhythm-regular.
- P waves precede each QRS.
- P-P interval constant.
- P-R interval constant.
- A QRS follows each P wave; normal QRS configuration; R-R interval is regular.
- Usually has gradual onset; gradual slowing; rate varies with activity or condition.

Look for yourself!

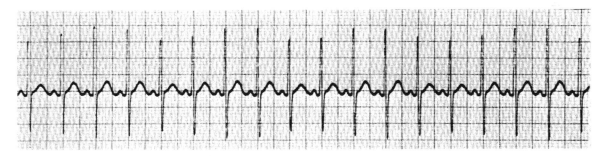

Sinus tachycardia in a three-year-old with an elevated temperature.

Some *culprits* that may be responsible for sinus tachycardia include agitation, fever, infection, anemia, hypovolemia, blood loss, low cardiac output, sepsis, decongestants, etc. The treatment for sinus tachycardia consists of *discovering the underlying cause and treating it!* As with all rapid rhythms, ventricular fill time is reduced, thus diminishing stroke volume and cardiac output. When related to hypovolemia, fluid replacement is the first line of treatment to restore hemodynamic stability.

Sinus Arrest

Sinus arrest or *sinus pause* is the result of momentary failure of the SA node to initiate an impulse. Since there is no SA stimulus, no atrial or subsequent ventricular activity occurs. So there's no _____ and no _____. (If you said P wave and QRS, you may go to the head of the class!) 🙂 The pause is usually of *short, but undetermined,* duration. Occasionally, an escape beat may interrupt the pause (a built-in safety device of the heart)! Let's take a look.

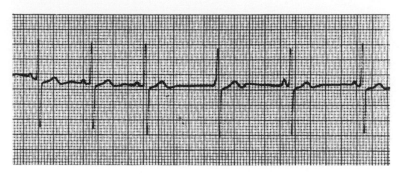

Notice the sinus pause following beat 3. A junctional escape beat interrupts the pause. The normal sinus pacemaker then resumes at a slower rate.

The specifics of *sinus arrest* are as follows:

- Baseline rate usually within normal bounds
- Rhythm irregular owing to pause(s)
- QRS follows every P wave; P-P interval regular and irregular
- QRS of normal duration, R-R interval regular and irregular

A close cousin of sinus arrest is *sinus block.* Although the sinus pacemaker fires on time, it is blocked somewhere within the conduction system . . . in other words, *it never gets out of the gate!* Usually the pause in sinus block is the duration of two normal sinus impulses as seen in the diagram below.

duration of 2 sinus impulses

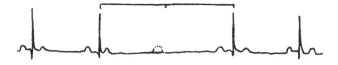

Sinus pause and sinus arrest are *most commonly caused* by increased vagal tone, hypoxia, and digitalis. Usually treatment is not required unless the pauses are pronounced or of frequent occurrence.

Sick Sinus Syndrome

Sick sinus syndrome was discussed back in Section 2. It is seen when the good ol' SA node fails to function as the dominant pacemaker of the heart. Consequently, one sees a variety of dysrhythmias that are *together* labeled as *sick sinus syndrome.* These dysrhythmias include:

- bradycardia
- SA block
- sinus arrest with junctional escape beats
- P.A.T. (remember paroxysmal atrial tachycardia?)
- slow or fast ectopic atrial or junctional rhythms

Though rare, sick sinus syndrome may be found in children who have undergone extensive cardiac surgery. This is especially true when the surgery involves the atria and atrial septum.

Oftentimes these children develop frequent episodes of tachycardia requiring drug therapy. Usually, the tachycardia episodes decrease as the child grows older. If bradycardia is pronounced, pacemaker therapy may be required.

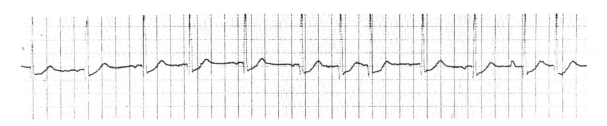

The above strip demonstrates a sick sinus syndrome, though the heart rate is within normal limits.

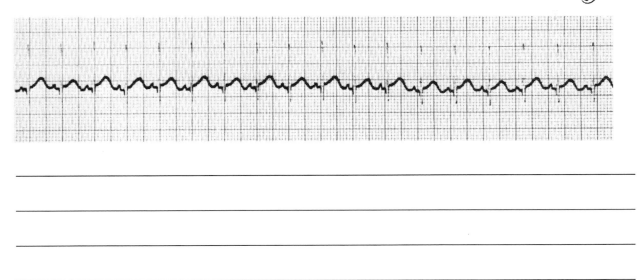

Practice Exercise 2

A. The easiest way to determine rhythm irregularity is to measure the P-P interval or the _____ interval.

B. Analyze the following rhythm strip. Bear in mind that the owner of this rhythm is six years old!

_____

_____

_____

_____

_____

C. Sinus bradycardia in a child is defined as a heart rate (circle the correct answer!)

less than 90
less than 70
less than 80
less than 60

 For Feedback 2, refer to page 392.

14.3 Atrial Dysrhythmias

With no further ado, we are going to begin exploring atrial dysrhythmias in children. You will remember that we are talking about pacemaker impulses that are generated in abnormal areas of the atria (outside the SA).

Atrial dysrhythmias are identified by P waves that may be premature or may vary in appearance from normal sinus P waves . . . or there may be multiple atrial deflections per QRS. Read on . . .

Premature Atrial Contractions (P.A.C.)

As the name implies, the P.A.C. is premature in its relationship to the sinus rhythm. You will recall that the premature P wave is different in appearance from the "normal" P wave.

Inspect this example!

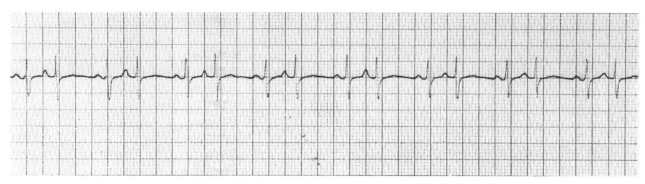

Look closely! Every other beat is a P.A.C. (Atrial Bigeminy). Notice that the P waves of the P.A.C.s look distinctly different from the sinus P waves.

Get out the check list. . . . **Rhythms interrupted by P.A.C.s have the following features:**

- Rate—usually normal rate . . . remember . . . the rate varies with age!
- Rhythm—irregular due to the interruption of the premature beats.
- P wave—of the P.A.C. is of different size and/or shape from normal P; P-R interval of normal beats is within normal limits; P-R of ectopic beats may vary from normal.
- QRS—normal duration; R-R interval irregular.
- Even though the P.A.C. is not initiated in the SA node, the SA node is depolarized by the early atrial activity. The SA node thinks it has done its job, so there is typically a "normal" R-R interval between the premature and following sinus beat (incomplete compensatory pause).

P.A.C.s are frequently observed in children with

- atrial enlargement
- electrolyte imbalances
- hypoxia
- hypoglycemia
- following atrial surgery

. . . and *surprise,* P.A.C.s are *common* in **healthy** children and newborns!!

The treatment of P.A.C.s depends on the underlying cause. If the cardiovascular system is healthy, no treatment is usually necessary. If the premature beats are frequent, multifocal, or seen in couplets (two or more together), continuous monitoring should be provided and a physician notified. Usually, digitalis or propranolol are the drugs of choice if treatment is deemed necessary.

Supraventricular Tachycardia (S.V.T.)

S.V.T. is the most common dysrhythmia of clinical significance encountered in pediatrics. One finds a hyperexcitable ectopic focus within the atria or junctional tissue discharging rapidly or, encounters a re-entry phenomenon. (If you need a "re-entry refresher," please review Section 2!) Basically, S.V.T. is a broad, descriptive category. In other words, when a definitive distinction cannot be made between atrial tachycardia and junctional tachycardia, the rhythm is termed *supraventricular tachycardia*. Supraventricular tachycardia has a sudden onset. And often, owing to the rapid rate, one cannot determine where in the cardiac cycle P waves are occurring (before, during, or after the QRS). Look at a strip of S.V.T.

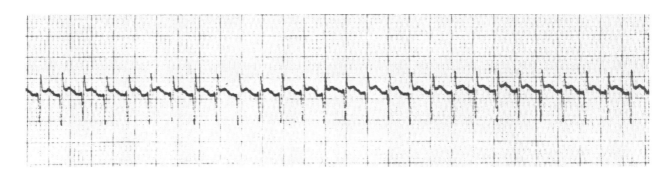

This rhythm strip demonstrates a supraventricular tachycardia at a rate near 300 beats per minute! It is impossible to determine whether the "bump" between QRSs is a P wave, a T wave, or both. In cases like this, the term supraventricular tachycardia is *most* appropriate! The term implies that the pacemaker is above the level of the ventricles. If the rhythm were ventricular in origin, the QRS would appear widened. (A widened QRS may occasionally be observed with a supraventricular rhythm, as well. This occurs when the AV conduction pathway has had insufficient time to recover between rapid fire stimulations, thus slowing ventricular depolarization. Slowed ventricular activation causes the QRS to widen.)

S.V.T. has the following identifying features:

- Ventricular rate—>220 in infants; >160 in children.
- P waves—difficult to distinguish owing to the rapid rate.
- QRS—usually normal in duration (the initiating pacemaker is somewhere above the ventricles).
- Abrupt onset and termination.
- Rate does not change with change in activity.

S.V.T. is *most often seen* in infants one to three months of age, but there are some *little ones* who like to begin life in the *fast lane* by demonstrating S.V.T. in utero. (Definitely type A personality babies!)

S.V.T. may also be associated with

- congenital heart disease
- infections
- following cardiac surgery
- adolescents—fatigue, stress, caffeine, tobacco, illicit drug use
- hypoxia
- hypovolemia
- hyperthermia
- Wolff-Parkinson-White (WPW) Syndrome
- no known reason—*unfortunately,* the greatest percentage!

The problem with S.V.T. is one we have already encountered *numerous* times—as demonstrated with the example of the toilet flushing in Section 2. The rapid ventricular rate causes decreased ventricular filling and thus, decreased cardiac output.

The treatment for S.V.T. depends on the severity of the episode. Sometimes the rhythm will spontaneously convert. Vagal stimulation (gagging, brief application of cold or ice water to the face) may convert stable S.V.T. to a sinus rhythm. When associated with cardiac compromise, more definitive treatment is required! Adenosine is the typical drug therapy of choice. If the situation is more acute, cardioversion may be used. (*0.5 to 1.0 joules per kg. of body weight.*) Whatever therapy can be accomplished most quickly should be initiated for S.V.T. with hemodynamic instability.

Atrial Tachycardia

First, a test of your short-term memory. Do you remember the *minimum* and *maximum* inherent rates of SA node discharge? Well, time's up . . . !

Age	Rate
0–1 month	100–180
1 year	80–180
5 years	70–150
10 years	60–125

In *atrial tachycardia,* the heart rate is usually in excess of 180 beats per minute, considerably *faster* than the inherent firing rate of the SA node (aren't you glad we reviewed those rate limits!). You will recall from Section 2, atrial tachycardia may be precipitated by (1) a single atrial ectopic site (P.A.C.) firing repeatedly, or (2) may result secondary to an aberrant circuitry within the atria, allowing an initiating ectopic stimulus (P.A.C.) to repeatedly re-enter and activate the atria in a circus-like fashion. (If you need a quick review of re-entry pathology, refer back to Section 2.

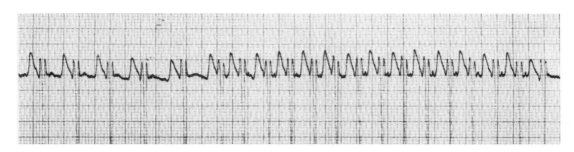

This rhythm strip demonstrates a child's sinus rhythm. The rhythm slows slightly after beat 4. Beat 6 initiates a burst of atrial tachycardia at a rate of approximately 200 per minute! Since there are definite P waves, we know the rhythm is atrial in orgin!

Atrial tachycardia has the following identifying features:

- Rate—greater than 220 beats/minute in infants less than 1 year; greater than 180 beats/minute in children.
- Rhythm—extremely regular; does not vary with change in activity.
- P wave—obvious before each QRS; if not obvious, but other features are met, the term supraventricular is utilized in lieu of atrial tachycardia.
- P-R may be prolonged owing to tissue refractoriness (the tissue must have sufficient recovery time if the next impulse is to conduct normally).
- QRS—usually of normal duration.

Atrial tachycardia with sudden onset is termed paroxysmal atrial tachycardia (P.A.T.). The term S.V.T., as above, is used more commonly in pediatrics. In essence, there is little difference between P.A.T. and S.V.T.; however, P.A.T. requires visible and identifiable P waves. The treatment for S.V.T. and P.A.T. is the same: Vagal maneuvers can be attempted for stable atrial tachycardias, synchronized cardioversion or IV adenosine for unstable atrial tachycardias.

Atrial Flutter

Remember the "Jaws" movies? Well, for those of you who are too young, or who have better taste in movies, sharks have a *sawtooth* type fin that protrudes above the water. Atrial flutter resembles a *convention of all Pacific coast great white sharks*—multiple sawtooth waves (sawteeth) with QRSs interspersed.

A Convention of Great White Sharks

Do not color sharks . . . ⟶   ← Water (Pacific Ocean)
they are white   Color this blue

P.S. We must humor the author . . .

Atrial flutter arises from an excitable ectopic site within the atria or occurs secondary to an anomalous atrial re-entry circuit. The atrial flutter rate is *usually* 240–360 beats per minute! However, not all of those impulses are passed through the AV junction. Commonly, one sees a 2:1, 3:1, or 4:1 conduction i.e., one QRS per four sawtooth waves). The sawtooth waves are flutter waves.

Atrial flutter has the following characteristics:

- Atrial rate 240–360 . . . therefore, the ventricular rate is usually ½, ⅓, or ¼, of 240–360.
- Atrial rhythm—regular.
- P waves—rather than P waves, there are continuous flutter waves.
- QRS is of normal duration; R-R interval may be regular or irregular depending upon the degree of physiologic block in the AV junction.
- Atrial and ventricular activity are related because the interval between a conducted flutter wave and its QRS is always constant.

> **NOTE:** Flutter waves may cause distortion of the QRS, ST segment and T wave, owing to their continuous nature.

Atrial flutter is seen *rarely* in children, but may be associated with

- chronic, severe rheumatic fever
- sick sinus syndrome
- hypoxia
- hypoglycemia
- following intra-atrial surgery

The following strip at the top of page 368 demonstrates a 2:1 atrial flutter . . . sometimes it's difficult to identify flutter waves. Try looking at the strip upside down to better view the flutter waves!

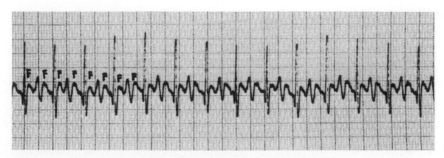

The atrial rhythm is regular at a rate of 300 per minute. Note the "SHARK" waves!

The object of treatment is to reduce the rapid ventricular response rate and restore the normal sinus mechanism. (A rapid ventricular rate reduces cardiac output owing to the reduced ventricular fill time.) With hemodynamic instability, synchronized cardioversion may be the initial treatment of choice. Digoxin and/or beta blockers can be used for chronic therapy.

Atrial Fibrillation

In *atrial fibrillation* there are no P waves, just bizarre, irregular, rapid deflections which distort the baseline. (The baseline *undulates* . . . remember?) The atrial activity has no rhythmic pattern. See for yourself!

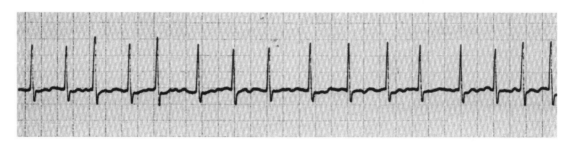

Note the varying R-R interval of atrial fibrillation.

You will notice that there is no coordinated effort in the atria. Some parts of the atria are in a state of excitation and some are refractory.

The specifics of atrial fibrillation include the following characteristics:

- Atrial rate—400–600 per minute (but who's counting—who could count that!).
- Rhythm—irregularly irregular (everything is irregular).
- P waves—none present; instead, wavy baseline.
- QRS duration normal, but the R-R interval varies continuously.
- Ventricular rate—usually rapid and irregular in uncontrolled atrial fibrillation.

In children, one may see atrial fibrillation associated with

- electrolyte imbalance
- hypoglycemia
- hyperthyroidism
- intra-atrial surgery
- structural heart defects

As with the adult, treatment is aimed at *reducing the rapid ventricular rate* and restoring sinus rhythm. When the ventricular rate is rapid, there is a reduced cardiac output owing to the decreased ventricular fill time. Similar to other rapid atrial dysrhythmias, cardioversion may be the first line of treatment, depending upon the child's tolerance of the dysrhythmia!

Wandering Atrial Pacemaker (W.A.P.)

The name says it all . . . the atrial pacemaker wanders! There is a gradual shifting between the SA node and other ectopic atrial foci to be the "big cheese" (site of impulse formation). A wandering atrial pacemaker may result when there is a slight slowing of the SA node impulse formation or when various sites within the atria have similar intrinsic rates.

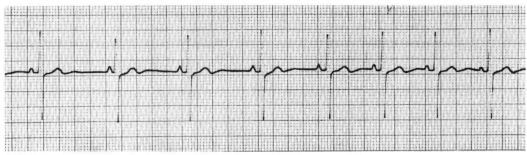

Notice the changing appearance of the P waves, the slight variation in the P-R interval and the variable heart rate.

The following are criteria which assist in identifying a wandering atrial pacemaker:

- Rate—within normal limits.
- Rhythm—slightly irregular.
- P wave—constantly changing, may be SA, atrial, or junctional in origin (if the pacemaker wanders out of the atria), or may not be visible. P-P interval irregular.
- P-R interval—varies continuously (though the variation is seldom marked).
- QRSs—are related to all P waves; QRS duration within normal limits.

Usually a wandering atrial pacemaker is a benign dysrhythmia and frequently is seen in *otherwise* healthy children. However, it may also be associated with the following conditions:

- acute rheumatic fever
- increased vagal tone (i.e., increased intracranial pressure, hypertension, etc.)
- drugs—digitalis, propranolol

No treatment is required when a wandering atrial pacemaker is found in a healthy child. When associated with other clinical conditions, it is the underlying clinical problem that may require treatment.

Practice Exercise 3

A. The aims of treatment for any rapid atrial dysrhythmia (i.e., S.V.T.) are:

1. _____

2. _____

B. What are the identifying characteristics of a premature atrial contraction?

1. _____

2. _____

3. _____

C. Analyze this strip:

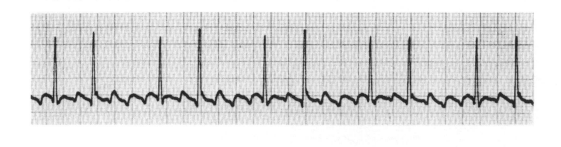

_____

_____

_____

_____

_____

D. Describe the identifying features of a wandering atrial pacemaker.

_____

_____

_____

_____

E. Describe the treatment for supraventricular tachycardia?

_____

_____

_____

_____

For Feedback 3, refer to page 392.

input section 14.4 Junctional Dysrhythmias and Rhythms

A little *junctional escape rhythm lore*—

Any cell within the heart can be a potential pacemaker. This includes the SA node, the atria, the AV junctional tissue, and the ventricles. Only the dominant or fastest pacemaker will normally control the heart rate. If the sinus pacemaker fails to fire, *or* if the impulse fails to be conducted, *or* if the sinus node discharges impulses slowly, a lower, more distal pacemaker will assume the role of pacemaker. Whew!

Junctional Escape Rhythm

If a rhythm originates in the AV junctional tissue, it is known as a *junctional escape rhythm* or an *idiojunctional rhythm*.

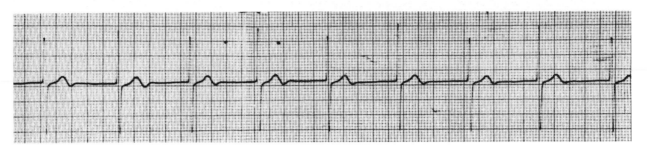

This strip demonstrates a junctional escape rhythm in a five-year-old female. The heart rate is approximately 64 per minute. Notice that there are no visible P waves occurring before or after the QRS. In this example, the atria and ventricles are being activated at approximately the same time ... thus, the P wave is *hiding* within the QRS. (If you need a refresher on hiding P waves, turn back to Section 3.)

The specifics of junctional escape rhythms:

- Ventricular rate—usually 50–90 in infants and 50–70 in children, though rates vary.
- Rhythm—regular ... (escape rhythms are almost always regular).
- P—may be observed before or after the QRS ... or may be hiding within the QRS. If visible, P waves will be inverted in leads II, III, and aVF. (If you need a refresher, refer back to Section 3.)
- QRS—duration normal.

How could this happen, you ask??? **A junctional escape rhythm may be associated with the following conditions:**

- children who have an otherwise normal heart
- sick sinus syndrome
- increased vagal tone
- following atrial surgery and/or any open heart surgery

If the ventricular rate is adequate, treatment is usually not necessary. Remember, however, not only does the slower heart rate compromise the child, so does the loss of *atrial kick*. Therefore, if the child is hemodynamically compromised, increasing heart rate with epinephrine, atropine or pacing may be necessary.

Junctional Escape Beats

A *junctional escape beat* is an impulse arising from the junctional tissue due to an interruption of the sinus pacemaker. Junctional escape beats will come later than anticipated normal beats (better late than never!). If a P wave is present, it does not initiate the junctional beat, and can occur before or after the QRS ... or be buried in the QRS.

The following tracing demonstrates a slowing of the sinus pacemaker which allows two junctional escape beats to come through. Remember ... escape beats will always come later in the cardiac cycle than anticipated normal beats.

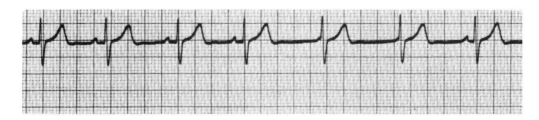

Single, infrequent junctional escape beats have no real significance. If the SA node persistently fires slowly or if the sinus impulse fails to conduct, a sustained AV junctional rhythm may be observed as demonstrated on page 371. Remember, escape beats or escape rhythms are *never* a primary phenomenon . . . they are *always* secondary to another event. They occur because of failure or disruption of the sinus apparatus. So, you would never want to eradicate escape beats or escape rhythms. It's the proverbial "you don't bite the hand that feeds you."

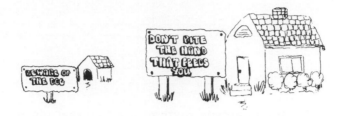

Premature Junctional Contractions (P.J.C.s)

Like P.A.C.s, *premature junctional beats* arise from an excitable focus. The P.J.C. arises within the AV junction, outside the normal conduction cycle, interrupting the underlying rhythm. The premature beats cause the rhythm to appear irregular. As with junctional ectopic beats, if a P wave is present, it may occur before, during, or after the QRS. There may also be retrograde conduction of the junctional impluse upwards to the atria causing a retrograde P wave. If you need a review of antegrade v.s. retrograde conduction, check out Section 3! Typically, the QRS duration of the premature beat is within normal limits.

Single, infrequent P.J.C.s in otherwise healthy children have no clinical significance. They may also be associated with

- surgery near the AV junction
- hypoxic conditions
- hypoglycemia

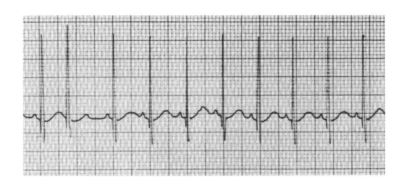

Look closely at the above strip! Beat 2 is a P.J.C. that interrupts the otherwise normal rhythm. In this instance, the P wave of the P.J.C. is "hiding" in the QRS.

Usually P.J.C.s require no treatment, though it is important to note their presence and frequency.

Junctional Tachycardia

In *junctional tachycardia*, a hyperirritable ectopic focus within the AV junction assumes control of the rhythm owing to its rapid rate of discharge . . . usually 160–200 discharges per minute. Junctional tachycardia may result after surgery near the AV node, or be associated with digitalis toxicity or myocarditis. You will remember that the patient with junctional tachycardia experiences a reduced cardiac output from both the rapid ventricular rate and the loss of atrial kick. Atrial activation must be synchronized with ventricular activation to maximize cardiac output!

Let's look at an example of junctional tachycardia.

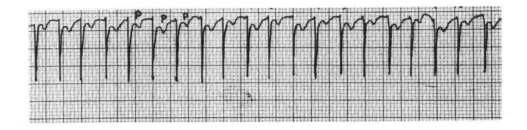

You will notice in this strip, retrograde P waves follow the QRSs indicating that ventricular activation precedes atrial activation. This is a junctional tachycardia with a rate of approximately 200 per minute.

Junctional tachycardia will have the following characteristics:

- Rate—160–220.
- Rhythm—regular (usually).
- P waves—may not be visible (buried in the QRS), or are inverted occurring before or after the QRS. **Often because it is difficult to establish definitive P waves, these rhythms are called supraventricular tachycardias.**
- P-R interval—if an inverted P wave occurs before the QRS, the P-R will be shorter than the lower limits of normal.
- QRS is usually of normal duration.

Treatment is aimed at decreasing the rapid ventricular heart rate and restoring the sinus pacemaker. If rapid treatment is required due to a deteriorating clinical condition, synchronized cardioversion is the treatment of choice (*0.5 to 1.0 joules per kg. of body weight*).

Anticipating that your energy may be on the downslope, practice exercise 4 will be relatively short!

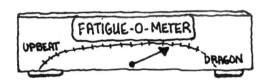

Practice Exercise 4

A. What is the difference between a junctional tachycardia and an atrial tachycardia? _____

_____

_____

_____

_____

_____

B. What is happening in this strip, and why?

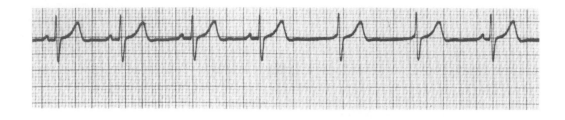

_____

_____

_____

_____

For Feedback 4, refer to page 393.

input section 14.5 **Ventricular Dysrhythmias**

Well, you're still with us, and I believe the worst—meaning the most confusing—may be behind us!

Premature Ventricular Contractions (P.V.C.s)

P.V.C.s are extra beats arising in an excitable focus or site somewhere in either ventricle (outside the normal conduction system). There is no failure of the normal rhythm, merely additional beats arising from an irritable site or focus.

Rhythms displaying P.V.C.s typically have the following features:

- Rate—within normal limits for age group.
- Rhythm—underlying rhythm usually regular, interrupted by premature beats.
- P waves—no P wave visible prior to the abnormal QRS; may be a P wave following the abnormal QRS. Do you remember why? For a thorough explanation, see page 107.
- QRS—the QRS of the P.V.C. is wide and *bizarre* in relation to the other QRS complexes. You will remember that the QRS is wide because the premature impulse originates and travels outside the normal conduction system. Thus, conduction is slow!
- T wave—the T wave of the P.V.C. usually appears directionally opposite to the T wave of the normal QRS. In addition, there may be a full compensatory pause following the P.V.C.!

Let's look at some pint-size P.V.C.s!

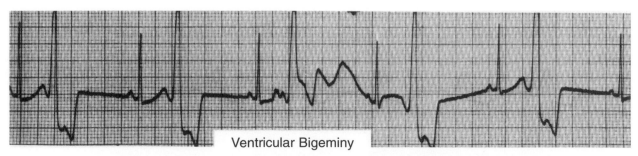

Ventricular Bigeminy

This strip is interesting! Notice the artifact that disrupts the baseline midstrip.
Ventricular Bigeminy is the order of the day!

The following two rhythm strips demonstrate frequent P.V.C.s and short bursts of ventricular tachycardia. These strips were taken from a thirteen year old overdose victim!

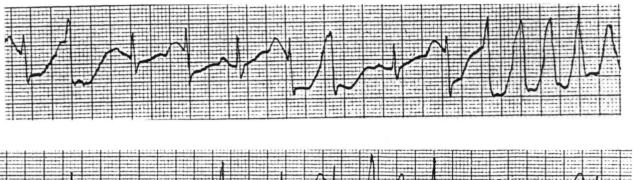

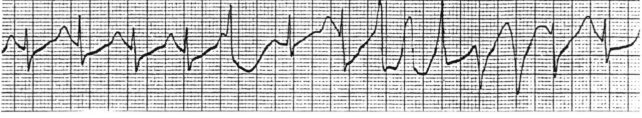

One may observe P.V.C.s in children with

- normal hearts
- congenital heart disease
- drug intoxication (e.g., digitalis)
- electrolyte imbalance
- hypoxia—of the patient or of the myocardium
- hypoglycemia

In a healthy child, occasional P.V.C.s are relatively harmless. When *associated* with an underlying cardiac condition, P.V.C.s represent *ventricular irritability* and may be the forerunner of ventricular tachycardia or ventricular fibrillation. *Not a good way to go!!* Additionally, multiformed, coupled, and frequent P.V.C.s and P.V.C.s precipitated by activity are usually significant. Treating any underlying causative factors as well as the P.V.C.s is indicated

P.V.C.s are usually treated with amiodarone (5mg/kg IV over 30–60 minutes) or lidocaine. Lidocaine therapy involves an initial loading dose—usually 1 mg/kg body weight, followed by a continuous drip (20 µg/kg/minute).

Ventricular Tachycardia

The following strip demonstrates ventricular tachycardia with a rate of slightly greater than 200 beats per minute.

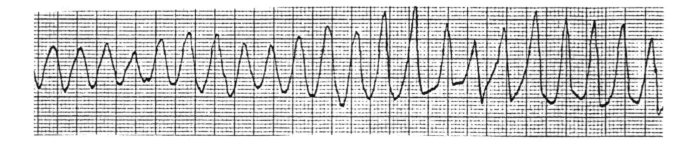

It is important to assess whether the patient has a pulse associated with these wide, aberrant QRSs. We will not dwell on *ventricular tachycardia* long, not because it isn't important, but because it is a *rare* finding in children. Typically, this rhythm rapidly deteriorates to ventricular fibrillation.

Identifying features of ventricular tachycardia:

- Ventricular rate—slower than P.S.V.T., usually 120–180.
- Rhythm—basically regular.
- P waves—usually not visible. (If visible, they bear no relationship to QRSs.)
- Wide slurred QRSs.

You may find ventricular tachycardia associated with

- hypoxemia
- hypovolemia
- severe digitalis toxicity
- myocarditis
- severe electrolyte imbalance and metabolic disorders
- anesthesia
- following cardiac surgery
- hypothermia
- thromboembolism

Amiodarone is the drug treatment of choice, although lidocaine may also be used. Magnesium sulfate should be administered if serum levels are low.

If drug therapy is ineffective, synchronized cardioversion should be instituted. You will remember that the usual current setting for cardioversion is *0.5 to 1.0 joules per kg. of body weight.* In severely compromised situations, cardioversion may be the first line of intervention. Treatment will also be aimed at correcting the underlying disorder.

Ventricular Flutter

Ventricular flutter is most commonly a brief *transition rhythm* from ventricular tachycardia to ventricular fibrillation. In ventricular flutter, cardiac output is minimal owing to the rapid, feeble ventricular contractions!

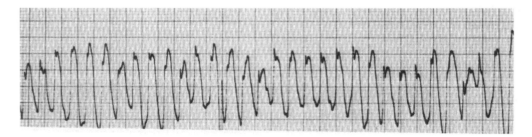

Ventricular flutter, rate 300 per minute.

Usually, the ventricular flutter rate is greater than 200 beats per minute. Ventricular flutter represents a *true* medical emergency. CPR and immediate cardioversion are the treatments of choice if the rhythm persists. Owing to its transition nature, however, immediate defibrillation may be employed.

Ventricular Fibrillation

Well, you ask, *what could be worse than ventricular flutter?* The answer, *ventricular fibrillation! Ventricular fibrillation* represents chaotic, uncoordinated ventricular depolarization. There is *no* effective cardiac output. In effect, the fibrillating heart muscle quivers, but there is *no coordinated* ventricular activity. Death will occur in minutes without emergency intervention.

One usually observes P.V.C.s or some evidence of myocardial irritability prior to ventricular fibrillation.

Ventricular fibrillation may be associated with

- hypoxia
- digitalis or quinidine intoxication
- anesthesia
- chest trauma
- cardiac catheterization
- hypothermia
- drug overdose
- severe electrolyte imbalance
- hypothermia

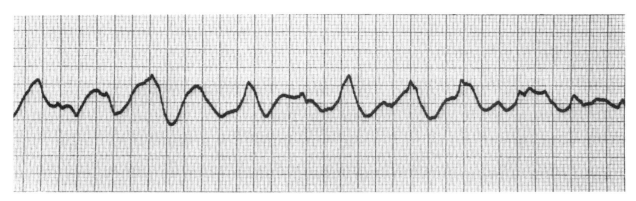

Coarse ventricular fibrillation

In ventricular fibrillation, one finds:

- Rate—no pulse.
- Rhythm—irregular, fluctuating baseline with no P, QRS, or T waves.

Ventricular fibrillation is a *medical emergency*. The treatment for ventricular fibrillation is CPR and defibrillation (two joules per kg) followed by intravenous amiodarone or lidocaine. If a normal sinus rhythm resumes, usually prophylactic drug therapy is initiated and the underlying electrolyte factors corrected.

> **NOTE:** Ventricular fibrillation is a **rare** finding in children. More commonly, terminal rhythms are bradycardic in nature.

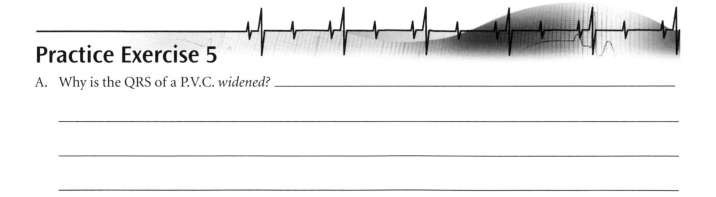

Practice Exercise 5

A. Why is the QRS of a P.V.C. *widened?* _____

_____

_____

_____

B. Ventricular fibrillation is a common / uncommon finding in children (circle one).

C. Draw a strip demonstrating ventricular fibrillation.

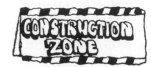

D. If electrical intervention is required for ventricular fibrillation one would use *synchronized cardioversion or defibrillation*. Why? _____

_____

_____

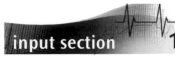 **For Feedback 5, refer to page 393.**

input section 14.6 **Complex Dysrhythmias**

Pulseless Electrical Activity (PEA)

Pulseless Electrical Activity (PEA) was previously known as electrical-mechanical dissociation (EMD). Essentially, meaningful cardiac contractions are absent, though cardiac electrical activity (wave forms) is present on the monitor. Cardiac contraction and perfusion does not follow electrical activity. The patient is pulseless, thus immediate CPR is required!

You will recall, in adults PEA is frequently the end result of cardiac insult caused by hypoxia and respiratory failure. **In children, the most common causes of PEA include:**

- severe hypovolemia
- prolonged hypoxia
- severe acidosis
- electrolyte imbalance
- hypothermia

- pulmonary embolism
- tension pneumothorax
- cardiac tamponade
- toxic ingestions

Initial treatment for PEA is high quality CPR. Treatment for PEA with visible ventricular tachycardia (VT) or ventricular fibrillation (VF) wave forms includes defibrillation (initially 2 J/kg). If ineffective, epinephrine is administered followed by repeat attempts to defibrillate. Antiarrhythmics, including amiodarone, may also be administered. Treatment for PEA associated with other visible rhythms or wave forms involves the administration of epinephrine in attempt to augment both the heart rate and myocardial contractility. Initial treatment (during the resuscitation procedure) must also focus on the identification and correction of the underlying causative condition(s).

There are four points to remember about PEA:

1. PEA is a descriptive classification rather than a distinct rhythm.
2. Pulselessness is a medical emergency requiring immediate CPR.
3. Visualization of a monitor rhythm does not assure patient well-being.
4. An underlying clinical condition(s) is responsible for PEA.

Inherited Long QT Syndrome (LQTS)

You will recall that the QT interval represents the total time for ventricular depolarization and repolarization. It encompasses the entirety of ventricular refractoriness (time when the ventricular myocardium is immune to further stimulation). On page 355, it was noted that in infants less than 6 months of age, the maximum QT interval is 0.45 seconds. In adolescents, the maximum QT interval is 0.425 seconds.

A prolongation of the QT interval (prolonged refractoriness) can be caused by drug effects or electrolyte imbalances. This type of QT prolongation is known as *acquired* long QT syndrome. It can also occur as an inherited disorder (*inherited or congenital long QT syndrome*). It is the inherited type that is commonly abbreviated LQTS. The inherited disorder is thought to relate to a mutation in genes that control sodium and potassium channels.

The presence of LQTS predisposes *the owner* to torsades de pointes (TdP) or polymorphic ventricular tachycardia which may lead to ventricular fibrillation and sudden death (refer to page 123 for a scholarly discussion of TdP! 😕) Though LQTS is believed to be relatively rare, children may present in the ER with syncopy, fainting or post cardiac arrest, and with no previous history of problems. Inconclusive, qualitative research has attempted to relate SIDS to LQTS.

In the presence of LQTS, dysrhythmias may be precipitated by the proarrhythmic effects of certain drugs (including certain bronchodilators and antibiotics), by adrenergic stimuli (like exercise or emotional upset) . . . or dysrhythmias may occur with no known precipitating event or condition! Unfortunately, congenital LQTS is often first identified after a ventricular fibrillation event.

Any concerns for LQTS should be immediately referred to a pediatric cardiologist or electrophysiologist for evaluation. There is no definitive treatment for long QT syndrome. Beta blockers may be utilized; an implantable defibrillator may be surgically implanted. Activities will be limited. The risk of sudden death persists despite therapy. Relatives of persons identified to have long QTS should be screened as well. Family members of the patient with LQTS must know CPR and use of the AED.

Now, on to complex practice!

Practice Exercise 6

A. Explain a PEA rhythm.

_____

_____

_____

_____

_____

B. Check (X) all of the true statements about QT intervals and LQTS.

❑ LQTS may predispose a child to polymorphic ventricular tachycardia.

❑ Pedi QT intervals vary principally with age.

❑ The QT interval represents the ventricular refractory period.

❑ LQTS is a genetic disorder.

For Feedback 6, refer to page 393.

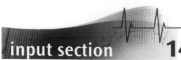

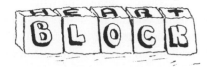

Conduction disturbances are defined as *delays,* or worse still, sometimes *failure* of impulse conduction through the AV junction, through the bundle of His, down the bundle branches to the Purkinje fibers. There are three levels of heart block: first degree heart block; second degree heart block; and, third degree heart block. (Clever names, huh?)

First Degree Heart Block

The only abnormality observed in *first degree heart block* is a prolonged P-R interval. Simple enough, huh!!

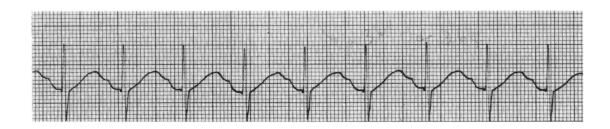

The above rhythm strip belongs to a five year old boy taking digitalis. Though it is somewhat difficult to measure here, the P-R measures approximately 0.18 seconds. A normal P-R interval for a five year old is 0.10–0.16 seconds. (If in doubt, check out the Pediatric P-R Interval chart on page 354.) So, for this little guy, we have a first degree AV block!

First degree AV block has the following identifying features:

*   Rate—normal for age group
*   Rhythm—usually regular
*   P waves—normal in appearance and duration; P-R interval prolonged (remember, the duration of the normal P-R interval *varies with age*)
*   QRS—normal duration

First degree heart **block may be associated with**

*   increased vagal tone (e.g., increased intracranial pressure, hypertension, gastric dilatation)
*   rheumatic fever
*   atrial septal defect
*   structural heart disease
*   following myocardia surgery
*   digitalis toxicity

First degree heart block usually does not require treatment. In infants, digitalis may be held if prolongation of the P-R interval is seen on the digitalis *predose* rhythm strip, or if, during the administration of digitalis, the P-R continues to increase in duration.

Well, that wasn't too complicated. Let's try second degree heart block. . . .

Second Degree Heart Block Mobitz Type I Second Degree Heart Block

In *Mobitz type I,* or *Wenckebach phenomenon,* there is a progressive prolongation of the P-R interval until a P wave is finally blocked (not conducted). In Wenckebach, as the P-R interval lengthens, the R-R interval shortens! Wenckebach may be observed in otherwise normal hearts or may be associated with underlying heart disease. There are several subsets of second degree blocks. Second degree blocks are characterized by at least some dropped beats; i.e., some P waves are not followed by QRS complexes.

The following are some of the *more frequent* causes of Wenckebach or Mobitz type I second degree heart block in children:

- increased vagal tone
- myocarditis
- structural congenital disease
- cardiac surgery near the AV junction
- digitalis toxicity

Let's have a look! Following is a strip of a four year old following recent atrial surgery.

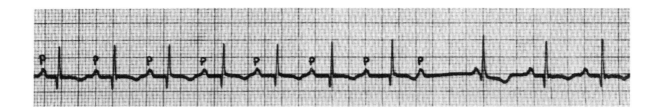

Notice (above) that the P-R interval lengthens until a P wave is finally blocked or not conducted. Let's analyze the above strip!

1. The heart rate is within normal limits, which is common.

2. The rhythm is irregular. If you look closely, you will notice that the non-conducted P wave principally accounts for the irregularity.

3. The P-R and R-R interval progressively lengthens until the P wave fails to conduct.

4. The duration of the QRSs are normal since there is no interference with ventricular activation.

Usually Wenckebach, or Mobitz type I, requires no treatment per se. Treatment is directed at the underlying cause.

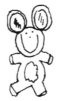

Would you believe me if I told you I had a teddy bear named WENCKEBACH?

2:1 (or higher) AV Block

In this type of block, a ventricular complex follows every second, third, or fourth P wave due to a block in conduction at the level of the AV node indicating 2:1, 3:1, or 4:1 block. The P-P interval is normal for age, as is the P-R interval of the conducted beats. The P waves are uniform and the ventricular rate is low.

Study the following rhythm strip **carefully!**

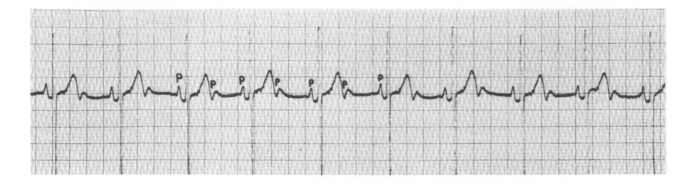

The above rhythm strip belongs to a ten day old infant, two days post cardiac surgery to correct a structural anomaly. Notice that the ventricular rhythm is regular at a rate of 75 beats per minute. There are two distinct P waves for every QRS. HOWEVER, the morphology of the conducting P wave is different from the non-conducting P wave. The P-R interval of the conducted beats is constant. In a *textbook* 2:1 AV conduction pattern, one would expect all P waves to be uniform in appearance and to occur regularly (constant P–P interval) throughout the strip. Here, there is variation in the P–P interval. So . . . while this rhythm represents a 2:1 conduction pattern, it is atypical. (Likely, this rhythm is a multifocal atrial tachycardia with a bigeminal block pattern . . . or, an atrial tachycardia with bigeminal blocked P.A.C.s!)

This rhythm strip is included to emphasize the importance of analyzing all facets of a rhythm and to reinforce the value of an accurate description (rather than struggling with naming terminology)!

In a true 2:1 conduction pattern, *the P-R interval of the conducted beats will always be constant.* By contrast, in a third degree heart block, the interval between the P wave and the QRS will always vary, since there is no relationship between atrial and ventricular activity (see below, complete Heart Block).

Mobitz Type II Second Degree Heart Block

Mobitz type II is a *rare* finding in children. For that reason, we will not address the subject here. However, the *finer* identifying features of Mobitz type II (adult version), are discussed on page 146. Should Mobitz type II be observed in children, it is usually related to surgery on or near the bundle of His or the bifurcation of the bundle branches. Cardiac pacing may be considered.

Third Degree Heart Block (*AKA Complete Heart Block)

In *third degree heart block,* all atrial impulses are blocked from reaching and activating the ventricular system. None of the atrial impulses are conducted through to the ventricles to initiate ventricular depolarization. Though the sinus mechanism fires at a normal regular rate and activates the atria normally, none of the impulses reach the ventricular conduction system. Lower pacemakers sense the absence of sinus impulses, so . . . as a self-protection mechanism, a lower, more distal pacemaker assumes control of the heart (*self-preservation* you might say). The lower (escape) pacemaker may be initiated from either the junctional or ventricular tissue.

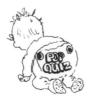

Circle the correct answer on the Pop Quiz found on the next page!

---

* AKA = *Also known as*

POP QUIZ!

1. If an escape rhythm is initiated in the AV junction, the QRS complexes will usually be:

   ❏ widened   ❏ normal duration

2. If the escape rhythm is initiated in the ventricles, the resulting QRS complexes will be:

   ❏ widened   ❏ normal duration

If you answered *of normal duration* to question number 1, go to the head of the class! If you answered *widened,* go to page 370 for some quick review.

All right, down to facts. We have a regular sinus P wave representing atrial depolarization, but then going nowhere . . .

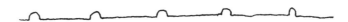

an escape rhythm originating in either the junctional tissue . . .

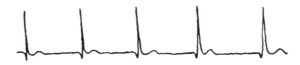

or ventricular tissue. . .

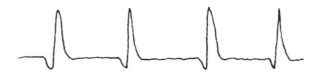

When the atrial activity is combined with the escape mechanism, you will see evidence of the *two independent pacemakers*—the atrial pacemaker and the junctional, or ventricular, pacemaker. These two pacemakers are *totally independent* of one another. In other words, the electrical and mechanical activity is unrelated or dissociated (hence, the term *AV dissociation*).

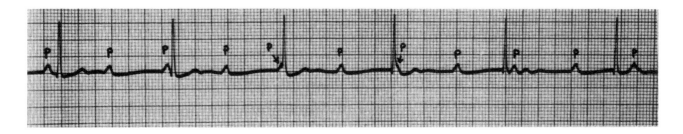

In the above rhythm strip, you will notice that the atria and the ventricles function independently. The atrial activity occurs regularly at a rate of 83 per minute. The ventricular activity is regular, but slower at a rate of 44 per minute. Atrial activity is unrelated to ventricular activity . . . *how do I know,* you ask. Look at the P-R interval . . . it *always* varies. *This variation implies AV dissociation.* (AV dissociation is a descriptive term meaning that the atrial and ventricular activity occur independent of one another!) Often, the P waves are said to be *marching through the rhythm!*

Third degree heart block has the following identifying features:

- The atrial and ventricular activity occur in a regular pattern.
- Atrial and ventricular rates are different, the atrial rate being faster than the ventricular rate (the atrial rate is usually normal for the age category).
- Atrial and ventricular activation are independent of one another. Therefore, the P-R interval is *never* constant.
- The ventricular rate is slow and regular.
- The QRS may be narrow (junctional) or widened (ventricular).

Complete heart block may be associated with the following conditions:

- congenital cardiac disease
- following cardiac surgery
- myocarditis
- digitalis toxicity

The aim of treatment is to restore hemodynamic equilibrium and an adequate ventricular rate. If ventricular activation is initiated by a junctional pacemaker, atropine may be the treatment of choice. Atropine inhibits vagal effect and, therefore, may speed up the junctional rate. Atropine *will not* eliminate the heart block . . . it may simply increase the rate of the junctional escape pacemaker! If the ventricles are activated by a ventricular pacemaker (widened QRS), epinephrine may be administered or external pacing may be initiated.

Occasionally, third degree heart block presents as a congenital anomaly, often associated with maternal lupus. Though certain infants develop congestive heart failure, others adjust to the slow ventricular rate through compensatory mechanisms (such as chamber hypertrophy and increased stroke volume).

Bundle Branch Block

Our section on blocks would be incomplete if we did not discuss bundle branch blocks. You will remember that the conduction system consists of three fascicles. For a quick review of right and left bundle branch conduction defects, turn back to page 156.

Right Bundle Branch Block

Right bundle branch block is the most common form of ventricular conduction disturbance seen in children. Commonly, however, the right bundle branch is intact. The delayed right ventricular activation is often due to *structural heart disease* that result in right ventricular volume overload (e.g., atrial septal defect). This volume overload and subsequent stretching of the right ventricle results in slower right ventricular activation!

In other cases, right bundle branch block patterns result secondary to right ventricular surgery, such as the repair of Tetralogy of Fallot. In most instances, there is interruption of the Purkinje system rather than the right bundle branch. Just thought you might want to know that!

Unlike the adult patient, the rsR' or "M" pattern is a common finding in a *healthy juvenile EKG specimen*, though the QRS is within normal limits! If you have forgotten the normal pediatric QRS durations, you may want to review page 355. However, in a right bundle branch block, you can expect to see:

Right Bundle Branch Block Criteria

- rsR' in lead V_1
- QRS duration greater than the upper limits of normal for age
- wide, slurred S wave in lead I, V_5, and V_6

Take a look!

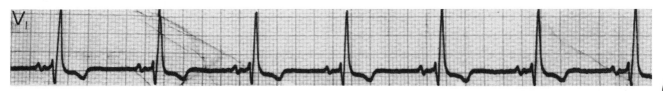

This is a sixteen-year-old female with right ventricular hypertrophy and a right bundle branch block. The heart rate is 62 per minute.

Left Bundle Branch Block

Left bundle branch block is extremely rare in children . . . in fact, so rare that we could not find a single example! We are told, however, that should *you* come across a *true* left bundle branch block, you can expect to see:

- wide S waves in leads V1 and V2
- QRS duration greater than the upper limits of normal for age
- slurred and wide R waves in I, aVL, V_5, and V_6
- QRS voltage may be larger than normal because of asynchronous depolarization of the ventricles

So much for bundle branch blocks . . . right? Carry on!

Practice Dead Ahead . . .

Practice Exercise 7

A. Describe the abnormality in this strip and the probable treatment. This is a five-year-old female with congestive failure.

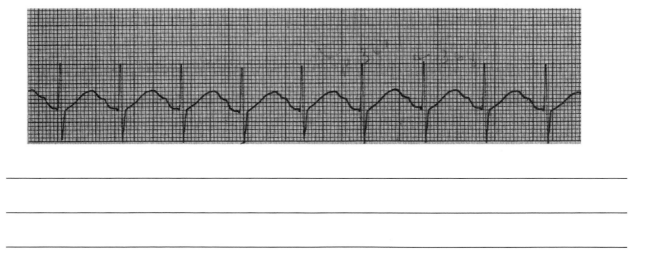

_____

_____

_____

_____

B. Draw a picture of Mobitz type I (Wenckebach).

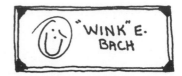

"WINK" E. BACH

C. This rhythm strip demonstrates complete heart block. Describe the findings that support a complete heart block classification.

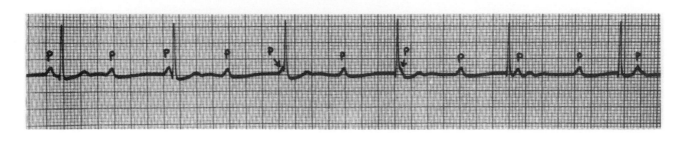

_____

_____

_____

_____

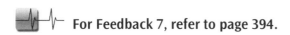 **For Feedback 7, refer to page 394.**

For Feedback 7, refer to page 394.

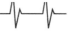

input section ## 14.8 **Drug and Electrolyte Induced Dysrhythmias**

Potassium (K^+) norms vary in accordance with chemistry analyzers and collection techniques. One should *always* verify accepted norm ranges in any pediatric setting!

Relative Serum Potassium Value

Age	Potassium Level Norms
Premie	4.0–7.2 mEq. per liter
Full term	3.0–7.0 mEq. per liter
2 days–3 mos.	3.5–6.0 mEq. per liter
3 mos.–1 year	3.6–5.6 mEq. per liter
1–16 years	3.5–5.0 mEq. per liter

You will remember from earlier sections, potassium (K^+) ions play an important role in the repolarization activities of the myocardial cells. Since the T wave represents repolarization, look for changes in the EKG near the T wave.

Hypokalemia

Hypokalemia is the term used for potassium levels below the suggested low norm. On the EKG, hypokalemia may produce *depressed ST segments, flat or diphasic T waves,* and *prominent U waves.*

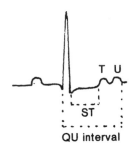

You will remember that the U wave is thought to represent late repolarization of the Purkinje fibers. Because of this add-on feature (the U wave), the QT interval appears prolonged. In reality, there is now a QU interval!

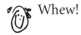 Whew!

Hypokalemia most commonly results from vomiting, diarrhea, or diuretic therapy. **Hypokalemia causes electrical instability** and may produce any of the following dysrhythmias:

- P.V.C.s
- atrial tachycardia or P.A.T.
- junctional tachycardia
- supraventricular tachycardia or P.S.V.T.
- ventricular tachycardia
- ventricular fibrillation

Unfortunately, U waves are *difficult* to spot . . . and we did not spot any! Usually, when an extreme hypokalemia is confirmed by lab values, one may be able to go back to a 12 lead EKG and discern U waves . . . though the U waves are never evident in all leads.

Happy Hunting!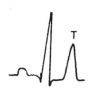

Treatment for hypokalemia involves the administration of potassium supplement, oral or intravenous, depending upon the severity of the hypokalemia.

Hyperkalemia

Hyperkalemia is the term used for potassium levels that exceed the upper limits of the suggested norms (refer back to the table, page 386).

In mild hyperkalemia, tall, peaked T waves may be observed.

As potassium levels increase, the QRS widens, the P-R interval prolongs, and P waves may disappear.

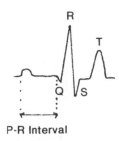

P-R Interval

In pronounced cases of hyperkalemia, ventricular fibrillation and cardiac arrest may follow. The widened QRSs may become diphasic ∧∨ . Look at this example!

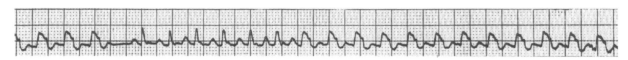

Neonate showing EKG manifestations of hyperkalemia (10.9 mEq./L.)

Hyperkalemia may be associated with kidney damage or infusions of *rapid or excessive amounts of potassium replacements.* Hyperkalemia *depresses* the normal electrical activity of the myocardial cells. So, the child with hyperkalemia is at risk for *sinus bradycardia, first degree heart block, escape rhythms, ventricular fibrillation, etc.*

Treatment for severe hyperkalemia (*greater than 7.0 mEq. per liter*) is aimed at reducing the serum potassium levels. Drug treatment may include calcium gluconate (counteracts effects on the neuromuscular system), sodium bicarb (shifts serum K^+ into the cells), or concentrated glucose (increases cellular uptake of K^+). *These drug solutions do not remove K^+ from the body!* Rather, they shift serum K^+ into the cell. Therapy may need to be repeated if the source of hyperkalemia persists. Oral or rectal administration of kayxalate can eliminate potassium from the body.

This is mostly a review . . . right?!

Digitalis Toxicity

High serum levels of digitalis may provoke characteristic EKG pattern changes and dysrhythmias. We will look at specific dysrhythmias momentarily. *Please remember,* there are certain **predisposing factors** the child to digitalis toxicity, such as the following conditions:

- renal impairment
- elevated serum calcium (Ca^{++})
- acute hypoxia
- decreased serum potassium (K^+)

Digitalis toxicity usually involves disturbances in the formation and conduction of impulses. As you remember, digitalis in excessive amounts retards AV conduction, producing various forms of heart block— *sinus block, first degree AV block, second degree AV block, blocked P.A.C.s, paroxysmal atria tachycardia with block, escape beats,* etc. Additionally, one may find supraventricular tachyarrhythmias, premature atrial and junctional beats, and P.V.C.s (the multiformed or multifocal variety) associated with digitalis toxicity.

Following is a discontinuous rhythm strip associated with digitalis toxicity.

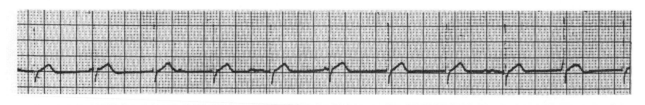

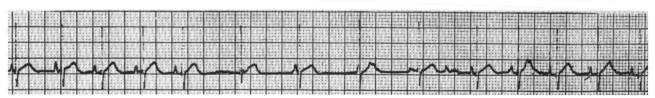

In the top strip, observe the junctional escape rhythm. In the second strip, the sinus pacemaker is evident for several beats, then gives way to the junctional escape rhythm. Finally, the sinus pacemaker resumes control. Remember . . . an escape rhythm will only be observed when there is failure or disruption of a higher pacemaker.

The most common EKG findings associated with *therapeutic* levels of digitalis are

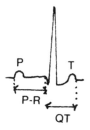

- shortened QT interval

- slowed heart rate

- slight prolongation of the P-R interval

- changes in the ST segment

You should remember, a child "isn't only a heart"—a digitalis toxic child may have anorexia, nausea, vomiting, or diarrhea. Usually digitalis is held if the P-R interval is increasing, new dysrthymias are occurring, or the pulse is below 100 in infants or 70–80 in children.

> **WARNING:** If a child is on digitalis, any new dysrthymia should be considered "suspect" for digitalis toxicity until ruled otherwise (by official "digitalis toxicity rulers" . . . otherwise known as physicians).

Practice Exercise 8

A. Abnormalities associated with potassium imbalance will be observed in the _____ segment of the EKG.

B. Construct an EKG complex demonstrating mild hyperkalemia.

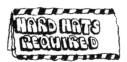

C. Check (✔) the dysrhythmias that may be related to digitalis toxicity.

❏ sinus bradycardia   ❏ Wenckebach

❏ first degree heart block   ❏ P.A.C.s

❏ blocked P.A.C.s   ❏ junctional tachycardia

❏ P.V.C.s

For Feedback 8, refer to page 394.

input section   14.9   Kids' Artifact

Last, but not least, we need to acknowledge that children's monitors, like adults' monitors, occasionally display *artifact.* You may find it helpful to review Section 6 (beginning on page 171). *Artifact,* you will recall, is an electrical signal appearing on the monitor that originates from sources other than the heart! Sound familiar?

    Owing to their high activity levels, children are prone to "creating" motion artifact. That means that special attention should be given to skin preparation. It is also helpful to secure the monitor cable and wires in a manner that reduces motion. (Tough job, right?)

    Since Section 6 is comprehensive, we will not belabor the point.

    Look at this rhythm strip (lead II) from a premie. Can you find the artifact? . . . And better yet, can you guess what is causing it?

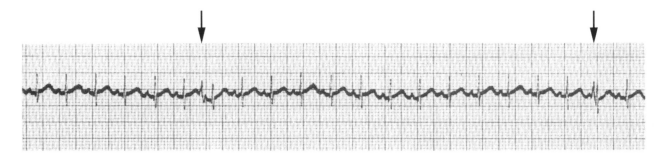

    Note the peculiar spiked waves occurring before complex 7 and before complex 20. These are hiccoughs! Neat, huh.   Baby hiccoughs!

    I thought about asking you to draw a baby hiccough . . . but, I reconsidered since this is the last input section!

    . . . And, here's one more baby rhythm strip to ponder. This one belongs to an eleven month old "*little lamb.*" See what you think!

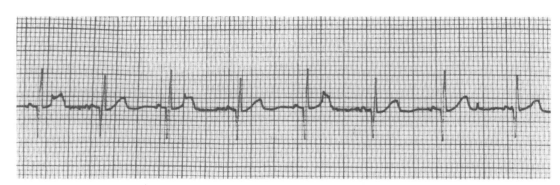

Notice that the T waves of beats 1, 3, and 5 are distorted. Grounds for blocked P.A.C.s, right?! Well, *not exactly*, because there will *always be* pauses following P.A.C.s (conducted or blocked P.A.C.s). This is just one more example of baby artifact that may be confused with certain dysrhythmias!

There is no practice exercise associated with Input 9 . . . just be on the **lookout** for artifact!

A Final Note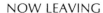

Pediatric dysrhythmias are generally classed as stable or unstable. Dysrhythmias are considered stable if the child remains asymptomatic, maintaining a good cardiac output, normal blood pressure, normal respiration and an unaltered mental status. Unstable dysrhythmias are associated with diminished cardiac output, decreased responsiveness, hypotension, and respiratory embarrassment or failure. **Generally, unstable pediatric dysrhythmias occur secondary to reduced cardiac contractility caused by extreme hypoxia and respiratory failure.**

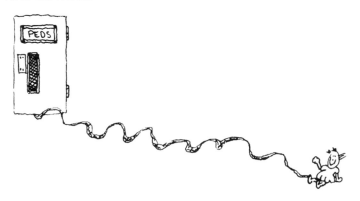

NOW LEAVING

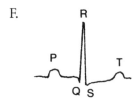 Feedback 1

A. The heart rate, the duration of P-R, QRS, and QT intervals all vary with <u>age</u>!

Circle the correct answer:

B. The heart rate increases / (decreases) with increasing age.

C. The P-R interval (lengthens) / shortens with increasing age.

D. The duration of the QRS is (greater) / lesser with increasing age.

E. The duration of the QT interval increases / (decreases) with increasing age.

F.

This is a normal cardiac complex with the exception that there is slight ST segment depression. Commonly, ST segment depression is associated with hypokalemia or digitalis administration.

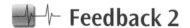 **Feedback 2**

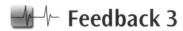

A. The easiest way to determine rhythm irregularity is to measure the P-P interval or the <u>R-R</u> interval.

B. This rhythm is a sinus tachycardia at a rate of 150. For a normal six year old, a heart rate should be approximately 100 per minute. One would need to *investigate* and treat the underlying cause of the tachycardia!

C. Sinus bradycardia in a child is defined as a heart rate of (less than 70) per minute. (Remembering heart rates is the most difficult part of this whole process!)

 Feedback 3

Hang in There

A. The aims of treatment for any rapid atrial dysrhythmia are:

   1. Reduce the rapid ventricular rate.

   2. Restore hemodynamic stability—restore a sinus rhythm!

B. The identifying characteristics of a premature atrial contraction are:

   1. The beat is premature, interrupting the underlying rhythm.

   2. There is a P wave before the premature beat and the premature P wave has a different configuration.

   3. There is a pause following the premature beat, allowing the sinus pacemaker to reset itself.

C. This strip demonstrates an atrial flutter with a variable ventricular response. You will remember that the ventricular response will be irregular if there is variable AV block. The identification of atrial flutter is confirmed by the rate and the regularity of the flutter (shark) waves. The atrial rhythm is regular at a rate of 300 per minute!

D. In a wandering atrial pacemaker, one finds:

   • a normal rate
   • a slightly irregular rhythm
   • P waves that constantly change in appearance since the pacemaker wanders around in the atria
   • a varying P-R interval
   • the QRS duration usually within normal limits

E. The treatment for supraventricular tachycardia consists of using measures to slow the ventricular rate and restore the sinus pacemaker. Vagal maneuvers (valsalva, gagging, ice water applied to the face) may *break* the rhythm. If these measures are ineffective, adenosine may be administered. In acute situations, synchronized cardioversion may be used. Cardioversion is usually applied using a current setting of 0.5 to 1.0 joules per kg. of body weight.

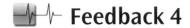 Feedback 4

A little lamb

A. The difference between a junctional tachycardia and an atrial tachycardia is slight when it comes to heart rate! However, cardiac output will be more significantly reduced in a junctional tachycardia owing to the loss of atrial kick.

B. The underlying rhythm here is sinus rhythm at a rate of 75 per minute. (If this strip belongs to a newborn, it is a sinus bradycardia!) When the sinus pacemaker slows, a junctional escape pacemaker (safety mechanism) takes over for two beats. Then, back to sinus rhythm.

Feedback 5

A. The QRS of a P.V.C. is wide and bizarre because the beat originates in the ventricular myocardium outside the normal conduction system. Because the electrical impulse travels cell to cell outside the normal conduction route, ventricular depolarization takes more time . . . therefore, the QRS is widened.

B. Ventricular fibrillation is a common / (uncommon) finding in children.

C. Your drawing of ventricular fibrillation should look something like this!

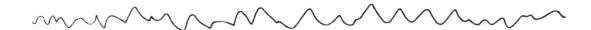

D. If electrical intervention is required for ventricular fibrillation, *defibrillation* is utilized because there is no effective cardiac activity. Synchronized cardioversion is only used when there is an effective underlying rhythm. (R waves are required to synchronize the patient's rhythm with the defibrillator unit). The usual current setting for pediatric defibrillation is two joules per kg.

Feedback 6

A. A PEA rhythm might be any rhythm. The electrical activity observed on the monitor is disassociated from the mechanical activity of contraction. Thus, the patient is pulseless. A PEA rhythm is a medical emergency requiring immediate CPR and other emergency interventions.

B. All of the statements about QT intervals and LQTS are true.

☒ LQTS may predispose a child to polymorphic ventricular tachycardia.

☒ Pedi QT intervals vary principally with age.

☒ The QT interval represents the ventricular refractory period.

☒ LQTS is a genetic disorder.

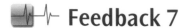 **Feedback 7**

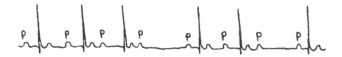

A. Since this is a rhythm strip from a five year old, the rhythm is a borderline sinus bradycardia. Normally the heart rate of a five year old would approach 100 per minute. In this example, the heart rate is approximately 94 per minute. Additionally, the P-R interval measures 0.18 seconds. The upper limits of normal for a five year old is 0.16 seconds. Thus, this is a borderline sinus bradycardia with a first degree AV block. Treatment probably is not warranted, but adequacy of cardiac output should be assessed.

B. Hope your Wink E. Bach looks something like mine! Note the increasing P-R interval until finally, a P wave fails to conduct.

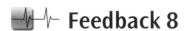

C. The ventricular rhythm is regular with a rate of 44 per minute. The QRS complexes are narrow, measuring 0.08 seconds. Atrial activity is regular occurring at a rate of 88 per minute. There is no relationship between atrial and ventricular activity (A-V dissociation). The narrow QRS indicates the escape pacemaker is of a junctional origin.

Feedback 8

A. Abnormalities associated with potassium (K^+) imbalance will be observed in the ST segment of the EKG.

B. Hope you were in compliance with all construction codes! Your EKG complex should look *something* like mine!

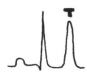

C. *All* of the following dysrhythmias may be related to digitalis toxicity!

☑ sinus bradycardia   ☑ P.A.C.s

☑ first degree heart block   ☑ junctional tachycardia

☑ blocked P.A.C.s   ☑ Wenckebach

☑ P.V.C.s

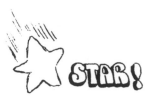

Notes

Notes

Test Your Skill

Objectives

Find a comfortable chair and complete this review exercise. And remember, it's okay to use the book to answer the questions . . . that's why the book is attached to the review exercise! 🙂

When you have completed Section 15 you will be able to determine

1. areas of learning and accomplishment
2. content areas requiring further review or study
3. your readiness for Advanced Dysrhythmia Interpretation Practice (Section 16)

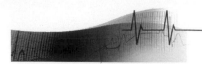

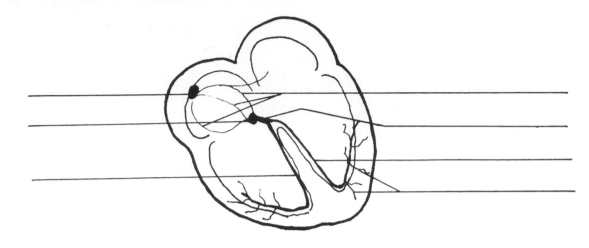

Review Exercise

This is an exercise to tie all the loose ends together. Try to answer each question on your own. If you get stuck, **cheat!** (That's why the book is attached to the review exercise!) ☺

1. Label the parts of the myocardial conduction system.

2. On EKG, the P wave represents _____.

   The normal P-R interval is _____ to _____ small boxes

   wide, or _____ to _____ seconds. The QRS represents

   _____ and should be *less* than _____

   small squares or *less* than _____ seconds. The _____

   represents recovery of the ventricles following depolarization.

3. Name two methods for calculating heart rate.

   a. _____

   b. _____

4. The treatment for sinus tachycardia consists of _____

   _____

   _____

   _____.

5. The patient with atrial fibrillation has a/an _____ pulse.

   The irregularity of the ventricular response is a result of _____

   _____

   _____.

6. In the normal heart, the AV junction is generally unable to conduct greater than _____ impulses per _____. The AV junction will _____ impulses greater than this rate. This is referred to as a _____ block.

7. "Saw-toothed" F waves are characteristic of _____. In this rhythm, there are actually two rates to calculate. The atrial or flutter rate may be between _____ to _____ per minute. Characteristically, the ventricular rate will vary between _____ to _____ beats per minute. Usually atrial flutter is a (regular/irregular) rhythm. What effect would digitalis have on atrial flutter? _____ _____ _____ _____.

If the heart rate (ventricular rate) is between _____ and _____ per minute, one should always *consider* atrial flutter.

8. What is an escape rhythm? When would one see an escape rhythm? What is the probable treatment?
_____
_____
_____
_____
_____
_____.

9. In order to qualify as a junctional beat, the P-R interval must be _____
_____.

10. Describe the criteria that must be met in order to identify a beat as a P.V.C.: _____
_____
_____
_____
_____
_____.

11. P.V.C.s may be harmful in patients with coronary disease; P.V.C.s indicate _____
_____, and may forewarn of _____.

12. Describe what is meant by "R on T" pattern when referring to P.V.C.s:
_____
_____
_____
_____.

13. What are the identifying features of ventricular tachycardia—and how should it be treated?

   _____

   _____

   _____

   _____ .

14. Describe myocardial activity and the EKG picture associated with ventricular fibrillation. What is the

   appropriate treatment? _____

   _____

   _____

   _____

   _____

   _____ .

And now, the fun part!

15. For each of the following rhythms, write one descriptive sentence that would help a new learner identify
   the rhythm. Then, draw a picture from what you have described!

   a. Mobitz type I (Wenckebach): _____

   _____

   _____

   _____ .

   b. Mobitz type II: _____

   _____

   _____

   _____ .

c. Complete (third degree) heart block: _____

_____

_____

_____.

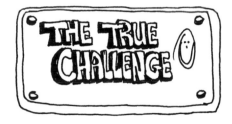 Whew!

16. When looking at a 12 lead EKG, which chest lead is most helpful in identifying bundle branch blocks?

_____.

17. Mild hyperkalemia may be suspected if _____

T waves appear on the EKG. Digitalis effect causes a _____

_____ of the ST segment.

18. With myocardial ischemia, the ST segment will appear _____.

ST elevation represents _____. The hallmark

finding on EKG indicative of a large scale myocardial infarction (tissue death) is the _____

wave in upright leads and the _____ wave in downwardly directed leads.

Describe the following EKG rhythm strips, including rate, regularity, etc. *If you feel comfortable,* apply a name.

19.

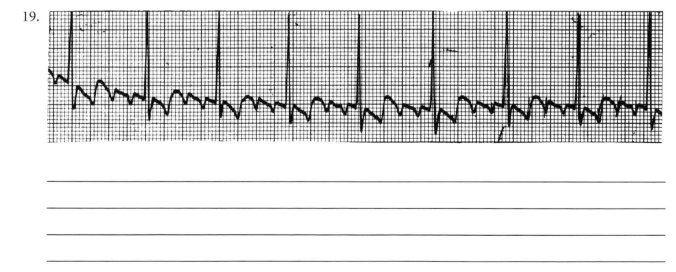

_____

_____

_____

_____

20.

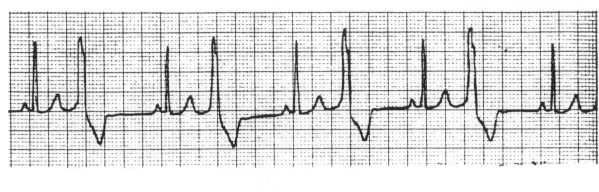

_____
_____
_____
_____

21.

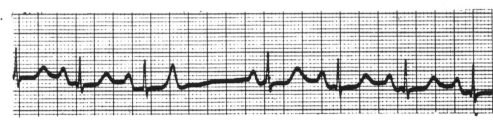

_____
_____
_____
_____

22.

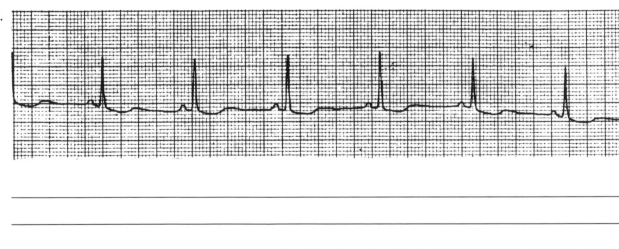

_____
_____
_____
_____

23.

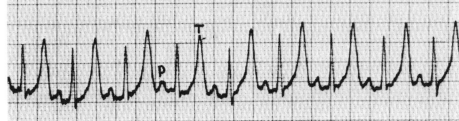

_____

_____

_____

_____

24.

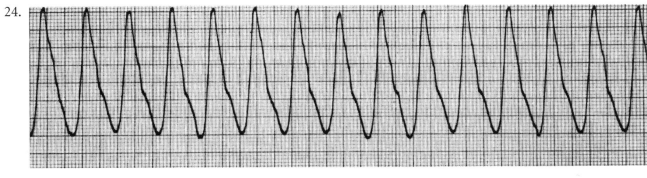

_____

_____

_____

_____

25.

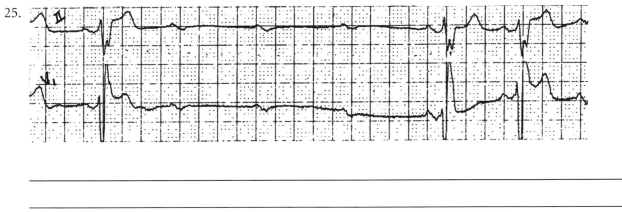

_____

_____

_____

_____

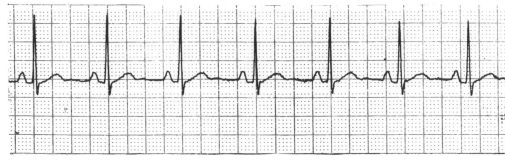

26.

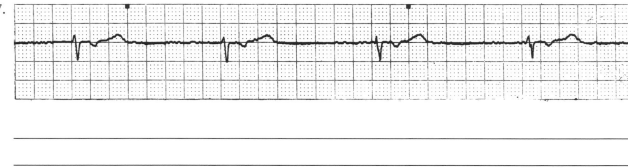

_____
_____
_____
_____

27.

_____
_____
_____
_____

28.

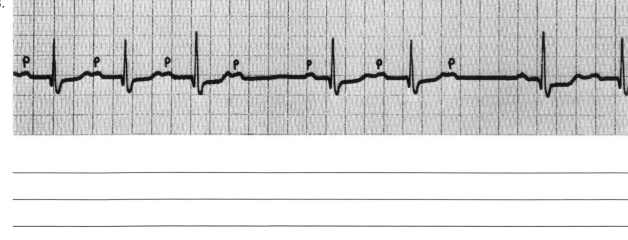

_____
_____
_____
_____

29.

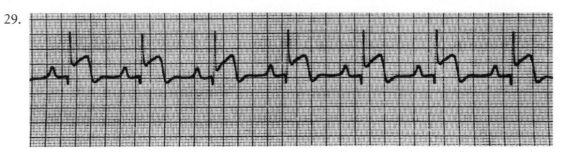

_____

_____

_____

_____

30.

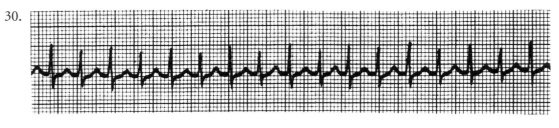

_____

_____

_____

_____

31.

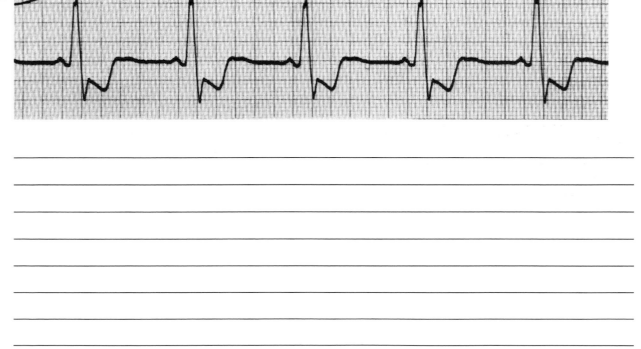

_____

_____

_____

_____

_____

_____

_____

32.

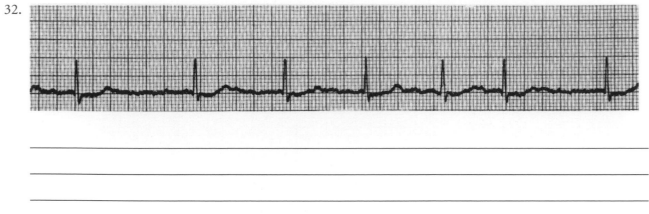

33.

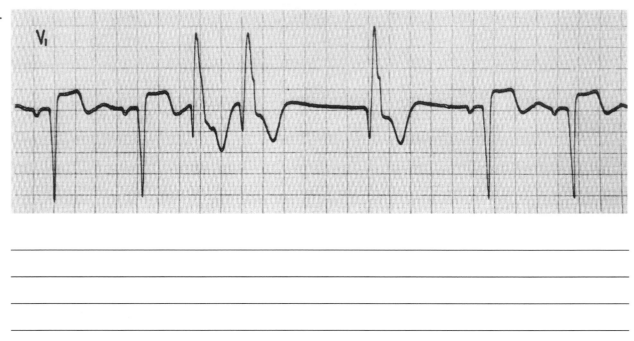

V₁

34.

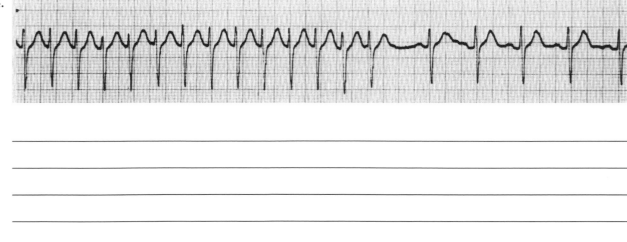

35.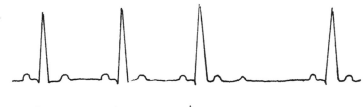

This is an example of motion artifact that masks the underlying rhythm. Describe actions that you would take to determine the significance of the rhythm disturbance. Then, describe methods for correcting the problem.

_____

_____

_____

_____

36. What are these two rhythms? Which dysrhythmia has the greater significance, and why?

A.

P-R = 0.14

QRS = 0.08

Heart Rate = 75

B.

P-R = 0.14

QRS = 0.08

Heart Rate = 75

_____

_____

_____

_____

_____

_____

37. 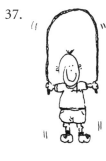 This is a _____. The major distinctions between a pediatric and an adult rhythm are:

a. _____ rate

b. duration of the _____ interval

c. duration of the _____.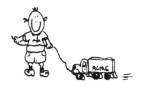

38. List three reasons or three conditions warranting the insertion of a temporary pacemaker.

a. _____

b. _____

c. _____

39. Pacemaker non-capture means that _____

_____

_____

_____

Draw a picture of ventricular non-capture.

40. Correctly match the following diagnostic abbreviations with the appropriate hemodynamic measurements. (☺)

CVP   left ventricular function

PCWP   myocardial contractile force

LVEDP   right heart preload

CO   left heart preload

41. Explain the differences between hospital defibrillators and AEDs (automatic external defibrillators).

_____

_____

_____

_____

42. Pulseless Electrical Activity (PEA) commonly results from _____ and _____.

Check (X) those statements that are true.

☐ PEA is diagnosed in part by EKG tracing.

☐ Defibrillation is the first emergency intervention.

☐ Secondary interventions include determining and treating the underlying cause.

☐ PEA is a true medical emergency.

43. When the major force of ventricular activation (depolarization) moves toward a positive ⊕ electrode, the resulting QRS will appear like which of the following? Circle the correct letter.

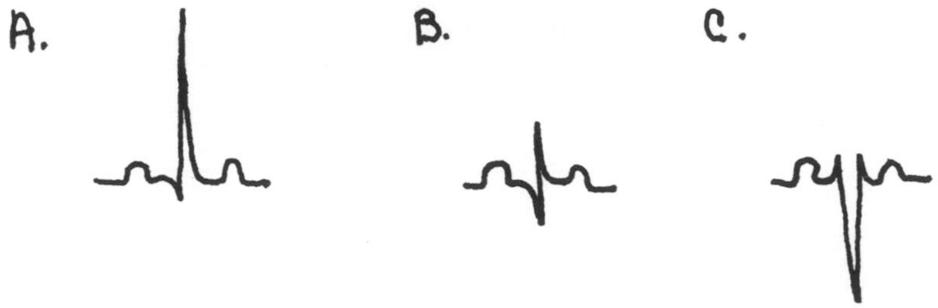

A.   B.   C.

44. Calculate the time elapsed for each of the following.

    a. 5 big squares and 4 small squares _____ seconds

    b. 6 small squares _____ seconds

    c. 17 small squares _____ seconds

    d. 15 big squares _____ seconds.

45. A demand-type pacemaker will generate a pacemaker impulse _____

_____

_____

_____

_____

_____

46. Beta-blocker drugs produce which of the following effects? (Check all that apply.)

☐ increased heart rate

☐ decreased automaticity of the SA node

☐ an increase in the AV node refractory period

☐ decreased heart rate

47. Hypokalemia increases/decreases (circle one) electrical instability. Name three rhythms that might be associated with moderate to severe hypokalemia.

    a. _____

    b. _____

    c. _____

48. Describe the following rhythm strip.

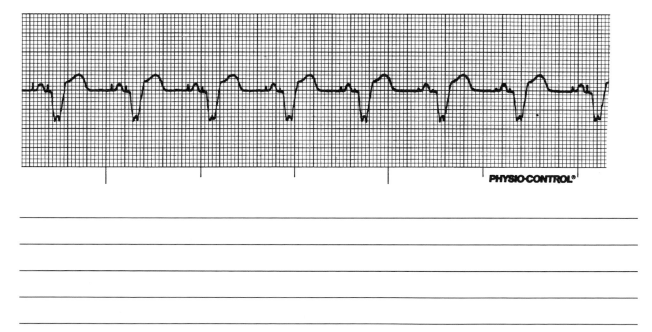

_____

_____

_____

_____

49. Describe the following rhythm strip.

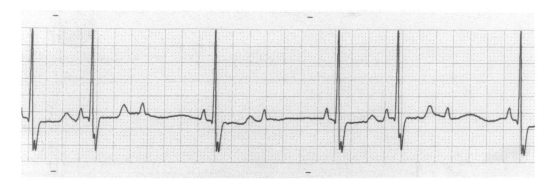

_____

_____

_____

_____

Great Performance!!

Remember, the major objective of this book was to assist you in describing EKG events . . . if you have learned some *jargon* and other facts along the way, that's a *bonus!* Just bear in mind that clinicians have a *great* tendency to disagree over terminology!

Answers for the review exercise begin below.

 **Review Exercise Answers**

The answers to questions 1 through 18 are strategically placed throughout the book . . . very clever, right? Since those questions have "concrete" answers, I will refer you to the appropriate page in the text. Then I will discuss the interpretations of the rhythm strips in detail!

1. Refer to page 16 to verify your answer.

2. Answers can be found on pages 17–22. If you had difficulty remembering any of these facts, you may want to reread Section I in its entirety.

3. Calculating heart rate is discussed beginning on page 24.

4. The treatment of sinus tachycardia is discussed on page 51.

5. If you had difficulty with this question, refer to page 71.

6. Look back to the discussion on physiologic block, page 66.

7. Atrial flutter is discussed on pages 66 through 71. Reread the entire section if necessary.

8. Escape rhythms are reviewed on pages 88 and 128.

9. Double check your answers on page 90.

10. How did you do with this one? P.V.C.s are wide and bizarre in appearance interrupting the underlying rhythm; the QRS of the P.V.C. measures a minimum of 0.12 seconds; there is no P wave preceding the abnormal QRS. Review page 136 if you had difficulty!

11. Verify your answers on page 108.

12. This one was easy! If you experienced a memory lapse, see page 110.

13. Ventricular tachycardia is always difficult to "definitely" identify. You may want to reread page 118.

14. The chaotic, uncoordinated ventricular depolarization of ventricular fibrillation is discussed on pages 125–126.

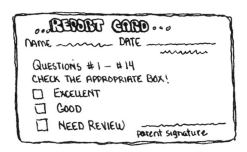

My favorite part of this review exercise is question 15 a, b, and c! The best way to learn is to draw!

15. a. Refer to page 145 for a textbook example and description of Wenckebach.

15. b. Page 147 clearly depicts Mobitz type II.

15. c. Complete heart block is discussed on page 153.

16. V_1 is the lead that most clearly identifies bundle branch block. See page 163.

17. Hyperkalemia and digitalis effects can be found on page 253.

18. ST segment depression connotes myocardial ischemia. ST elevation represents injury. And, the development of a pathologic Q wave in upright leads and the loss of R wave in negative leads represents myocardial necrosis. For a quick review see Section 11.

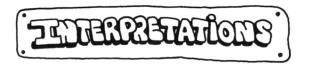

Before we begin to discuss the various rhythm strips, I need to repeat myself. The important aspect of dysrhythmia interpretation is accurately describing the electrical events. Do not compare how *I've written the interpretation* with how *you've written it!* Rather, make certain you have described what I have described! And remember, it is possible that you and I may see the same electrical events differently!

19. The rhythm appears regular. There is more atrial activity than ventricular activity. Atrial waves are "saw-toothed" in appearance and occur at a rate of 300 per minute. The QRSs are of normal duration and occur regularly at a rate of 75 per minute. Atrial waves (F waves) march through the rhythm. This is atrial flutter with 4:1 conduction (four flutter waves for every QRS). The fourth flutter wave is buried in the QRS—I know it is there however, because flutter waves are continuous, never stopping. If you need review, turn to page 66.

20. This one is easy! A normal sinus beat is followed by a P.V.C., then the whole cycle repeats. This is ventricular bigeminy. The heart rate should be determined by counting the patient's pulse for one full minute. It is helpful to count both apical and radial pulses because not all abnormal beats will be adequately perfused. The P-R interval of normally conducted beats is approximately 0.10 seconds.

21. The rhythm is irregular. There is a pause noted after the third beat. The underlying rhythm is a sinus rhythm with an approximate rate of 80 beats per minute—however, when a rhythm is irregular, it is important to count the rate over one full minute! The P-R interval is constant and measures 0.20 seconds; the QRS is constant and measures slightly less than 0.10 seconds. Looking closely at the pause, you will notice the preceding T wave is abnormally peaked. AH-HA! There must be a P wave sitting on top of the T wave! This is a P.A.C. that does not conduct. And as always, when a P.A.C. occurs, there is a pause allowing the sinus mechanism to reset itself. If you need review, turn to page 57.

22. The rhythm is regular with a ventricular rate of slightly less than 60 per minute. The P-R is constant measuring approximately 0.16 seconds; the QRS is constant measuring approximately 0.08 seconds. There is slight depression of the ST segment. This is a sinus bradycardia with a slightly depressed ST segment.

23. The rhythm is rapid and regular. The ventricular rate is approximately 120 per minute. The P-R is constant measuring 0.16 seconds; the QRS is constant measuring approximately 0.08 seconds. Giant, peaked, "tentlike" T waves are evident throughout. This is a sinus tachycardia with tall, peaked T waves (suggestive of hyperkalemia). If you need review, turn to page 253.

24. The rhythm is rapid and fairly regular with a ventricular rate of approximately 125 per minute. There is no obvious atrial activity; the QRSs are wide and bizarre. Though the rate is slower than a typical ventricular tachycardia and though there are no fusion or capture beats to confirm the "diagnosis," this is most likely ventricular tachycardia. This could, however, represent an accelerated idioventricular rhythm. For review, reread pages 118 and 128.

25. This is a poor quality rhythm strip, but a *great* thinking exercise! The rhythm is irregular. The atrial rate is regular occurring at a rate of approximately 68 per minute. The ventricular rate is slow and interrupted. The QRS is widened, measuring 0.14 seconds. Thus, a left a bundle branch block exists (check out lead V*1*). The ominous finding in this strip is the 3.6 seconds of ventricular standstill! (This rhythm does *not* demonstrate A-V dissociation; a constant P-R interval is evident in all conducted beats). Intermittant ventricular standstill requires intervention. There is no assurance that ventricular conduction will continue. In ventricular standstill, *complete* bundle branch block exists (blockage of both the right and common left bundle branches).

26. You guessed it!!! Normal sinus rhythm. The ventricular rate is approximately 75 beats per minute. The P-R is constant measuring approximately 0.16 seconds; the QRS is constant measuring approximately 0.08 seconds. *I hope you don't need review!*

Whew!

27. Here we have a regular, slow rhythm with a heart rate of 38 beats per minute. The QRS is within normal limits measuring 0.10 seconds. No P waves are visible prior to the QRS complexes. However, an inverted P wave follows each QRS. This is a junctional escape rhythm. For review, see page 88.

28. The rhythm is irregular, so to determine the rate, I would need to count the pulse for one full minute. The P waves all appear uniform in appearance but the P-R interval gets progressively longer until a P wave fails to conduct. Then, the cycle repeats, though irregularly. This is good ol' Wenckebach (Mobitz type I second degree heart block). If you need review, turn to page 145.

29. The rhythm is regular with a ventricular rate of approximately 60 per minute. The P waves are uniform in appearance. The P-R is constant measuring almost 0.28 seconds. The QRS is narrow followed by significant ST elevation. So, this is a sinus rhythm with a first degree heart block and ST elevation. One would need to do a 12 lead EKG to determine in which leads the ST elevation is present. ST elevation is suggestive of injury, and appears in the leads overlooking the area of injury. If you need a quick review, turn to pages 276.

30. The rhythm is regular and rapid with a ventricular rate of approximately 185 beats per minute. (I used the cheat guide on page 39.) It is difficult to identify any clear P waves, but the QRS is constant measuring 0.08 seconds. Therefore, I know the rhythm is not of ventricular origin. Since I am uncertain of P waves, I'm simply going to describe this strip as "supraventricular tachycardia, rate 185, QRS = 0.08 seconds."

31. The underlying rhythm here is sinus bradycardia with a rate of 50 per minute. The QRSs are wide *but* there is a P wave preceding each QRS. The P-R interval measures 0.16 seconds. The QRSs measure almost 0.20 seconds in duration! This is a bundle branch block. To know whether this is right or left bundle branch block, I would need to inspect lead V_1. So, in summary, this is a sinus bradycardia with bundle branch block! For review, see page 162. A depressed ST segment suggests ischemia.

32. Everything about this rhythm is ***irregular!*** There is lots of atrial activity, but no definitive atrial wave forms. The QRS complexes are uniform in appearance, occur irregularly, and measure 0.08 seconds. This is our *old friend* atrial fibrillation. For a refresher, see page 71.

33. *OOOOOh!* Well, the underlying rhythm is a sinus rhythm with a rate of 70 per minute. The P-R interval is of normal duration though the P waves appear inverted. (For a better view of atrial activity, one would need to view lead II.) The R waves are absent and there is marked ST segment elevation suggestive of an acute anterior wall injury! Beats 3, 4, and 5 are P.V.C.s. It is important to place this rhythm in context. Is the patient ischemic with resulting ventricular ectopy? Treatment may include interventions to improve blood flow and drugs to reduce ventricular irritability.

34. The beginning of this rhythm strip shows a supraventricular tachycardia at a rate of 166 per minute. I am calling it a supraventricular tachycardia because there is no clear evidence of P waves and the QRS duration is within normal limits. The rhythm then converts *spontaneously* to a sinus tachycardia with a rate of slightly greater than 100 per minute. The P-R interval of the sinus beats measures approximately 0.16 seconds. The QRS of the sinus beats measures approximately 0.08 seconds.

35. The significance of the disturbance can be determined by comparing the patient's pulse with the rhythm strip. When artifact is present, the pulse (rate and sequence) will assist one in locating QRS complexes. Motion artifact can often be eliminated or reduced by correct skin preparation and an ample quantity of gel on the electrode patches. To prevent cable wire movement, the cable may be clipped to the patient's clothing. If motion artifact relates to respiration, reposition the lead away from the diaphragm. For review, see Section 6.

    Note: Attaching the electrodes over bony areas will reduce motion artifact!

36. A *toughie!* Diagram A is a sinus rhythm with a blocked P.A.C. (notice that the non-conducted P wave occurs *early* or prematurely in the cycle and is different from the normal P wave). There is a pause following the blocked P.A.C. Frequently, blocked P.A.C.s are observed in digitalis toxicity. Diagram B represents a Mobitz type II second degree AV block! In Mobitz type II, a P wave is suddenly blocked without warning. The blocked P wave is neither early nor late . . . it occurs *right on time.* Mobitz type II occurs because of intermittent block and is almost always associated with myocardial damage. Oftentimes, a pacemaker is prophylactically inserted when Mobitz type II is observed. ***Always determine if non-conducted P waves occur early, late, or right on time!*** For review, see pages 56 and 146.

37. This is a kid. The major distinctions between a pediatric and an adult rhythm are:

    a. <u>heart rate</u>

    b. duration of the <u>P-R</u> interval

    c. duration of the <u>QRS</u>

38. A temporary pacemaker may be inserted to treat any of the following conditions:

    a. Mobitz type II second degree AV blocks associated with acute myocardial infarction
    b. drug-induced bradyarrhythmias
    c. third degree heart block
    d. symptomatic bradycardia

39. Pacemaker non-capture means that <u>a pacemaker generated impulse fails to produce the desired effect</u> (<u>atrial depolarization or ventricular depolarization</u>). See page 207 for a quick review of noncapture!

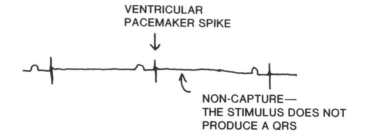

VENTRICULAR
PACEMAKER SPIKE

NON-CAPTURE—
THE STIMULUS DOES NOT
PRODUCE A QRS

40.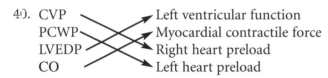

    CVP ———→ Left ventricular function
    PCWP ———→ Myocardial contractile force
    LVEDP ———→ Right heart preload
    CO ———→ Left heart preload

    For a refresher, review section 13 beginning on page 319!

41. **Hospital Defibrillator**

    - mobile
    - used in hospitals
    - capable of defibrillation, cardioversion, pacing
    - may require manual programming by trained clinician
    - requires clinician to interpret rhythm

    Automatic External Defibrillator (AED)

    - lightweight, portable
    - available in the community
    - used by first responders
    - uses algorithms to "read" rhythm
    - automatically determines current setting

42. Pulseless Electrical Activity (PEA) commonly results from *hypoxia* and *respiratory failure*. The following statements are true.

    ☒ PEA is diagnosed in part by EKG tracing.

    ☐ Defibrillation is the first emergency intervention.

    ☒ Secondary interventions include determining and treating the underlying cause.

    ☒ PEA is a true medical emergency.

43. When the major force of ventricular activation (depolarization) moves toward a positive ⊕ electrode, the resulting QRS will appear like diagram A.

    For a quick review, refer to Section 1.

44. a. 5 big squares and 4 small squares <u>1.16</u> seconds

    b. 6 small squares <u>0.24</u> seconds

    c. 17 small squares <u>0.68</u> seconds

    d. 15 big squares <u>3.0</u> seconds.

45. A demand-type pacemaker will generate a pacemaker impulse on an as-needed basis, working in synchrony with the underlying rhythm.

    See page 204 for a quick refresher.

46. Beta-blocker drugs produce the following effects.

    ☐ increased heart rate

    ☒ decreased automaticity of the SA node

    ☒ an increase in the AV node refractory period

    ☒ decreased heart rate

47. Hypokalemia increases electrical instability. Three rhythms that might be associated with moderate to severe hypokalemia include

    a. <u>atrial tachycardia</u>

    b. <u>junctional tachycardia</u>

    c. <u>ventricular tachycardia/ventricular fibrillation</u>

    Pages 253–255 provide an overview of hypokalemia.

48. This rhythm strip demonstrates an AV sequential pacemaker rhythm. Both atrial and ventricular activity are controlled by the two lead pacemaker. The atrial and ventricular rates are approximately 75 per minute.

    For a quick review of AV sequential pacemakers, refer to page 204.

49. This is an example of a second-degree AV Block (aka Mobitz II). Note the P waves all look the same. However, the second, fourth, and seventh P waves are not followed by a QRS complex. When the P wave does conduct to a QRS the PR is fixed at .20. Without warning a P wave is not conducted through to the ventricles, resulting in a pause.

15

Notes

The Final Analysis: Advanced Arrhythmia Interpretation Practice

Objectives

The purpose of this text has been to aid learners in gaining basic EKG interpretation competence. However, complicating rhythm strip interpretation is the fact that few "live" rhythms resemble their "textbook" cousins. Frequently, multiple anomalies can be found in one tracing. For

Textbook Cousins

Non-Textbook Cousins

example, ectopic activity may complicate conduction disturbances, or multifocal impulses may obliterate an underlying rhythm.

The analysis and interpretation of complex or "difficult" rhythms is aided by:

- knowledge of a patient's physical findings and overall sense of well being.

- review of the patient's underlying pathology, including current drug therapy and lab values (electrolytes, serum markers).

- observing the rhythm pattern over time (a six second strip is often too short to distinguish patterns)

- "tete to tete" consultation with a colleague

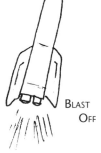

BLAST OFF

> **REMEMBER**: In all instances, the diagnosing of dysrhythmias is far less important than an accurate description of electrical events!

The following practice strips are included for their "less than textbook" quality. Use your best analysis skills and describe what you see! My analysis follows at the end of this section, beginning on page 468.

> **IMPORTANT NOTE:** A symbol precedes certain interpretations of mine. That symbol indicates the *advanced* nature of that rhythm. In a scholarly spirit, feel free to debate my interpretation!

Advanced Practice Exercise

Review each strip carefully. Describe all that you see!

1.

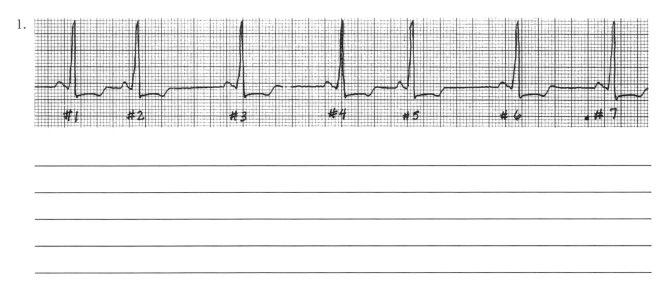

_____

_____

_____

_____

_____

2.

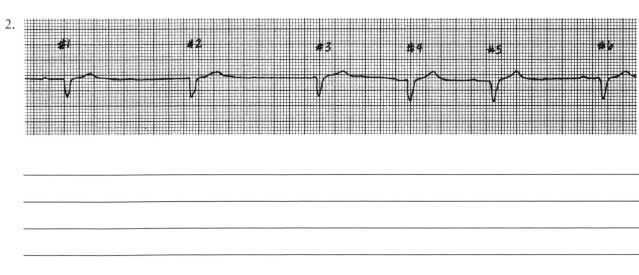

_____

_____

_____

_____

_____

3.

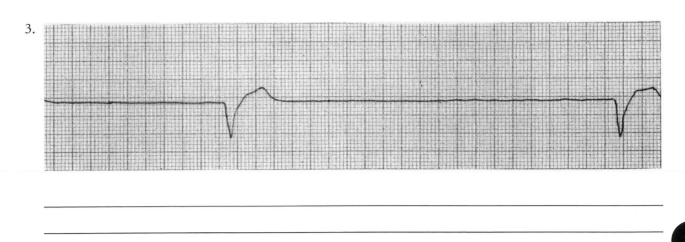

_____

_____

_____

_____

4.

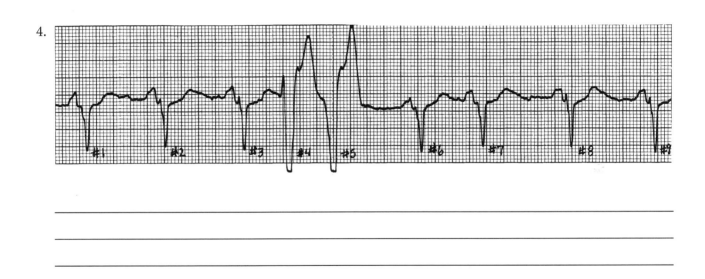

_____

_____

_____

_____

5.

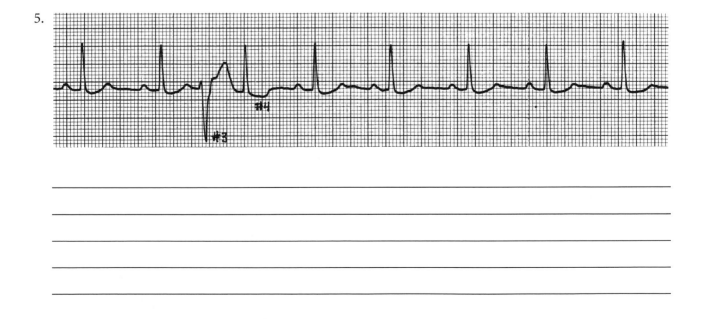

_____

_____

_____

_____

_____

_____

6.

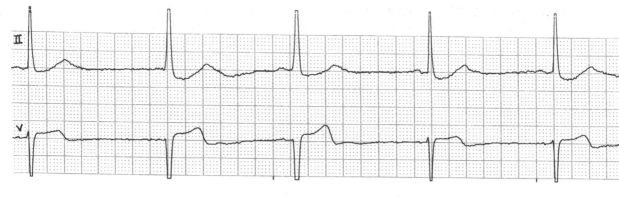

_____
_____
_____
_____
_____

7.

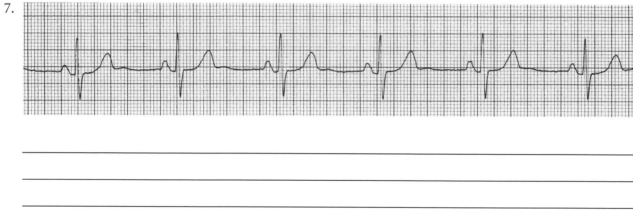

_____
_____
_____
_____
_____

8.

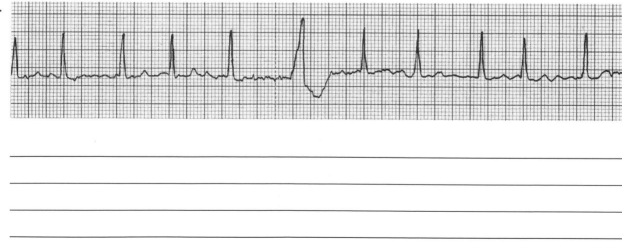

_____
_____
_____
_____
_____

9.

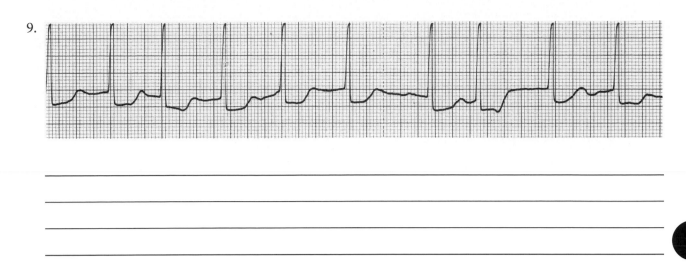

_____
_____
_____
_____
_____

10.

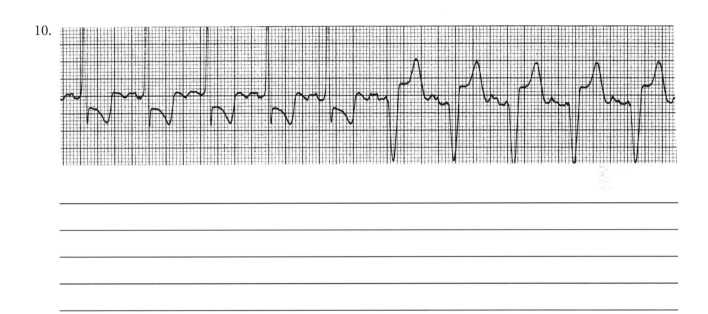

_____
_____
_____
_____
_____

11.

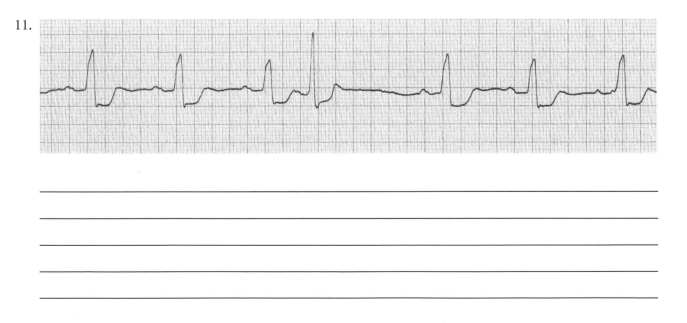

_____
_____
_____
_____
_____

12.

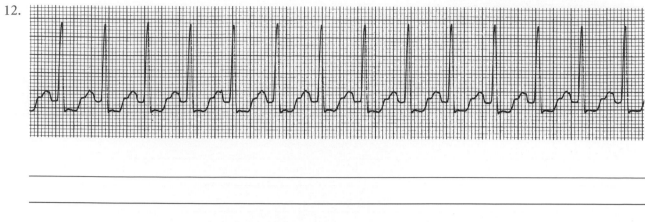

_____

_____

_____

_____

13.

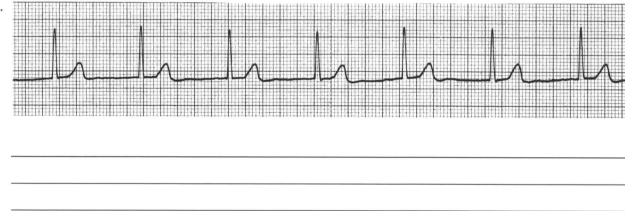

_____

_____

_____

_____

14. A.

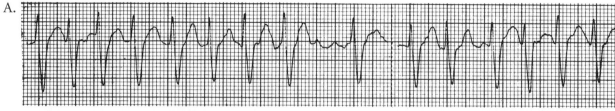

B.

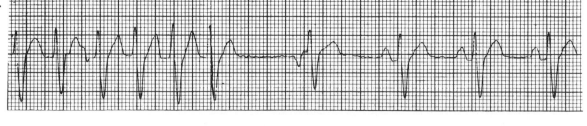

_____

_____

_____

_____

15. A.

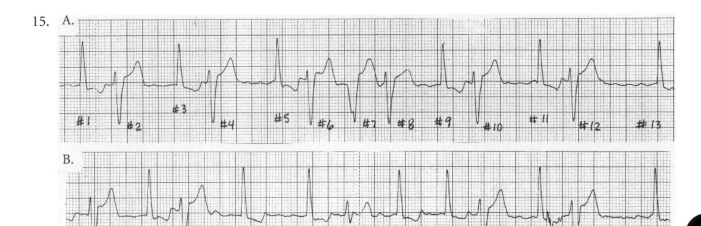

#1 #2 #3 #4 #5 #6 #7 #8 #9 #10 #11 #12 #13

B.

#1 #2 #3 #4 #5 #6 #7 #8 #9 #10 #11 #12

_____
_____
_____
_____

16.

_____
_____
_____
_____

17.

_____
_____
_____
_____

18.

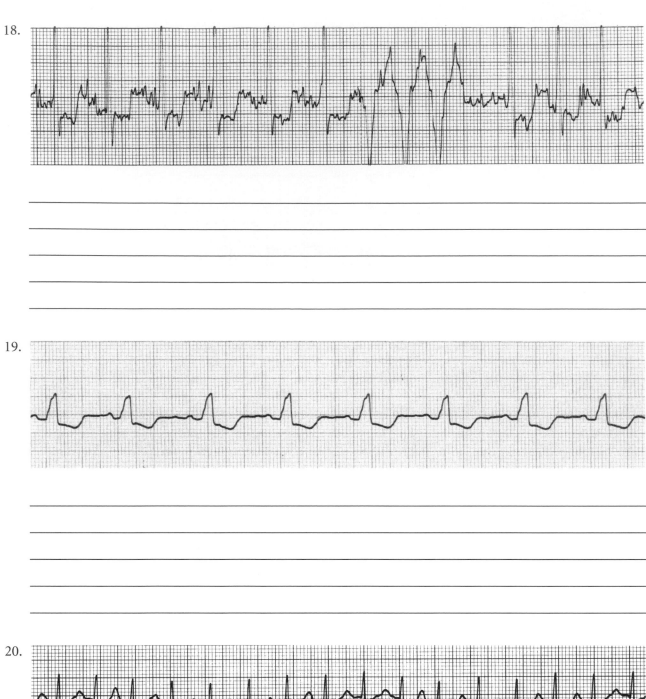

_____

_____

_____

_____

_____

19.

_____

_____

_____

_____

_____

20.

_____

_____

_____

_____

_____

21.

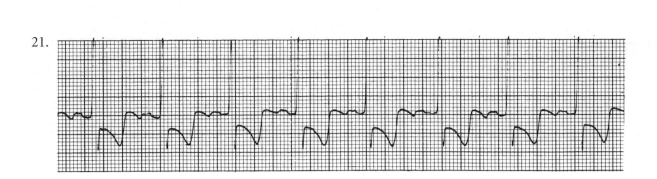

_____

_____

_____

_____

_____

22.

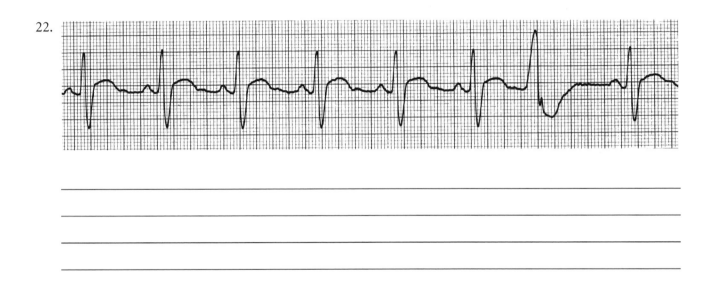

_____

_____

_____

_____

_____

23.

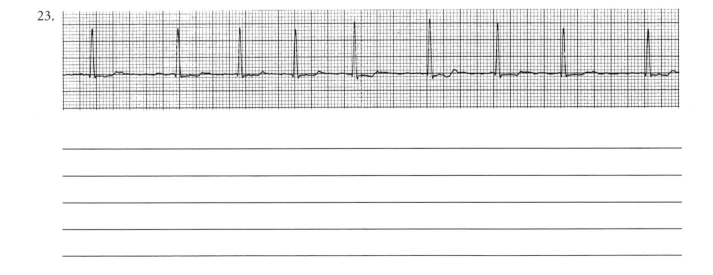

_____

_____

_____

_____

_____

24.

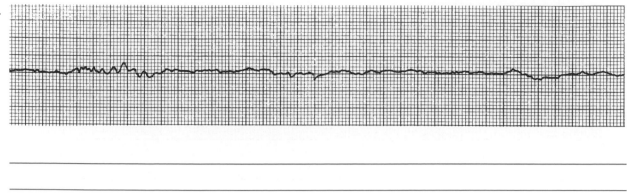

_____

_____

_____

_____

25. A.

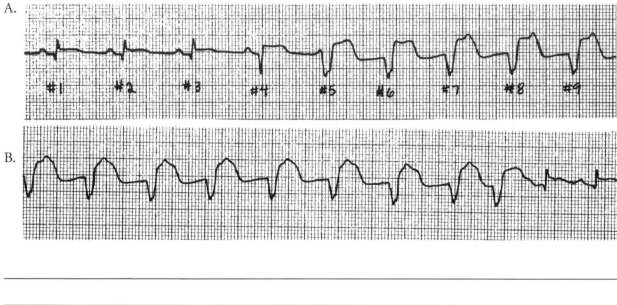

B.

_____

_____

_____

_____

26.

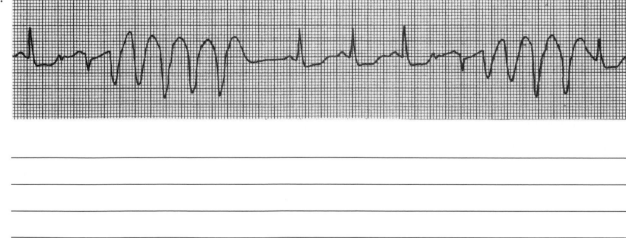

_____

_____

_____

_____

27.

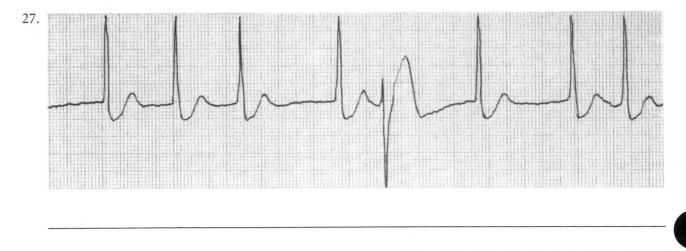

_____
_____
_____
_____

28.

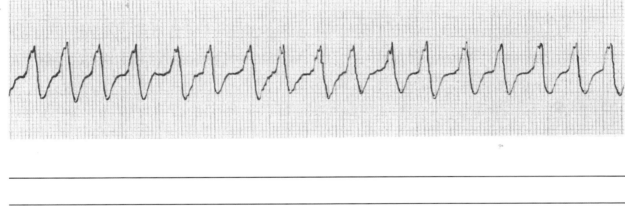

_____
_____
_____
_____

29.

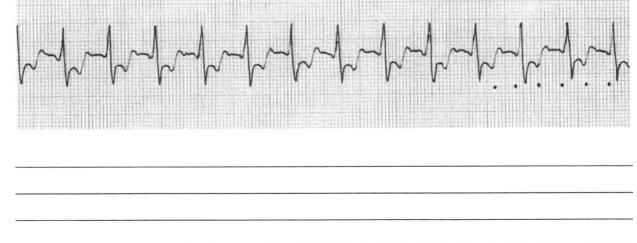

_____
_____
_____
_____

30.

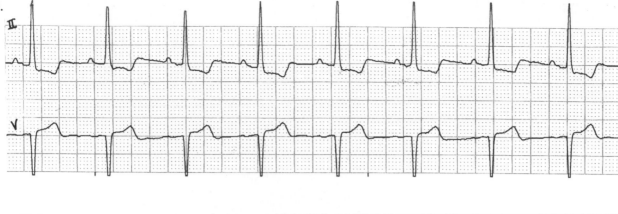

_____

_____

_____

_____

31.

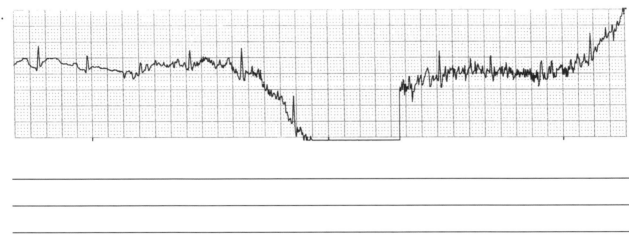

_____

_____

_____

_____

32.

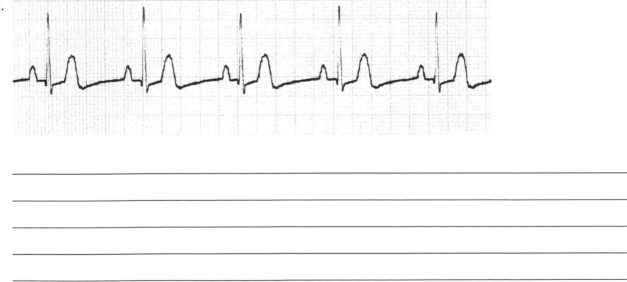

_____

_____

_____

_____

_____

33.

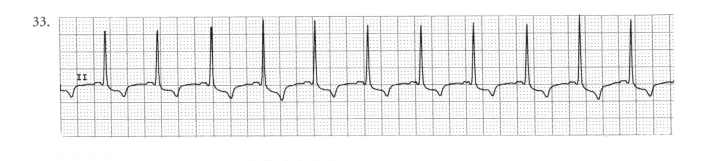

_____
_____
_____
_____
_____

34.

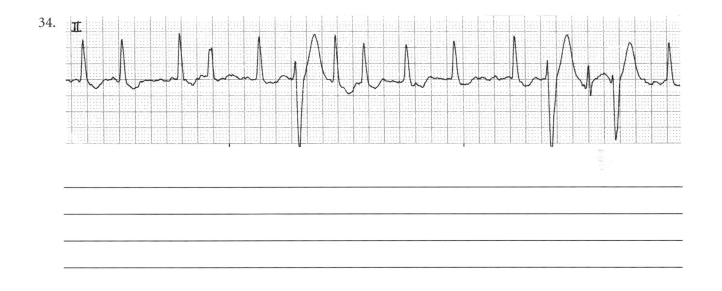

_____
_____
_____
_____
_____

35.

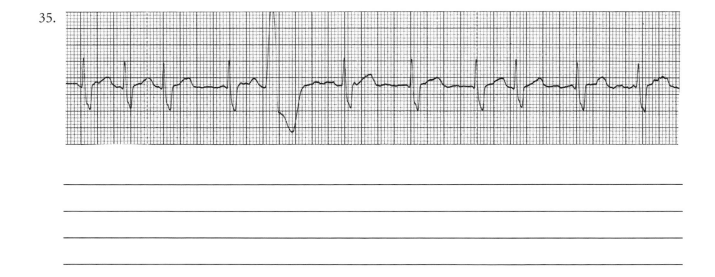

_____
_____
_____
_____

36.

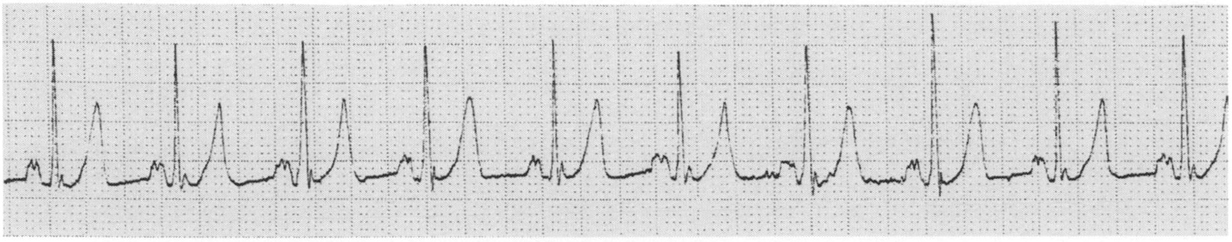

_____

_____

_____

_____

_____

37.

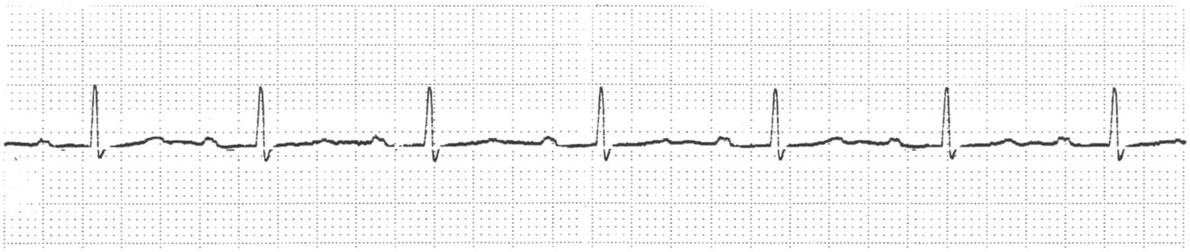

_____

_____

_____

_____

_____

_____

38.

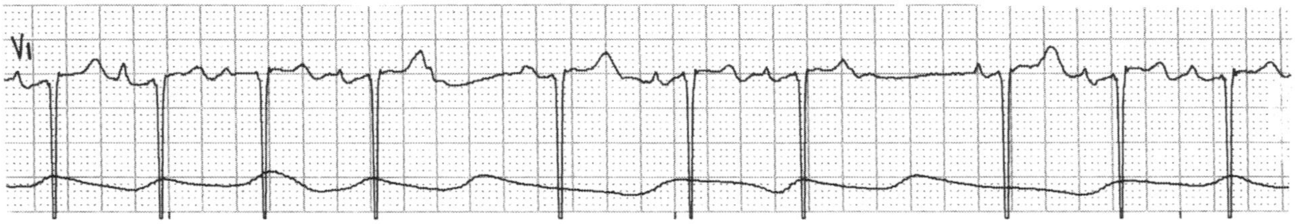

Note: The lower wave form is produced by a CVP monitor.

_____

_____

_____

_____

_____

39. V_1

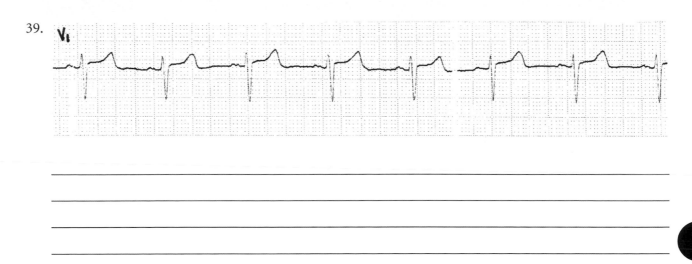

_____

_____

_____

_____

_____

40. II

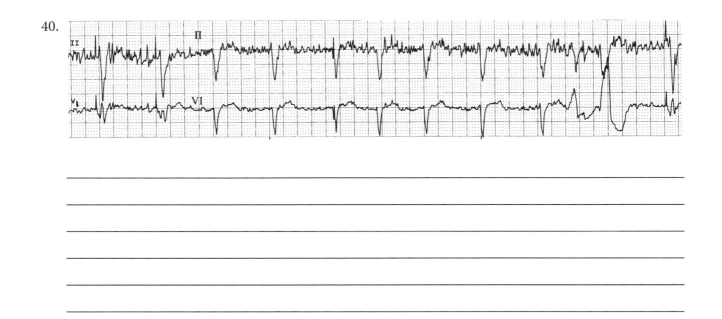

_____

_____

_____

_____

_____

_____

41.

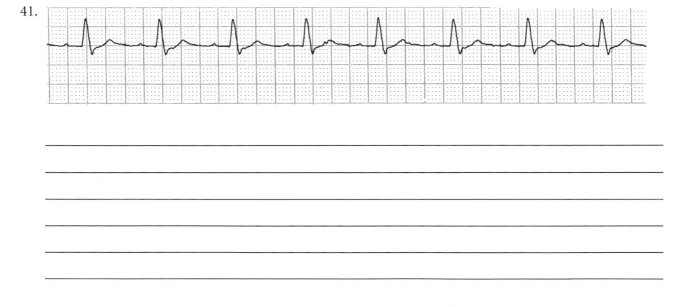

_____

_____

_____

_____

_____

42.

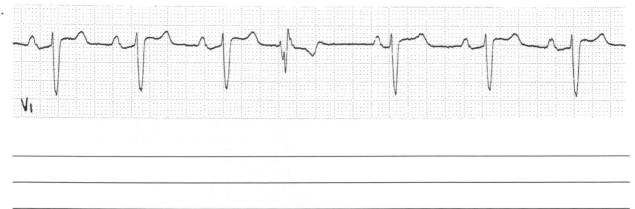

V₁

_____

_____

_____

_____

_____

43.

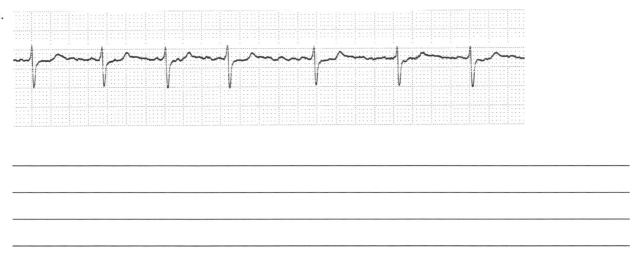

_____

_____

_____

_____

_____

44.

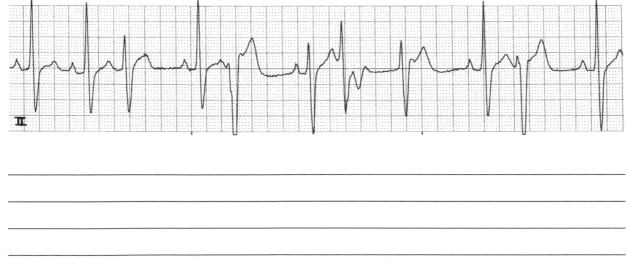

II

_____

_____

_____

_____

_____

45.

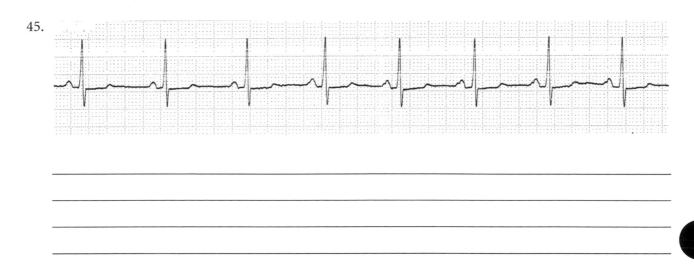

_____
_____
_____
_____
_____

46.

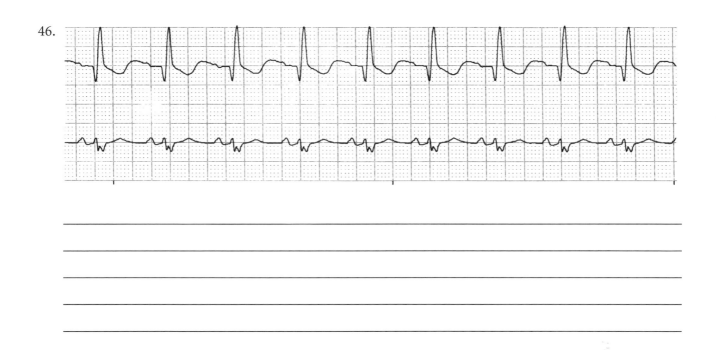

_____
_____
_____
_____
_____

47.

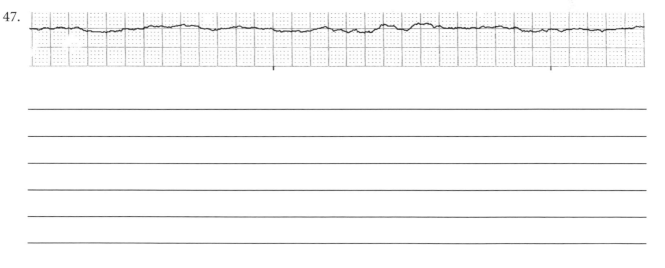

_____
_____
_____
_____
_____
_____

48.

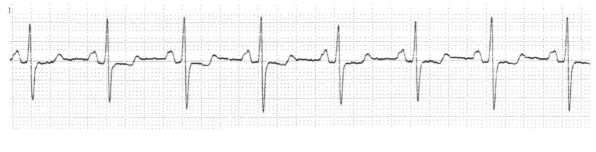

_____

_____

_____

_____

49.

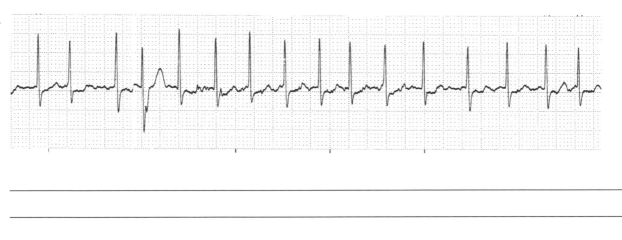

_____

_____

_____

_____

50.

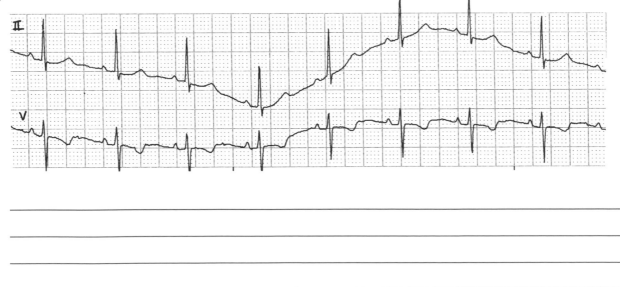

_____

_____

_____

51.

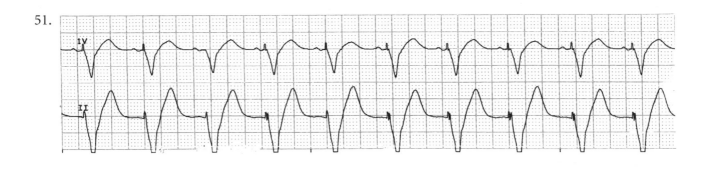

_____

_____

_____

_____

_____

52.

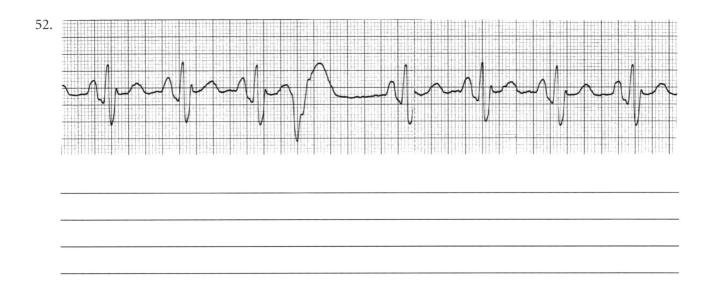

_____

_____

_____

_____

53.

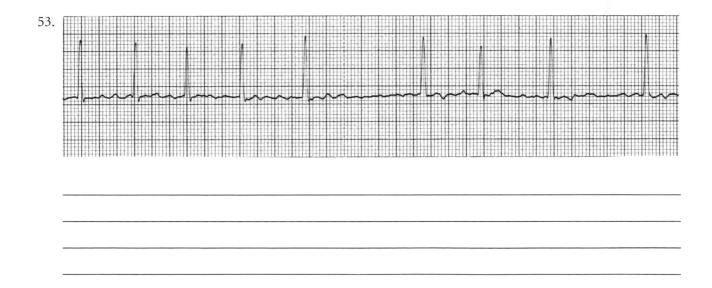

_____

_____

_____

_____

54.

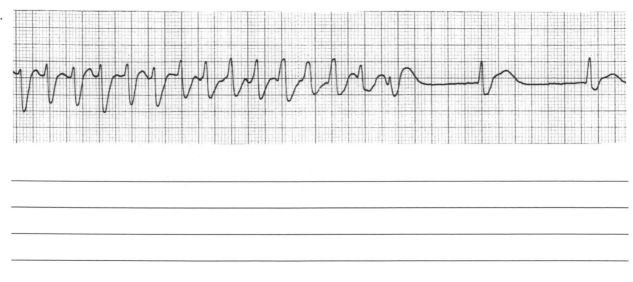

55.

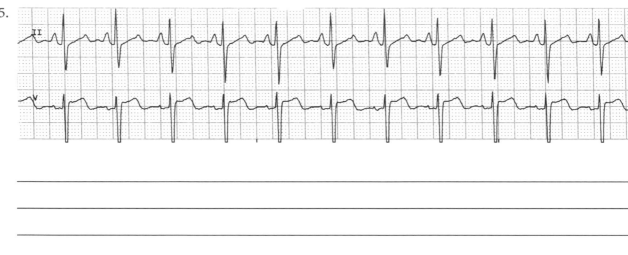

56.

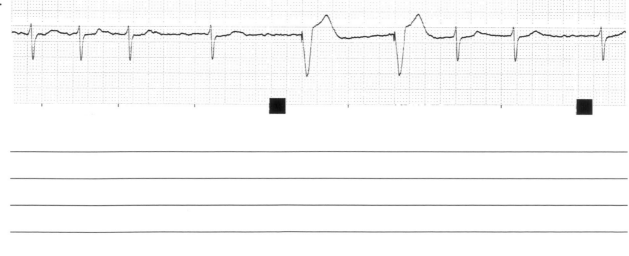

57.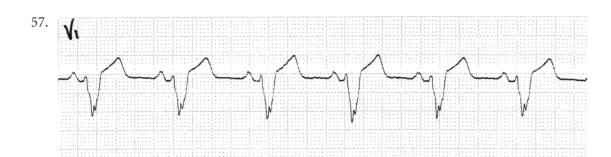

_____

_____

_____

_____

58.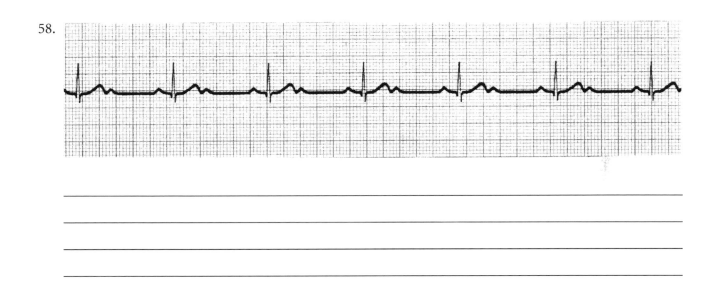

_____

_____

_____

_____

_____

59.

_____

_____

_____

_____

_____

60.

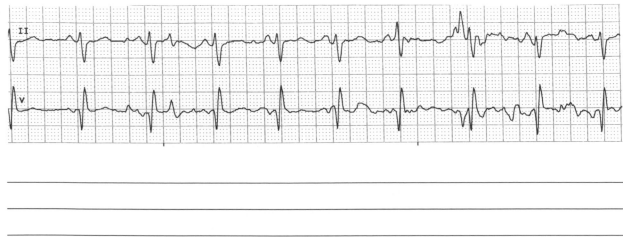

61.

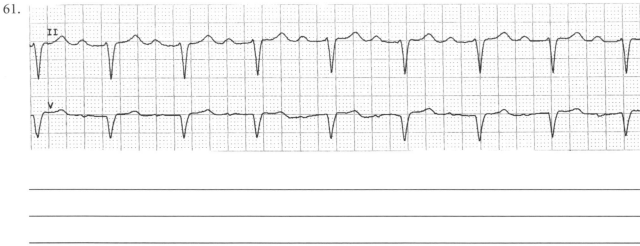

62.

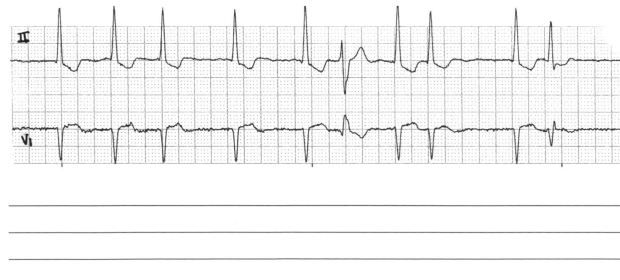

63.

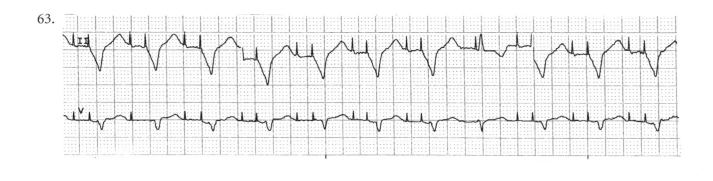

64.

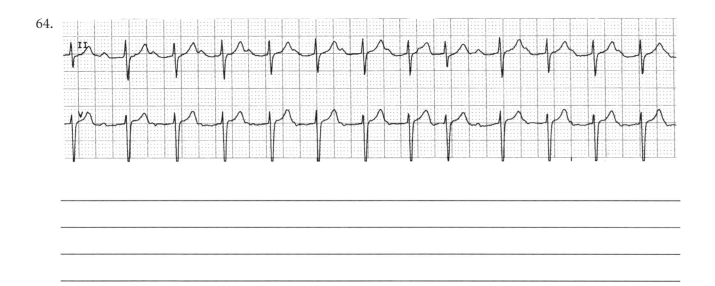

65.

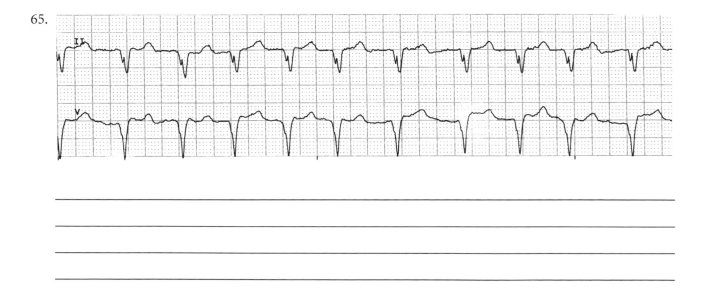

66.

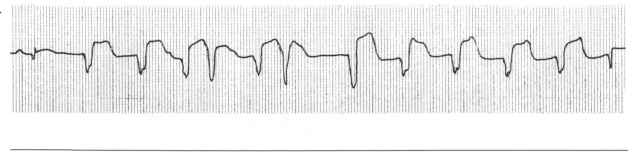

67.

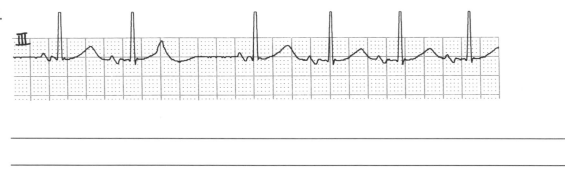

68.

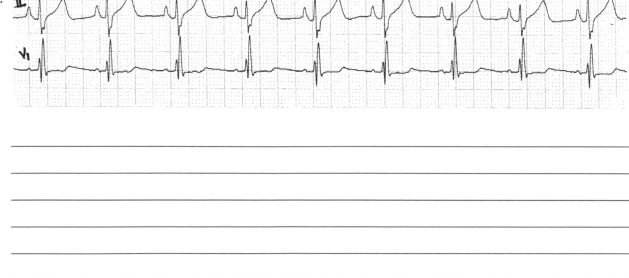

69.

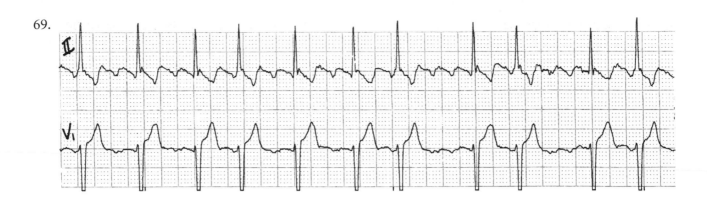

70.

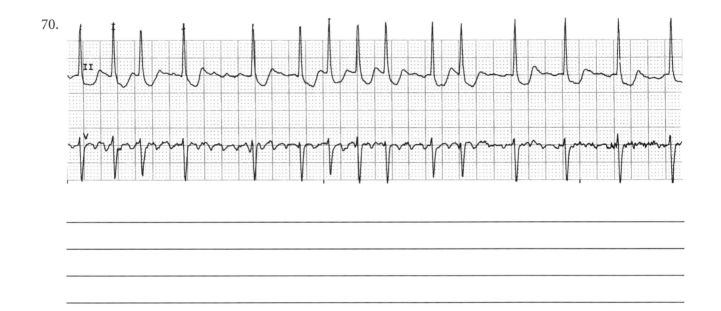

71.

72.

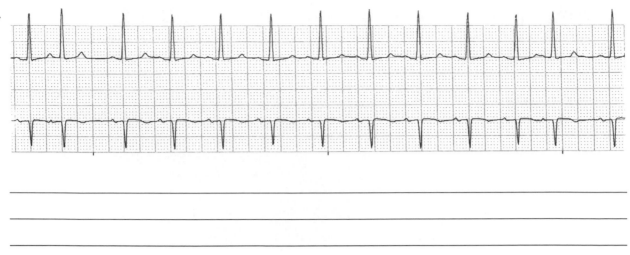

_____

_____

_____

_____

73.

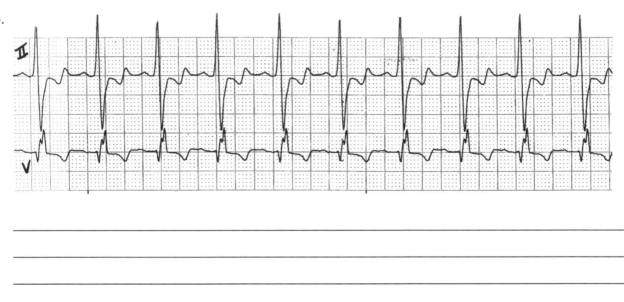

_____

_____

_____

_____

74.

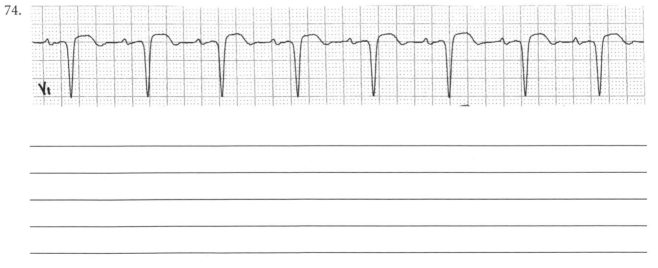

_____

_____

_____

_____

75.

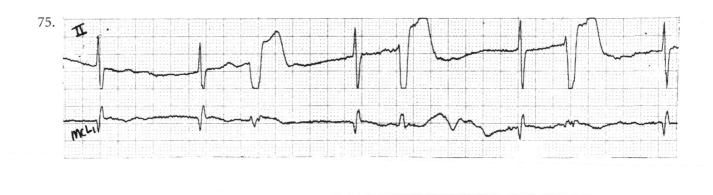

76.

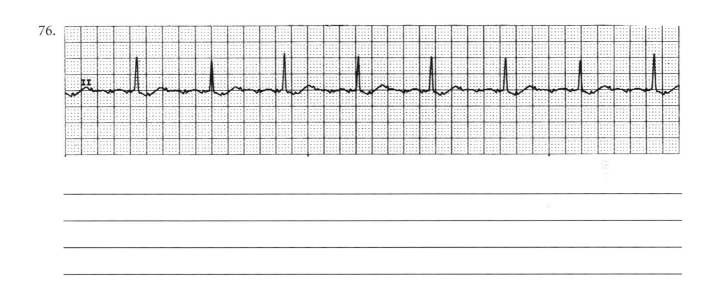

77.

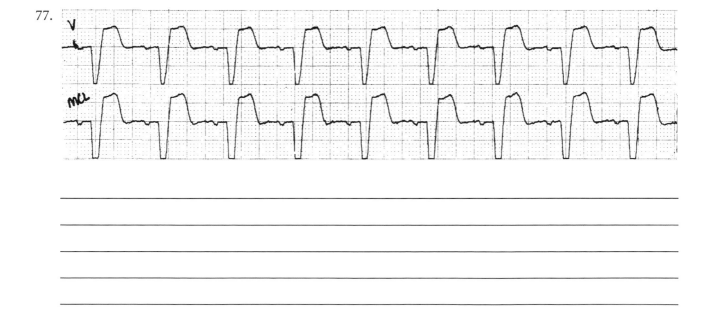

78.

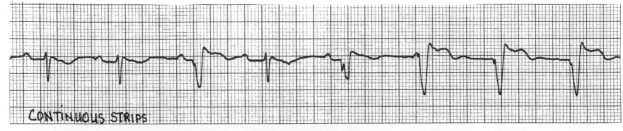

CONTINUOUS STRIPS

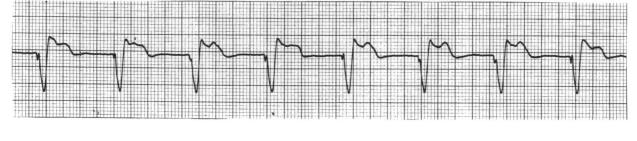

_____

_____

_____

79.

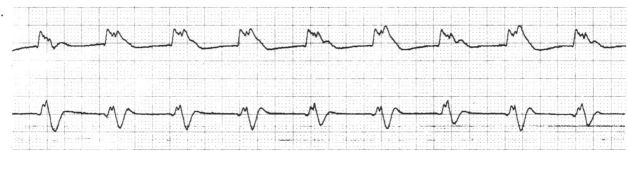

_____

_____

_____

80.

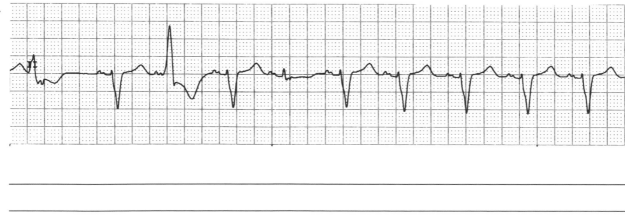

_____

_____

_____

81.

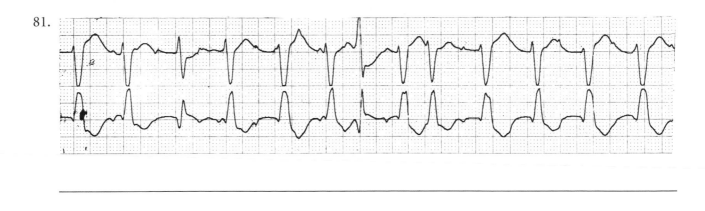

_____

_____

_____

_____

82.

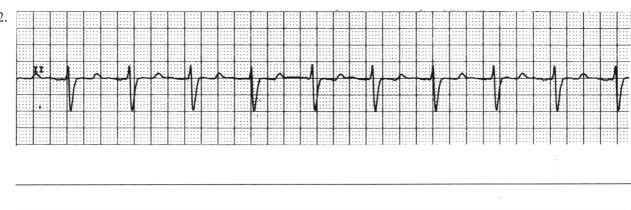

_____

_____

_____

_____

_____

83.

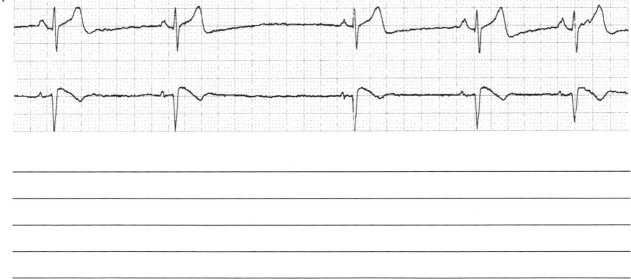

_____

_____

_____

_____

84.

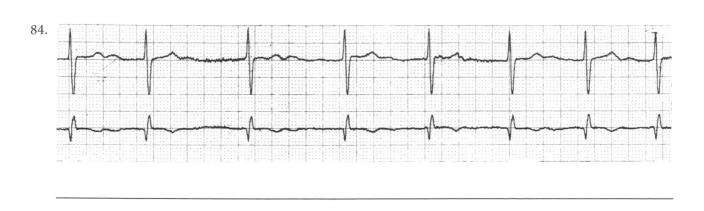

85.

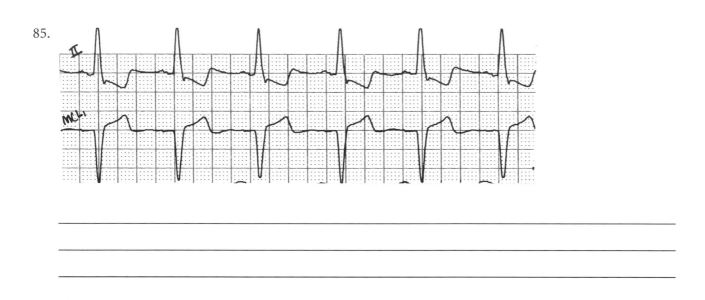

86.

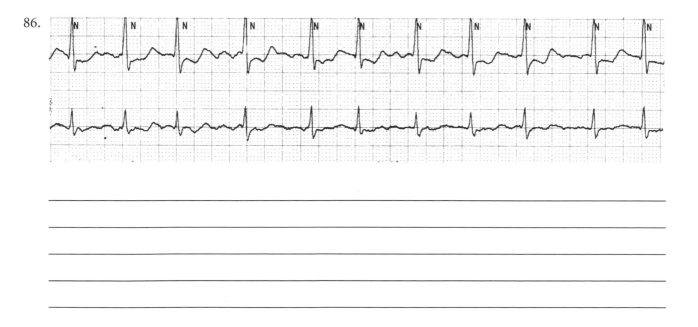

87.

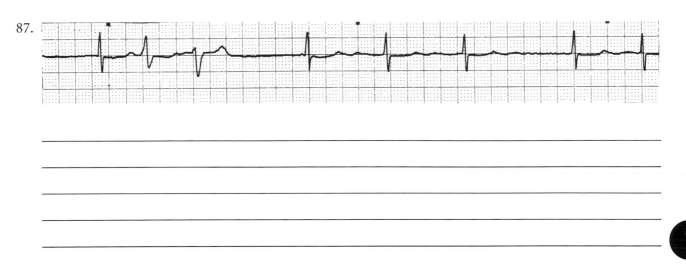

88.

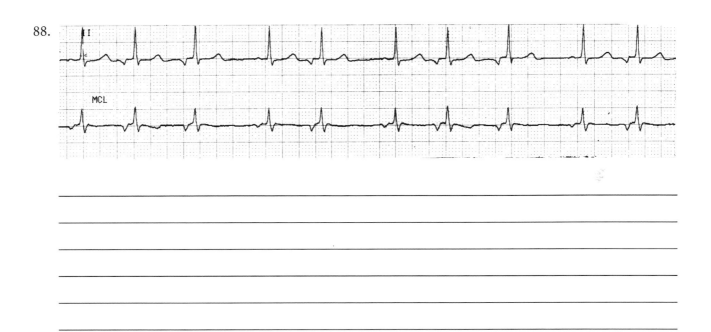

89.

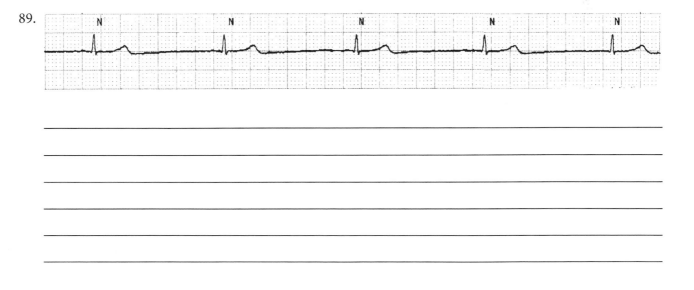

90.

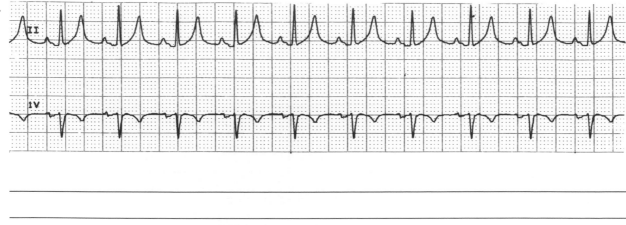

_____

_____

_____

_____

91.

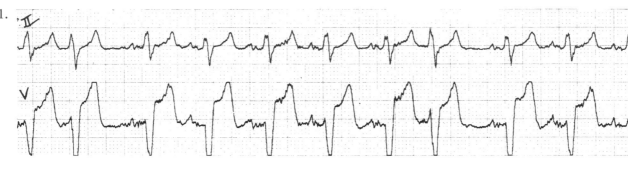

_____

_____

_____

_____

92.

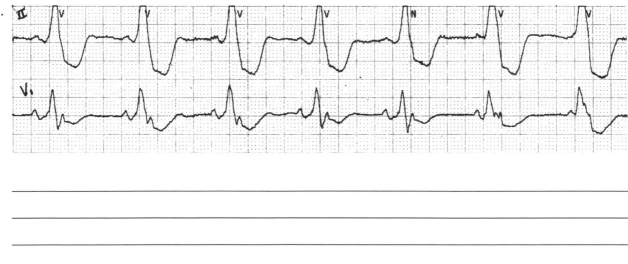

_____

_____

_____

_____

93.

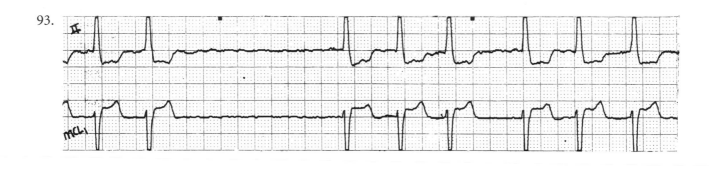

94.

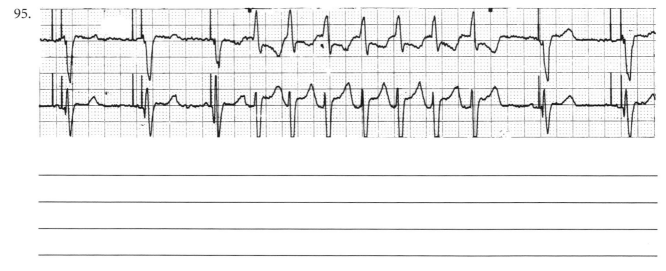

95.

96.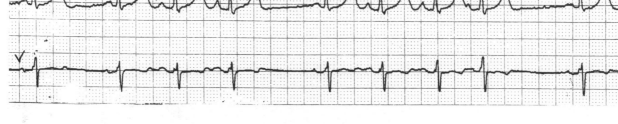

_____

_____

_____

_____

_____

_____

97.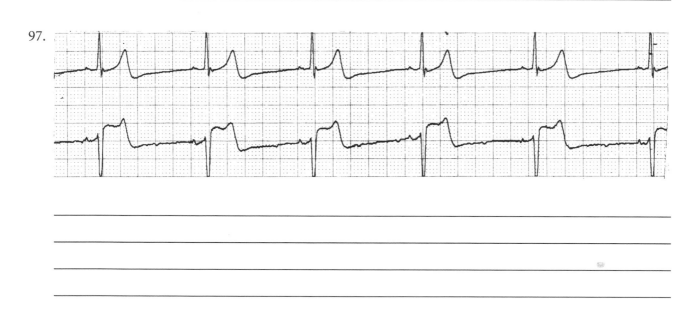

_____

_____

_____

_____

_____

_____

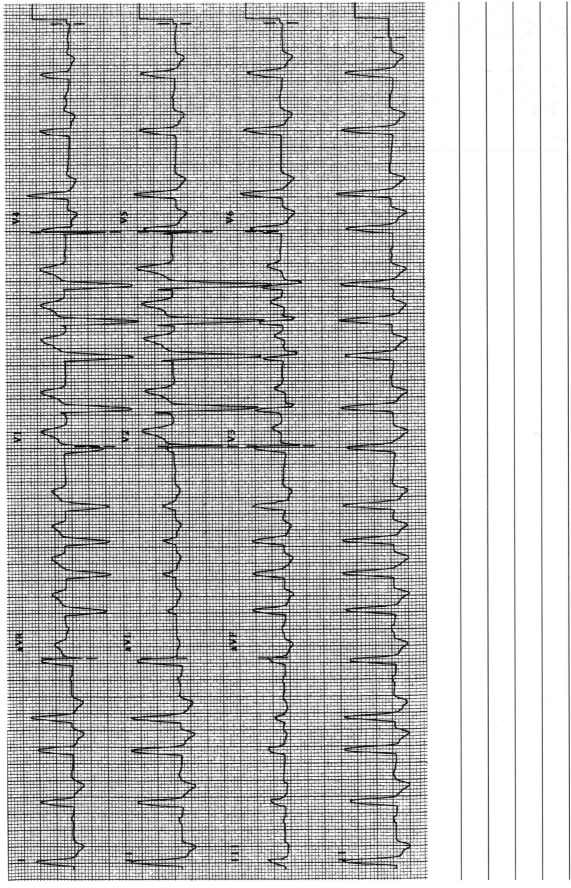

98.

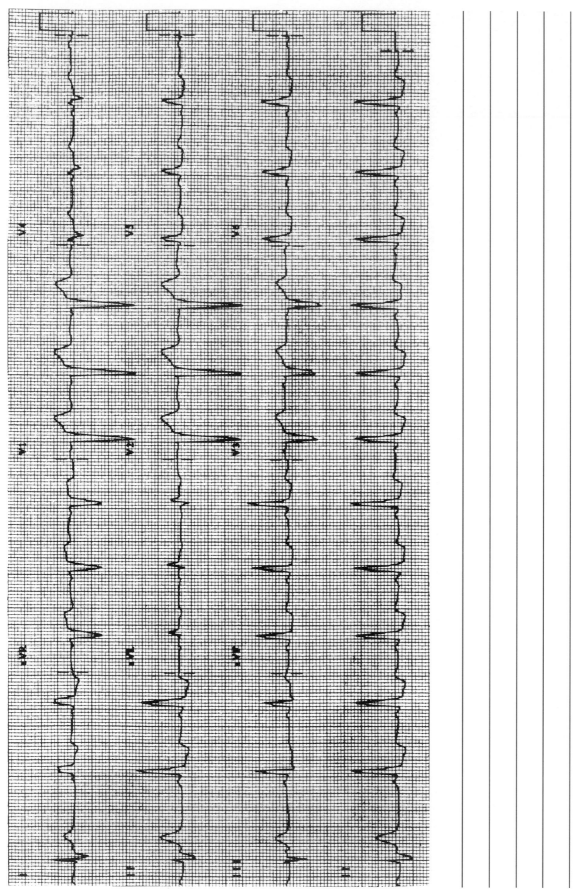

99.

100.

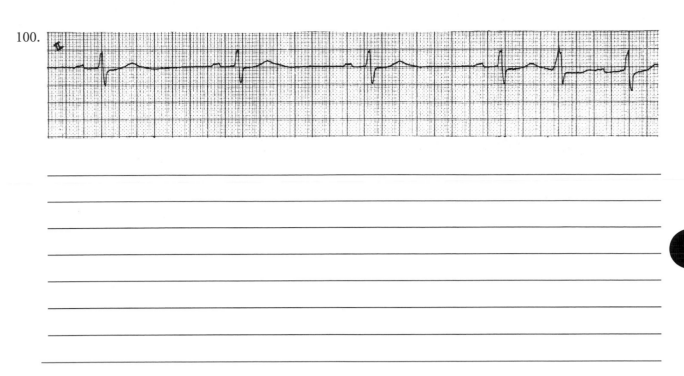

_____

_____

_____

_____

_____

_____

_____

_____

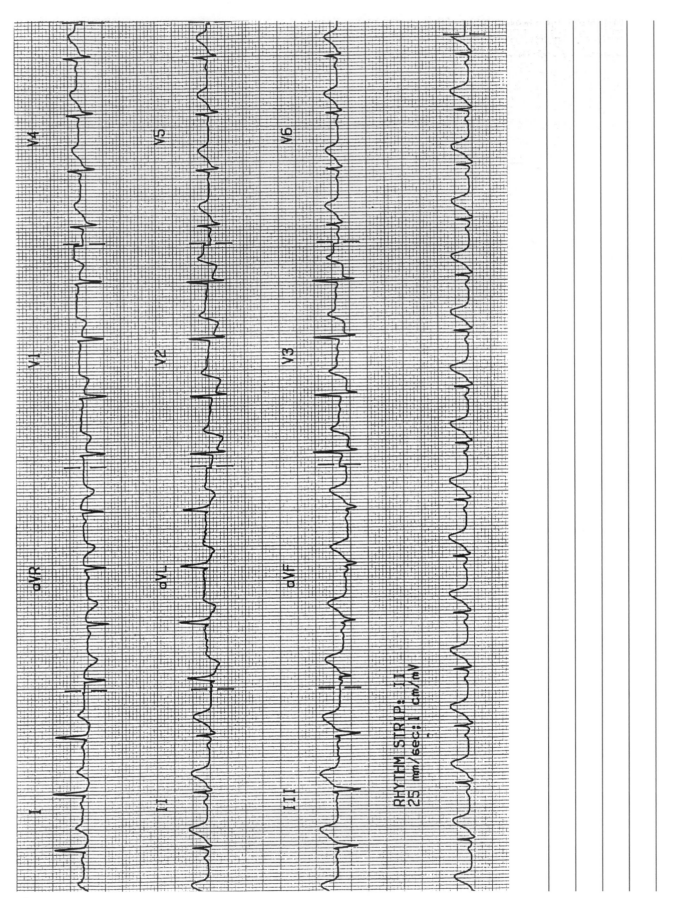

101.

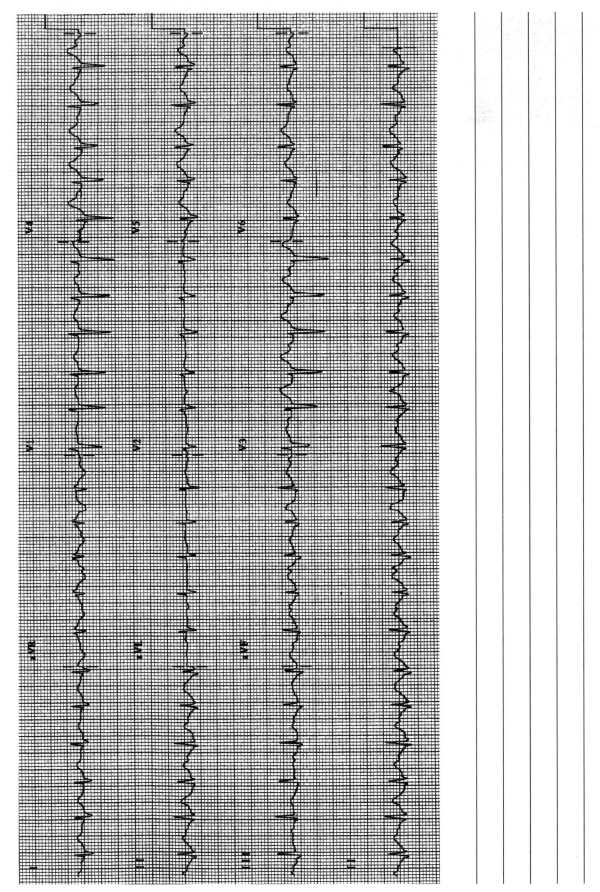

102.

103.

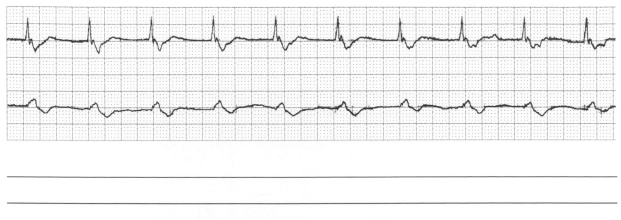

_____

_____

_____

_____

_____

104.

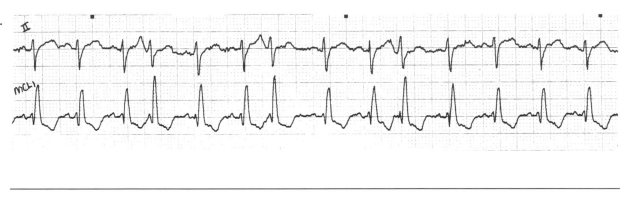

_____

_____

_____

_____

_____

105.

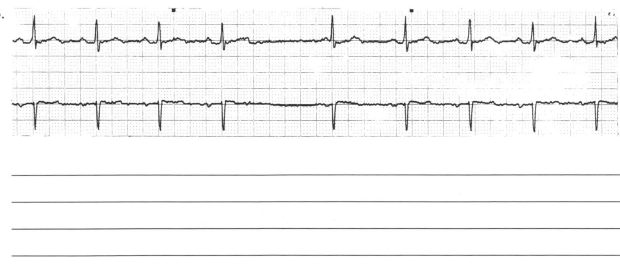

_____

_____

_____

_____

_____

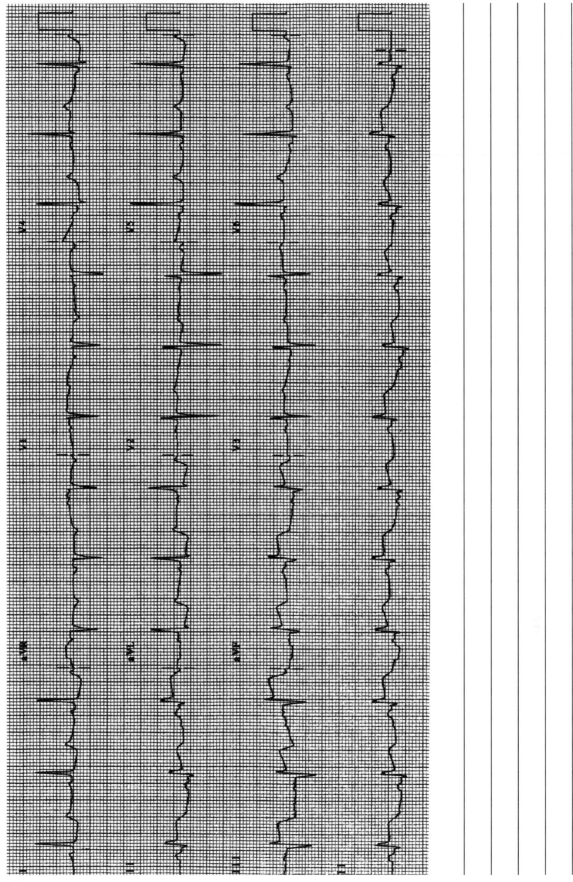

106.

107.

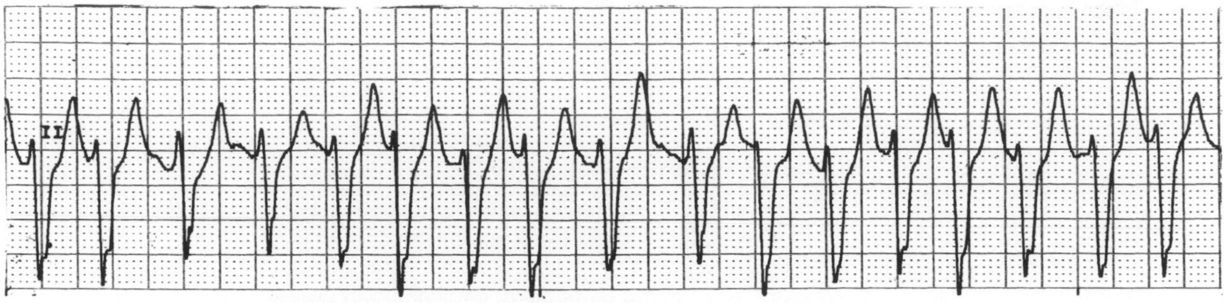

_____
_____
_____
_____
_____
_____
_____
_____
_____

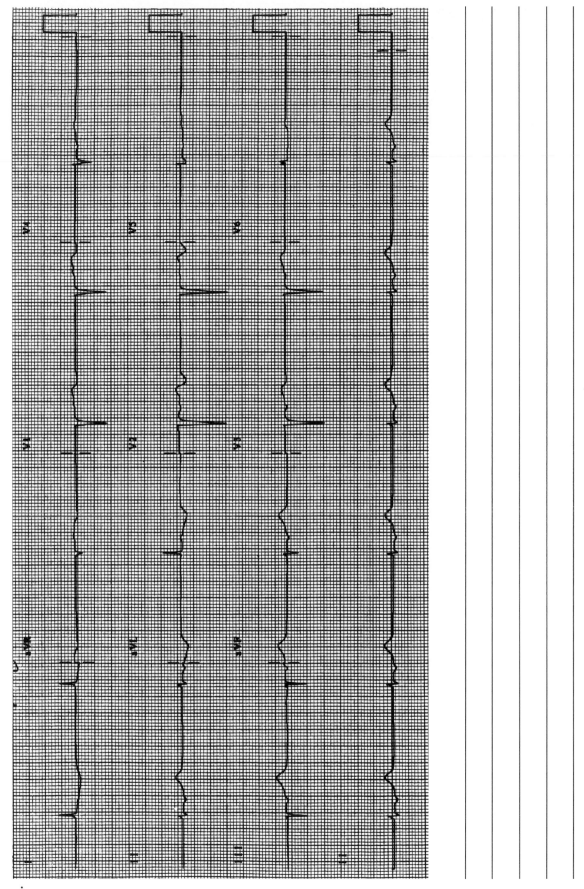

108.

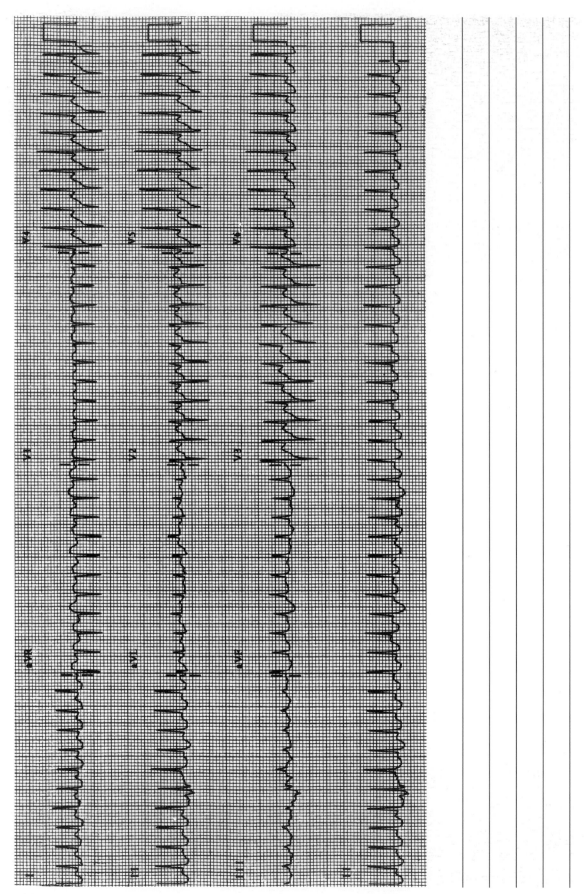

109.

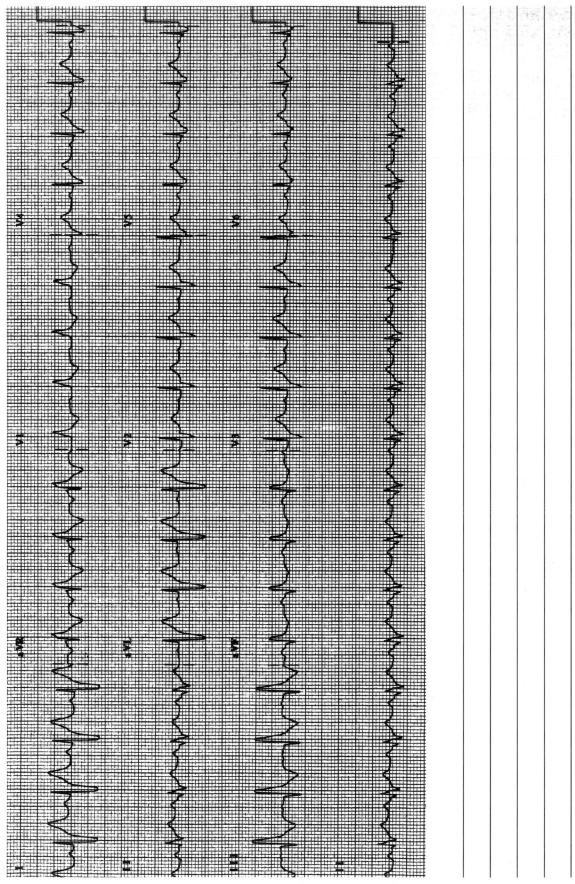

110.

111.

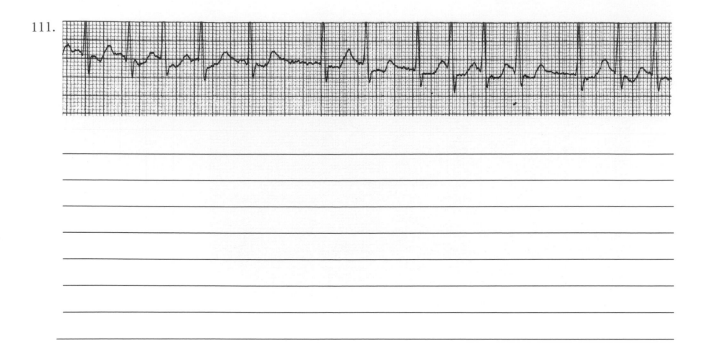

_____

_____

_____

_____

_____

_____

_____

_____

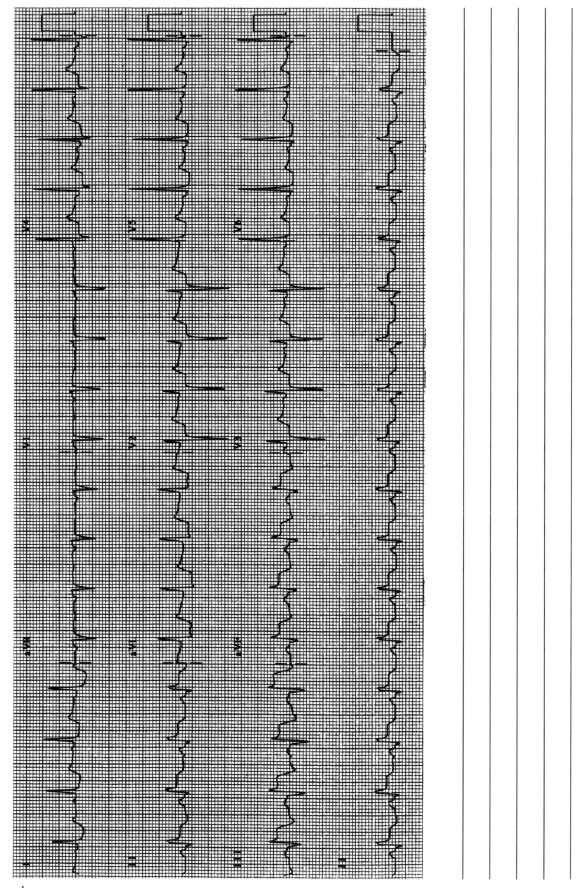

112.

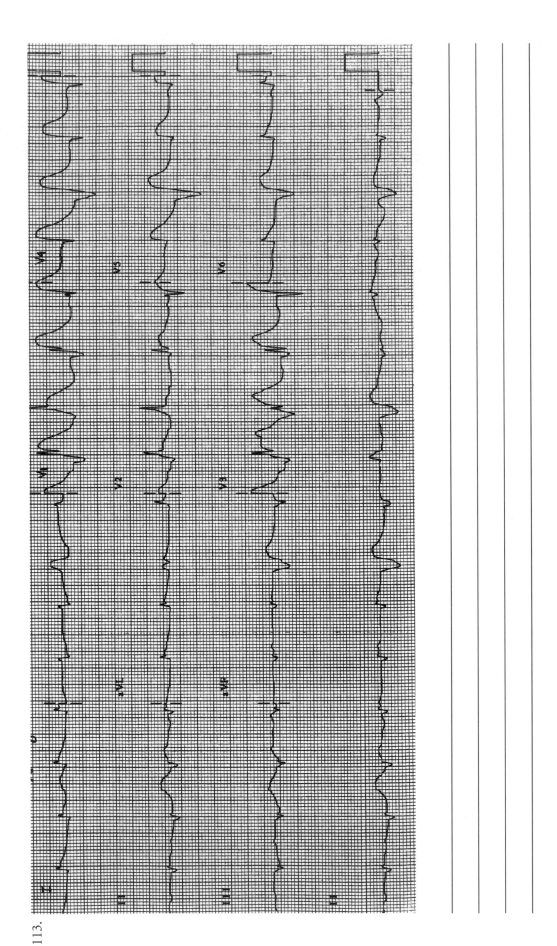

113.

114.

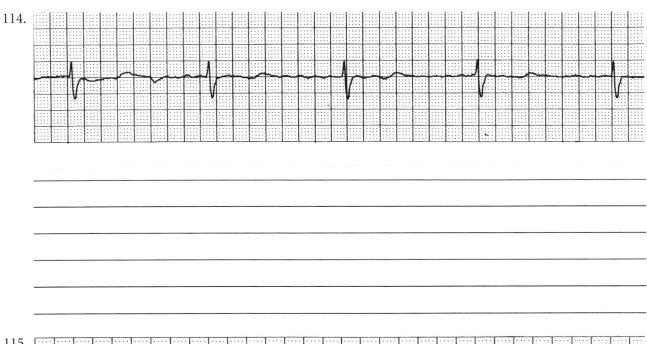

_____

_____

_____

_____

_____

_____

115.

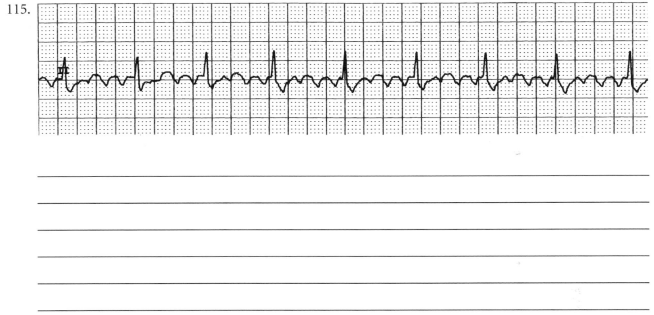

_____

_____

_____

_____

_____

_____

16

116. (Continuous Strip)

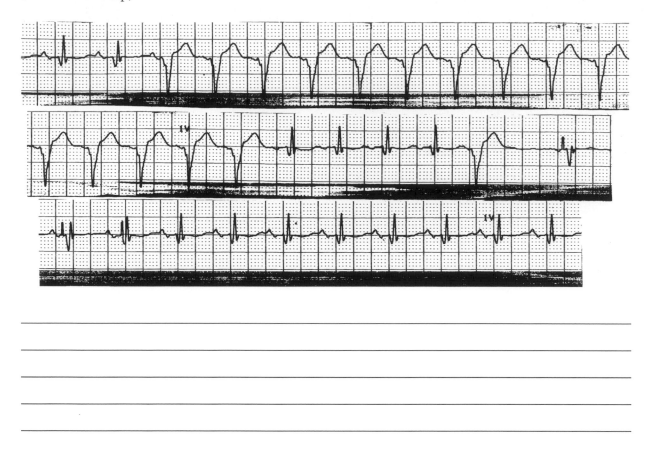

_____

_____

_____

_____

_____

_____

117.

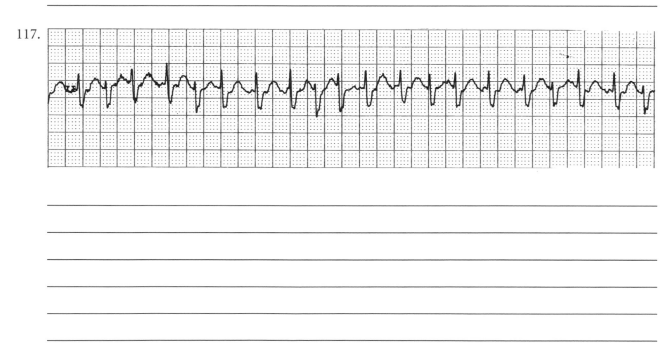

_____

_____

_____

_____

_____

_____

118.

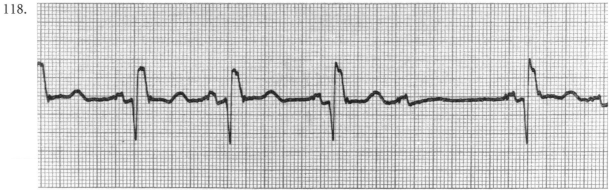

_____

_____

_____

_____

_____

_____

119.

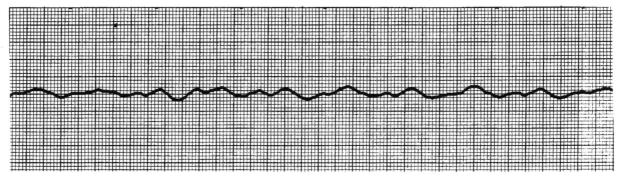

_____

_____

_____

_____

_____

_____

Interpretations

No two individuals analyze rhythm strips in the same manner. Thus, I do not expect your verbage to match mine!! Be certain, however, that your descriptions contain the "fundamentals."

1. By eyeball analysis, this rhythm is irregular. Every QRS is preceded by a P wave. Certain P waves appear different in configuration. My tendency is to identify something familiar and work backwards. Beats #3 and #4 appear similar—slow sinus beats. Beats #3 and #4 have identical upright P waves and the P-R interval of those two beats measures 0.16 seconds. The QRS complexes measure slightly less than 0.12 seconds. The ST segments are significantly depressed and the T waves are inverted. Beat #5 occurs earlier than expected in the cycle, the P wave is of a different configuration, and the P-R interval is shorter in duration. This is a P.A.C. Following the P.A.C. is the normal anticipated pause allowing the sinus mechanism to reset itself. Beats #6 and #7 appear to be sinus beats. Now back to the beginning of the strip. Beat #1 is a sinus beat. (Note the constant P-R interval of beats #1, #3, #4, #6, and #7.) Beat #2 is a P.A.C., coming earlier than anticipated, and followed by a pause. Viola! The underlying rhythm is a sinus rhythm interrupted by P.A.C.s (beats #2 and #5). The ST depression and inverted T waves noted throughout are suggestive of ischemia. How did you do?

2. This rhythm is slow and irregular. Beats #1, #5, and #6 all look alike in that they have clearly identifiable P waves appearing before the QRSs. The P-R interval measures approximately 0.28 seconds—grounds for first degree AV block. The QRS complexes throughout measure a "hair less" than 0.12 seconds. Beats #5 and #6 represent the underlying rhythm, a pronounced sinus bradycardia (rate approximately 40) with first degree AV block. Measure the interval between beats #5 and #6 and compare that to the interval between beats #1 and #2. You will notice that beat #2 is inscribed later than expected. Beats #2 and #3 represent an escape rhythm generated from the AV junctional tissues (the QRSs are not preceded by a P wave and the QRS duration is within normal limits). Beat #4 may have a P wave, though the P-R interval is shorter than beats #5 and #6. (Limb leads would better display atrial activity.) Note the slight ST elevation throughout. In summary, the underlying rhythm is a *slow* sinus bradycardia with first degree AV block. There is a period of sinus arrest (a failure) and a resulting junctional response. The sinus pacemaker resumes near the end of the strip. This patient was in the recovery phase of an acute M.I.

3. S L O W, irregular, ineffective ventricular rhythm. This is known as an agonal or dying heart rhythm. This rhythm strip followed an unsuccessful resuscitation.

4. First, I have scanned the strip to determine that beats #1, #2, #3, #6, #7, #8, and #9 appear similar. The P-R interval of those beats measures approximately 0.18 seconds. There is obvious artifact throughout the strip. Though somewhat difficult to measure precisely, the QRS appears to be 0.12 seconds in duration (normal duration is *less* than 0.12 seconds). The underlying rhythm is sinus rhythm (rate somewhere in the mid-sixties) with slightly delayed ventricular conduction. I would need to view lead V_1 for a better analysis and to distinguish right vs. left bundle branch block. Beats #4 and #5 are coupled P.V.C.s with the first P.V.C. falling near the vulnerable T wave of beat #3. Couplets may signify increasing ventricular irritability. In summary, this is a sinus rhythm with bundle branch block with coupled P.V.C.s.

5. The underlying rhythm is slightly irregular, probably secondary to a slight sinus arrhythmia (related to respiration). The approximate rate is 70 beats per minute. With the exception of beats #3 and #4, all P waves and QRS complexes appear identical. There is a "slight" first degree AV block present since the P-R interval measures approximately 0.21 seconds. Beat #3 is a P.V.C. though it does not interrupt the rhythm of the underlying pacemaker. This is an interpolated P.V.C. with the same significance of any other P.V.C.. Beat #4 is probably a sinus beat. Interpolated P.V.C.s typically cause a prolongation of the P-R interval of the next beat. I suspect a P wave is hidden in the recovery phase of the interpolated P.V.C. In any event, this is a sinus rhythm with borderline first degree AV block interrupted by a P.V.C. (interpolated). Generalized ST depression is present throughout.

6. Here is a two lead view of a sinus rhythm. Note the ST depression in lead II and the ST elevation present in the V lead. The ST elevation represents injury. The ST depression seen in lead II is a reciprocal change. One would want to view a 12 lead EKG to identify the location and extent of damage.

7. This rhythm is slow and regular with a rate near 50 beats per minute. Identically appearing P waves precede each QRS. The P-R interval is constant and measures 0.18 seconds. The QRSs are uniform in appearance and measure 0.11 seconds. This is a sinus bradycardia. T waves sometimes appear tented. Check the patient's potassium to rule out hyperkalemia.

8. Here we find an irregularly irregular rhythm. There are no clear P waves. The baseline appears to undulate. A lone ectopic beat breaks the ranks. This rhythm is atrial fibrillation with an Ashman's beat. One would need to count the rate for one full minute to accurately determine heart rate.

9. This strip presents another irregularly irregular rhythm with ST depression. Though T waves are pronounced following the ST depression, there are no definitive P waves preceding the QRS complexes. QRS complexes measure within normal limits. For a better view of atrial activity, I would monitor on leads II, III, or aVF. This rhythm strip is fine atrial fibrillation with ST depression. If you think rhythm interpretation is tedious and frustrating, you are correct!

10. **Never panic!** Always make the monitor believe *you* are in control! My first eyeball analysis reveals that P waves come before every beat! Thus, I can relax. This is *not* a ventricular anything. I am going to begin my analysis at the beginning of the strip. The first five beats occur regularly with an approximate rate of 85 per minute. Though some notching exists, the P waves appear uniform and the constant P-R interval measures 0.20 seconds. (Notching of the P wave may represent atrial hypertrophy.) The QRS complexes measure 0.12 seconds in duration, grounds for bundle branch block. An analysis of the second half of the strip reveals an approximate rate of 85 beats per minute. The P-R interval measures 0.22 seconds. The QRS complexes measure 0.12 seconds in duration. The second half of the strip also reveals a bundle branch block. My best guess is that this rhythm represents alternating right and left bundle branch blocks—no doubt a function of severe myocardial ischemia/damage. Both the right and left bundle branch blocks produce ST-T wave distortion. To be certain, more information is warranted and a 12-lead EKG is in order!

11. Another strange rhythm strip! The underlying rhythm is regular (approximate rate 62) with a premature beat appearing midstream. A P wave presents before each QRS of the underlying rhythm. The P-R interval is prolonged, measuring 0.24 seconds. Thus, a first degree AV block is present. The QRS complexes of the underlying rhythm measure approximately 0.14 seconds, signifying bundle branch block. To determine right vs. left bundle branch block, one would need to view lead V_1. The underlying rhythm is a sinus rhythm with both first degree AV block and bundle branch block. The premature beat interrupting the rhythm has a QRS measuring 0.14 seconds. Is it ventricular or supraventricular in origin? If possible, look at this ectopic beat in different leads to determine origin. I did not describe ST depression because, in the face of bundle branch block, it is impossible to diagnose in one lead.

12. The rhythm is regular with a rate of 125 beats per minute. P waves are present before each QRS and begin on the downstroke of the preceding T wave. The P-R interval is constant and measures slightly less than 0.20 seconds. The QRS duration is constant and measures slightly greater than 0.08 seconds. This rhythm is a sinus tachycardia with ST depression.

13. Here is a nice, pretty, regular rhythm with an approximate rate of 58 beats per minute. The QRS duration is within normal limits and the T waves are peaked in appearance. No P waves are obvious prior to, or following, the QRS. This rhythm is a junctional (escape) rhythm. A potassium level may be in order since prominent peaked T waves are a primary feature of hyperkalemia. Also, hyperkalemia depresses normal electrical activity and may precipitate conduction disturbances such as junctional rhythms!

14. This is a tough one, so I thought two consecutive rhythm strips (A and B) might be helpful! I always look for something "known" when I begin analysis. The last three beats of the second strip (B) demonstrate a sinus rhythm with an approximate rate of 75 per minute. The P-R interval measures 0.18 seconds and

the QRS is greater than the normal limits, measuring 0.14 seconds. So, the last three beats represent a sinus rhythm with bundle branch block. One would need to view lead V1 to determine right vs. left bundle branch block. Now back to the beginning, Strip A. At first glance, the rhythm resembles a ventricular tachycardia. The rhythm is irregular, the QRSs are widened, and there are no clearly distinguishable P waves. However, in the middle of Strip A there appears to be two consecutive P waves. Presumably the second P wave conducts through to the ventricles (a sinus beat). The QRSs of the rapid rhythm are similar in appearance to those at the end of the second strip, suggesting a bundle branch block. So, what is the rapid rhythm? I'm not certain either! Rather than risk confusion, I would simply describe this strip as a supraventricular tachycardia. The rapid rhythm breaks in the bottom strip. There is a pause, followed by a beat with an inverted P wave, then on to sinus rhythm. The pause might indicate a vagal maneuver resulting in a pause that allows the sinus to regain control.

Whew!!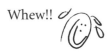

15. Another difficult strip for consideration! I hope having two consecutive rhythm strips helped. To be certain, this is an irregular rhythm. In beginning my analysis, I look for beats similar in appearance! In the second strip (B), beats #2, #4, #5, #7, #8, #10, and #12 look reasonably similar, as do beats #1, #3, #9, and #11.

First, I'll consider beats #2, #4, #5, #7, #8, #10, and #12 (B). No clear (obvious) P waves precede these beats, but the baseline undulates. The QRS complexes are within normal limits, measuring 0.10 seconds and the R-R interval varies. Note the ST segment depression and biphasic T wave following those QRSs. The underlying rhythm here is atrial fibrillation with ST segment depression.

Now back to beats #1, #3, #9, and #11 in Strip B. One can easily be misled believing these are sinus beats with a bundle branch block configuration! However, there are *no* P waves preceding these prolonged QRS complexes (QRS measures 0.16 seconds)! Look back at the ST segment and T waves of beats #4, #5, and #7 of Strip B. What appears to be P waves preceding the widened QRSs are in fact the biphasic T waves of the previous beat. *Ugh!* So, these wide beats (#1, 3, 9, 11 in strip B) are most likely P.V.C.s. Beat #6 (Strip B) is also a P.V.C. but of a different configuration (signifying irritability of different ventricular focus).

Now back to Strip A. Beats #2, #4, #6, #7, #8, #10, and #12 are likely P.V.C.s! This rhythm is an atrial fibrillation with *extreme* ventricular irritability as is evidenced by frequent P.V.C.s, multifocused ventricular excitability, and consecutive P.V.C.s. Clearly, amiodarone therapy would be in order.

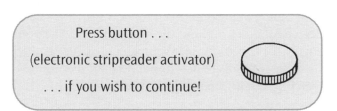

Press button . . .

(electronic stripreader activator)

. . . if you wish to continue!

16. This strip demonstrates a pacemaker generated ventricular rhythm. Note the pacemaker spikes initiating each QRS. The ventricular pacemaker rate is approximately 75 per minute.

17. The underlying rhythm is a sinus rhythm with an estimated rate of 70 beats per minute. The P-R interval of the sinus beats measures 0.18 seconds and the QRS measures less than 0.12 seconds in duration. The rhythm is interrupted by unifocal P.V.C.s occurring in a bigeminal pattern. Note the artifact at the end of the rhythm strip.

18. This strip first demonstrates a regular underlying rhythm, rate 100 beats per minute. The atrial activity is masked by artifact evident throughout the tracing. The QRSs of the underlying rhythm measure 0.12 seconds. Though distorted, there is evidence of significant ST depression. There is a probable run of P.V.C.s in the second half of the strip. As a first course of action, I would attempt to diminish the artifact. This rhythm is a sinus rhythm with bundle branch block interrupted by a short burst of ventricular tachycardia!

19. This strip seems simple compared to some of the previous examples! The rhythm is regular at an approximate rate of 66 beats per minute. The P-R interval is constant and measures 0.16 seconds. The QRS is abnormally wide, measuring almost 0.16 seconds. This is a sinus rhythm with a bundle branch block. One would need to review lead V_1 to accurately distinguish right from left bundle branch block.

20. The rhythm is regular with a rate of 136 beats per minute. When P waves cannot clearly be distinguished, I tend to use the term *supraventricular*. There may be P waves occurring on top of the T waves, but I am uncertain. Because the QRS is within normal limits (0.08 seconds), I know the rhythm cannot be of ventricular origin. Thus, we have a supraventricular tachycardia with a rate of 136 beats per minute. In all probability, this is a sinus tachycardia. P waves can be seen more distinctly when monitoring on leads II, III, or aVF.

21. The rhythm is regular, occurring at an approximate rate of 80 beats per minute. A widened P wave precedes each QRS (suggesting atrial hypertrophy) and the constant P-R interval measures 0.20 seconds. The QRS measures 0.11 seconds. Before naming this rhythm, I would want to view leads II, III or aVF to be assured that an atrial flutter is not hiding! Otherwise, this is NSR with ST depression.

22. Here we have a sinus rhythm with a rate of 75 beats per minute. The rhythm is interrupted by a lone P.V.C. (note the retrograde P wave following the widened QRS). The P-R interval measures 0.20 seconds and the QRS of the sinus beats measures 0.20 seconds (major conduction delay). There is evidence of ST elevation; however, abnormal ventricular depolarization causes abnormal ventricular repolarization. One would need to view a 12-lead EKG for further analysis. This is a sinus rhythm with a bundle branch block and ST elevation interrupted by a P.V.C.

23. The rhythm is irregularly irregular with an undulating baseline. This is an atrial fibrillation with an approximate rate of 80 beats per minute. The QRS measures 0.08 seconds.

24. This rhythm strip demonstrates an undulating baseline with no evidence of P, Q, R, S, or T waves. With no patient to observe, one would assume this is ventricular fibrillation and grounds for immediate resuscitation. However, the truth of the matter is that this patient lost his electrodes! In fact, the patient had a normal sinus rhythm once the leads were reattached! Always check the patient first!

25. Two continuous rhythm strips were presented to assist in rhythm interpretation. The first three beats in Strip A demonstrate a sinus rhythm with a rate of 75 beats per minute and ST elevation. The P-R interval measures 0.20 seconds and the QRS measures approximately 0.08 seconds. The P wave of beat #4 occurs on time, though the P wave is slightly more pronounced than in the previous three beats. The QRS of this beat is configured differently, but measures less than 0.12 seconds in duration. The pacemaker for this beat is located within the atria, but obviously travels a different pathway, resulting in a QRS with a different configuration. However, looking ahead to the next series of beats, I suspect that beat #4 is a fusion beat—partly formed by a sinus impulse and partly formed by an ectopic ventricular impulse. The remainder of Strip A demonstrates an accelerated ventricular rhythm, rate of 79 beats per minute. Fortunately, near the end of Strip B, the sinus pacemaker again resumes pacemaker control! This type of rhythm presents somewhat of a treatment dilemma. Depending upon the underlying pathology, aggressive clinicians might elect to treat based on the premise that, if the faster ventricular rhythm is abolished, a slower sinus rhythm will prevail. Conservative clinicians may refrain from aggressive therapy if the patient tolerates the rhythm. The rationale behind conservative treatment is the concern that this may be a ventricular escape mechanism, and, if abolished, there may be no underlying sustaining rhythm. To me, the strongest clue supporting an ectopic vs. escape origin is beat #4, the fusion beat. It is helpful to know that this patient had an acute inferior wall myocardial infarction in progress. Whew!!

26. The underlying rhythm is sinus rhythm (see mid-strip) with a rate of 80 beats per minute. The P-R interval and QRS measure 0.16 seconds and 0.11 seconds, respectively. Note the ST segment depression suggesting myocardial ischemia. The sinus rhythm is interrupted by bursts of ventricular tachycardia, rate approximately 160 per minute. You will note each "run" of ventricular tachycardia begins with a

"funny-looking beat" that has a P wave, and a QRS less wide than those of the ventricular tachycardia. These funny-looking beats are fusion beats and strongly support a ventricular tachycardia classification. Clearly, there is pronounced ventricular irritability!

How are you doing? I'm stopping for dinner!

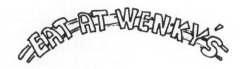

27. This rhythm is irregularly irregular and is interrupted by an Ashman's beat (a wide complex seen in atrial fibrillation). This is a "fine" atrial fibrillation. The QRS measures 0.12 seconds. This ventricular conduction delay probably accounts for the early distortion (ST segment depression) of ventricular repolarization.

28. This is one of those "treat now and ask questions later" strips. This looks like a ventricular tachycardia at a rate of 166 per minute and a QRS width of 0.16–0.20.

29. This strip demonstrates a rapid rhythm with a rate of approximately 120 beats per minute. The QRS duration is 0.12 seconds. This *may* be a sinus tachycardia with a first degree AV block (P-R measures almost 0.24 seconds) and a bundle branch block. However, I am a suspicious character by nature. Any time I see a "sing-song" rapid, regular rhythm, it makes me suspect an atrial flutter. (Sometimes, turning the strip upside down assists me in detecting atrial flutter waves.) I would want to see a rhythm strip of leads II, III, or aVF where atrial activity is more pronounced. I have drawn dots on the strip where I suspect flutter waves. If I am correct, this is a 2:1 atrial flutter. If I am wrong, this is a sinus tachycardia as described above.

30. This rhythm is viewed from both a lead II and lead V_1 perspective. You will note the rhythm is approximately 72 beats per minute. The baseline reflects patient movement. P waves are evident and the P-R interval is within normal limits. The QRS measures slightly less than 0.12 seconds. In lead II, there is pronounced ST depression. In lead V_1, ST elevation is present suggesting injury. So, this is a sinus rhythm with evidence of injury in lead V_1. One would want to view a 12-lead EKG to determine an overall pattern and location of injury. The ST depression in lead II probably represents reciprocal change. Need review? Refer back to Section 11.

31. Here we have classic artifact. If you observe closely, you can walk regularly occurring QRSs through the strip. The first two complexes suggest that this is a sinus rhythm.

32. This is a borderline sinus bradycardia with tall peaked T waves. I would want to check out the serum potassium level!

33. The presence of P waves tells me the rhythm is atrial in origin. However, the notching of the P wave is suggestive of left atrial hypertrophy. The T waves are inverted. I would want to inspect a 12-lead EKG. Note that the P-R is very short at 0.08. This is probably a borderline sinus tachycardia, but could be an atrial dysrhythmia as well.

34. Looking closely, you will note that no definitive P waves are evident. The baseline is chaotic and QRSs appear irregularly. This rhythm is atrial fibrillation interrupted by Ashman's beats.

35. This rhythm strip is similar to the previous example with one exception. In this strip, the QRS of the underlying rhythm is widened, measuring greater than 0.12 seconds. This is atrial fibrillation with bundle branch block interrupted by one Ashman's beat. One would want to view a V_1 lead to distinguish right from left bundle branch block.

36. Here we have a sinus rhythm with evidence suggesting left atrial hypertrophy and hyperkalemia. Note the tall, tent-like T waves!

37. This is a sinus rhythm with a first degree heart block. The P-R internal measures 0.28 seconds.

38. The rhythm is irregular. At first glance this looks like Wenckebach where one would expect to see an increasing P-R interval until finally, a P wave does not conduct. However, upon closer inspection and measurement, one notes that the P waves vary in size and configuration and the P-R interval, while slightly variable, does not conform to Wenckebach standards. Likely, this rhythm represents a wandering atrial pacemaker interrupted by blocked P.A.C.s. Notice the variation in the T waves preceding the pauses. I think there is a P wave sitting on top of those T waves. The P.A.C.s may not be conducting owing to refractoriness from the previously conducted impulses.

    P.S. The wave line at the bottom of the strip is a C.V.P. pressure tracing.

39. You are probably an expert by now! This is a sinus rhythm exhibiting slight ST elevation. One would want to inspect a 12-lead EKG to determine in which leads an injury pattern might be evident.

40. Here baseline artifact makes rhythm detection difficult, at best! Because QRS complexes are relatively discernable, I can see that the rhythm is irregular. A quick measurement of the R-R interval confirms this. I also note (see lead V_1) that when the rate slows, a pacemaker spike is visible. However, removing the source of artifact is important. Then re-evaluate for the presence of spikes. Measuring the R-R intervals, I note that when the rate drops below approximately 70, the pacemaker kicks in. V_1 shows the first two QRSs are upright. These may be the patient's own rhythm (unpaced).

41. This is a sinus rhythm with a bundle branch block. One would want to look at lead V_1 to distinguish right from left bundle branch block. P-R appears to be long, but is borderline at 0.20.

42. Here is a sinus rhythm with a first-degree AV heart block (P-R = 0.24 seconds) interrupted by a lone etopic beat (perhaps a premature junctional beat). Also note the slight ST elevation suggestive of injury.

43. This rhythm strip demonstrates a classic atrial fibrillation.

44. Never panic. Remember, the first pulse you take is your own! The first two complexes appear to be sinus beats (rate approximately 80). The QRS measures almost 0.20 seconds, grounds for bundle branch block. Following is a premature beat with a widened QRS and no obvious P wave. Because this premature beat's QRS is upright as the previous two sinus beats, I think this is a premature junctional beat. Its QRS is widened because of the existing bundle branch block. Complex 4 is also a sinus beat followed by a P.V.C. This is a P.V.C. for two reasons: First, the QRS is directionally opposite to the sinus beats; second, a small retrograde P wave follows the complex. Then the patterns repeat. Interestingly, beat 7 is a premature junctional beat followed by a late (escape) junctional beat. For descriptive purposes, I would say that this is a sinus rhythm with bundle branch block (I would need to inspect V_1 to determine right or left) interrupted by both premature and escape junctional beats and a P.V.C. Often times, complex rhythm strips require a beat by beat analysis!

45. This is a sinus rhythm with slight ST depression.

46. Here we have a sinus rhythm with evidence of bundle branch block. The QRS measures approximately 0.14 seconds. One would need to view leads V_1 and V_6 to determine right from left bundle branch block.

47. This is a ventricular fibrillation! Hope you did not miss this one! It seemed timely to give you a break.

48. Again, this is a sinus rhythm with notched P waves suggestive of atrial hypertrophy.

49. This is a rapid and irregularly irregular rhythm. Though baseline artifact makes precise interpretation difficult, this is most likely atrial fibrillation with one aberrantly conducted beat occurring early in the tracing.

50. Here we have sinus rhythm during deep slumber. The artifact is from the rise and fall of the chest. Note the flipped T waves evident in the chest (V) lead. One would want to inspect a 12-lead EKG to gauge the significance of the T wave inversion.

51. This rhythm is fairly regular. Pacemaker spikes are evident throughout the rhythm strip producing a paced rate of 83 per minute. It would appear that the underlying rhythm is a sinus rhythm.

52. Here we have a regular sinus rhythm interrupted by a P.V.C. However, the P waves are pronounced and the QRSs are wide, measuring 0.16 seconds. So, this is a sinus rhythm with bundle branch block interrupted by a P.V.C. Note the expected pause following the P.V.C. allowing the sinus pacemaking mechanism to reset. The pronounced P waves suggest atrial hypertrophy.

53. This strip is irregularly irregular. The baseline appears to undulate. This is atrial fibrillation! Despite the long pause, the rate is still approximately 70.

54. Yikes!! This is a *grab-the-cart-and-a-defibrillator-quickly* rhythm. This is a ventricular tachycardia (rate 187 per minute) that terminates spontaneously, giving way to a ventricular escape rhythm. The object of treatment is to abolish the ventricular irritability and then support the underlying rhythm. This patient is gravely ill!

55. This is a two-lead view of sinus rhythm. Note the ST elevation present in the V lead. One would want to inspect a 12-lead EKG to determine other leads reflecting injury pattern.

56. Here is another interesting strip demonstrating the proper functioning of a pacemaker. The underlying rhythm is atrial fibrillation. When the rate of conduction slows, the ventricular pacemaker (rate 50) responds.

57. Here we have a sinus rhythm with evidence of a classic left bundle branch block. The QRS measures a touch less than 0.16 seconds.

58. This looks like a sinus bradycardia, rate approximately 50 per minute. However, upon closer inspection, one notes that a non-conducted P wave follows every T wave. One can *walk* the P waves through the strips, meaning that P waves occur regularly at a rate of approximately 100 per minute. The important question to answer is whether the atrial activity bears any relationship to ventricular activity. To determine that, I measure the P-R interval of the conducted beats. The P-R interval is constant, so this is a 2:1 AV conduction pattern. Because the P-R is constant, this is a manifestation of Mobitz II (second degree block type II).

59. This is a ventricular tachycardia at a rate of approximately 300.

60. This is a sinus rhythm with lots of motion artifact!

61. Here we have a sinus rhythm with pronounced first degree AV block. Note that the P-R interval measures 0.32 seconds.

62. This is an atrial fibrillation interrupted by an Ashman's beat. Notice the QS pattern and slight ST elevation in lead V_1 and the reciprocal ST depression in lead II.

63. Some motion artifact complicates this rhythm strip. I presume this is an A-V sequential pacemaker. Having two leads to inspect is helpful given that all pacemaker spikes are not clearly evident in either lead. However, I would want to determine the type of implanted pacemaker and would want to verify two (dual) wires by chest x-ray.

64. Here we have a sinus tachycardia (rate 107) with a first degree heart block. The P-R interval measures 0.28 seconds. The rhythm is interrupted by a premature beat of uncertain supraventricular origin. I know the premature beat is not a P.V.C. because the QRS duration is within normal limits.

65. This is a bit of a perplexing strip. Despite the fact that two leads are demonstrated, I would want to view a 12-lead EKG. Though at first glance the rhythm appears fairly regular, if one measures the R-R interval, rhythm irregularity is evident. The R-R interval always varies and there are no discernable P waves. Thus, the underlying rhythm is atrial fibrillation. Typically, one would expect QRSs within normal limits when associated with a reasonable heart rate. In this example, however, the QRS complexes are widened,

measuring slightly greater than 0.12 seconds. Thus, a left bundle branch block (inspect lead V_1) exists, meaning that the conducted fibrillation waves travel in an antegrade (forward) fashion, but encounter delay secondary to a conduction disturbance in the left bundle branch.

66. Bummer. This one is tough! The very first complex is a sinus beat exhibiting a first degree block and ST elevation. After that, hold on to your hat. Because of the long pause following the initial sinus beat, it appears that an accelerated idioventricular pacemaker kicks in for three beats, and then is disrupted by a P.V.C. falling on the T wave of the preceding beat. That pattern occurs twice, then back to the probable idioventricular rhythm. If the patient is relatively stable, I would want to observe a 12-lead EKG. It is possible that the patient has a bundle branch block confounding a junctional escape rhythm with interspersed P.V.C.s. Whatever be the case, the owner is in a compromised position. Most likely, treatment would consist of a transcutenous pacemaker followed by amiodarone.

67. First notice the notched (bi-phasic) P waves. The P-R interval increases slightly in the second beat. There is a non-conducted P wave sitting on top of the second T wave. Note the distortion of the T wave prior to the pause. This is a non-conducted P.A.C. interrupting a sinus rhythm at a rate of 75.

68. This is a normal sinus rhythm with a QRS of 0.10–0.12, or a marginal right bundle branch block.

69. This rhythm is irregular and there is evidence of saw-toothed atrial activity. Though there is a bit of base-line artifact, one can *walk* the F waves through the strip (lead II). The flutter waves are occurring at a rate of 300 per minute. This is atrial flutter with variable A-V block. One would need to count the complexes for one full minute to determine an accurate heart rate. Note that flutter waves are most obvious in leads II, III, and aVF.

70. This rhythm looks somewhat similar to the previous tracing in that saw-toothed waves are evident in the V lead. However, when one tries to *walk* those waves through the rhythm strip, they tend to fizzle out. In other words, try as I might, the saw-toothed waves are not quite regular. Often times this type of rhythm is referred to as atrial fib-flutter. Some would argue that it is a course atrial fibrillation. Since treatment is essentially the same, it does not really matter!

71. Here again is a sleeping pattern, reflecting deep respiration. The rhythm is a sinus rhythm with first degree block (P-R = 0.28 seconds) and a bundle branch block. Respiratory artifact can be diminished by altering lead placement.

72. This is a sinus rhythm interrupted by a P.A.C.

73. This is a two lead view of a borderline sinus tachycardia with a bundle branch block. Do you remember that repolarization (ST and T wave) is anomalous secondary to bundle branch block? If not, refer to Section 5.7.

74. This is a sinus rhythm with first degree AV block. Note the ST elevation (injury pattern) and the absence of an R wave (QS infarct pattern). One would want to inspect a 12-lead EKG to determine the location and scope of injury and infarct.

75. Clearly, one would want to see a longer rhythm strip in order to determine if three or more narrow complex beats occur consecutively. If so, one could determine the regularity or irregularity of those complexes. If regular, one could assume an underlying junctional rhythm (owing to the relatively slow rate and the absence of visible P waves). If irregular, one could assume that the underlying rhythm is atrial fibrillation. The bottom line is that one cannot determine the underlying rhythm from this short tracing. Thus, the best one can do is describe the rhythm as an undetermined rhythm interrupted by bigeminal P.V.C.s. The underlying rhythm demonstrates no clear P waves; atrial fibrillatory waves versus artifact exists. The QRS complexes of the base rhythm measure just slightly less than 0.12 seconds.

76. The rhythm is regular and the narrow QRS (<0.08 seconds) ventricular rate is approximately 65 beats per minute. The *eye catcher* here is the regular atrial waves occurring at a rate of 250 per minute ($1500 \div 6 = 250$. The critical question is whether the atrial activity is related to ventricular activity. A

close measurement indicates that the atrial activity is related to ventricular activity. This may be atrial flutter, but I would still want to look at this rhythm in other leads. It is also possible that this is artifact.

77. This rhythm appears to be a classic left bundle branch block (LBBB) with a heart rate of approximately 80. The P-R interval measures 0.20 seconds. However, I would want to view this rhythm in multiple leads to ensure it is not a paced rhythm.

78. Here is a partially pacemaker (demand-type) generated rhythm. Beats 1, 2 and 4 represent the patient's own complexes, sinus beats with evidence of first degree AV block (P-R = 0.28 seconds). The heart rate of the first two beats is approximately 72 (1500 ÷ 21 small squares = 72). As the patient's heart rate slows below 68, the demand pacemaker assumes control (measure the distance between two pacemaker generated complexes (1500 ÷ 22 small squares = 68). You will notice throughout the strip, various complexes are fusions of the patient's and the demand pacemaker's QRSS (most obvious in beats 3 and 5, somewhat less obvious in beats 6, 8, 10, 11, 14, 15). This type of phenomenon is observed when the patient's actual heart rate is at or near the pacemaker set rate.

79. Here is a regular rhythm (heart rate approximately 80 per minute) with a widened QRS measuring greater than 0.20 seconds. The QRS morphology is bizarre, making precise QRS measurement difficult! There may be an inverted P wave (short P-R interval) occurring before the QRS. If so, this is a junctional rhythm with bundle branch block. More likely, however, there is no P wave occurring before the QRS. Thus, the rhythm is an accelerated idioventricular rhythm (ventricular escape rhythm).

80. The underlying rhythm (viewed from the last half of the rhythm strip) is a sinus rhythm (rate 88) with a bundle branch block (QRS measures 0.14 seconds). The P-R interval measures 0.16 seconds. Various ectopic beats interrupt the rhythm. The first beat originates in the AV junction as evidenced by the retrograde P wave following the QRS. Beat 2 is a sinus beat followed by a fusion beat. (The P wave before the fusion beat occurs on time and the P-R interval is short; thus, the beat is both formed by a normal antegrade impulse colliding with a P.V.C. traveling a retrograde path). Beat 5 is a FLB (funny looking beat). The P wave occurs on time and the P-R interval is consistent with the sinus beats. This beat is a normally conducted sinus beat (no bundle branch block). Notice the biphasic P waves throughout, a classic finding of bi-atrial hypertrophy.

81. This is an ominous rhythm in appearance, but remember, check the patient first! The rhythm is irregular and the rate is slightly tachycardic. P waves can be seen, but have different shapes. This may be a multifocal atrial tachycardia with an underlying bundle branch block.

82. Here is another rhythm for debate! The non-controversial points of the rhythm are these: the rhythm is regular, the heart rate is approximately 84 beats per minute. The QRS is widened measuring approximately 0.16 seconds. This rhythm is likely one of two rhythms: (1) sinus rhythm with a first degree heart block (P-R interval measuring 0.40 seconds) and a bundle branch block or (2) a junctional rhythm (with a hidden P wave in the QRS) and a pronounced T wave, resulting in a prolonged QT interval of 0.44 seconds, in part owing to the widened QRS. (The normal female QT interval is 0.39; the normal male QT is 0.41). Clearly a 12 lead EKG and a clinical history (including pharmacologic agents) would be helpful. What do you think?

83. This rhythm is slow and irregular. A P wave precedes each QRS. The P-R is consistent, measuring 0.16 seconds, though the P wave morphology varies. The QRSs are within normal limits measuring 0.08 seconds. This is a pronounced slow sinus arrhythmia (the R-R interval of beats 1 and 2 is equal to the R-R interval of beats 3 and 4). This rhythm would likely be treated as a sinus bradycardia and may be related to toxic drug effects, electrolyte imbalances, or ischemia involving the sinus node.

84. Here we have an irregularly irregular rhythm, atrial fibrillation. Notice the fine atrial oscillations. Though one would need to view a longer rhythm strip to accurately determine the ventricular rate, this would appear to be a controlled rate atrial fibrillation.

85. The rhythm is regular at an approximate rate of 70 beats per minute. The P-R interval measures 0.16 seconds. The QRS is widened measuring slightly greater than 0.12 seconds. This is a sinus rhythm with a left bundle branch block (note the V pattern in lead MCL_1). The repolarization abnormalties occur secondary to the bundle branch block.

86. This rhythm is also an atrial fibrillation with coarse atrial fibrillatory waves. Notice the irregular irregularity. The "N" notations at the top of the rhythm strip are the computerized monitor notations, signaling that ventricular conduction (QRSs) are narrow, conducting normally (N).

87. As always, it is easier to identify the *known,* than work backwards to identify the unknown! The last four complexes represent a fine atrial fibrillation. (It is unlikely that the "bump" before beat 4 is a P wave). The two unusual beats (#2 and #3) are aberrantly conducted beats, resulting in a widened QRS complex.

88. This is an interesting strip requiring some thoughtful analysis. Begin by noticing that the P waves vary (two different morphologies). As always, interpretation would be easier if a longer rhythm strip were available! The two different P wave configurations suggest that one is likely "normal" (sinus) and one is likely of ectopic origin. The positive (upright) P waves in complexes 1, 4, 6 and 9 identify sinus beats. The first sinus beat (beat 1) is followed by two ectopic atrial beats (beats 2, 3). A pause follows the third beat, allowing the sinus pacemaker to reset. Throughout the strip, the ectopic atrial pacemaker interrupts the normal rhythm. Very likely the ectopic pacemaker has a rate similar to the sinus rate; thus, the two pacemakers compete for control of the rhythm. The P-R interval of both presentations measures 0.16 seconds.

89. Here we need to check and possibly change leads to better visualize the baseline! The rhythm is regular at a rate of 44 per minute. The QRS complexes measure 0.08 seconds. Assuming that the diminished amplitude is not obscuring upright P waves occurring before each QRS, this is a junctional rhythm with P waves hidden within the QRS complexes.

90. Here, a borderline sinus tachycardia (rate 100) presents with tall "tent-like" T waves, often suggestive of hyperkalemia. The corresponding V lead demonstrates flipped (inverted) T waves suggestive of ischemia. One would definitely want to observe a 12 lead EKG. The P-R interval is this strip measures 0.16 seconds.

91. Artifact always makes rhythm strip interpretation interesting! Despite the motion artifact, portions of this rhythm (complexes 4–7) occur regularly with distinguishable P waves. The P-R interval of those beats measures slightly less than 0.20 seconds. However, the QRS measures slightly greater than 0.12 seconds. thus the underlying rhythm here is a sinus rhythm (approximate rate 85) with a bundle branch block. It is helpful that the V lead is also included which identifies the block as a left bundle branch block. Complex 8 is a premature beat followed by a characteristic pause. The last two complexes are sinus beats with LBBB. Though somewhat obscured, the initial complex (beat 1) is probably a sinus beat followed by a premature beat and pause. It is difficult to identify the origin of the premature beats given both the artifact and the LBBB. However, given that the appearance of the premature beats is distinctly similar to the normal beats, my guess is that they are of atrial origin with the P wave masked by the preceding T wave! Whew!

92. **IMPORTANT NOTE:** Some computerized monitors identify QRS configurations or patterns (V = wide). Here we have a sinus rhythm (rate 62) with a right bundle branch block (RBBB). The P-R interval measures approximately 0.14 seconds.

93. The *eyecatcher* in this strip is the unexpected pause measuring slightly greater than 2.0 seconds. The underlying rhythm is irregular and artifact obstructs the ability to easily identify atrial activity. On *first pass,* this looks like an atrial fibrillation with a left bundle branch block . . . and a long pause possibly relating to drug therapy Vs. ischemia Vs. vagal stimulation Vs. blockage of both the right and left bundle branches (bilateral bundle branch block). Remember, there is no perfusion during the pause!

94. Hope you did not miss this one! This is a ventricular tachycardia (rate 250) that terminates spontaneously. Evidence in support of ventricular tachycardia includes probable fusion beats (see MCL$_1$, beats 7 and 8).

95. Here we have an AV sequential pacemaker (rate 60) evident at both the beginning and end of the rhythm strip. Beat 3 and the second to the last beat appear to be jointly formed by the atrial pacer and the patient's own pacemaker. A *patient-generated* fairly regular, rapid (approximate rate 125) ectopic rhythm emerges beginning with beat 4, terminating at beat 10. The QRS is widened (0.12 seconds) in the ectopic sequence. Owing to baseline artifact, one cannot determine the presence or absence of P waves. Thus, this burst of ectopic activity could be of either a supraventricular origin (supraventricular tachycardia) with a bundle branch block or ventricular origin.

96. This rhythm strip can be a fooler. At first glance, one thinks of a *classic* Wenckeback rhythm. However, close inspection reveals a varying P wave morphology (the P waves appear different) with only slight variation in the R-R interval (the R-R interval becomes only incrementally shorter). This is likely a wondering atrial pacemaker with "blocked" atrial beats. (Blocked beats are *assumed* because of the pause. The assumed blocked beats do not conduct secondary to block in the AV node.

97. This is a sinus bradycardia (rate 50) with a sinus dysrhythmia likely associated with respiration. Peaked T waves are evident in Lead II. Lead MCL1 demonstrates ST elevation suggestive of injury. One would want to observe a 12 lead EKG to look for further evidence of injury/ischemia. The P-R interval (0.14) and QRS (0.08) are within normal limits.

98. Starting with the known, this is a relatively rapid, irregular rhythm with a left bundle branch block (lead V$_1$) pattern (QRS measures 0.12 seconds). Most obvious in the lead 2 rhythm strip, identifiable P waves are periodically visible (see beats 2, 5, 6, 12, 15), though the P morphology and the P-R interval changes slightly in the latter part of the rhythm strip. Presumably the rhythm is a sinus rhythm with left bundle branch block interrupted by short bursts of ectopic activity. The sinus mechanism, however is not dependable (notice the absence of P waves in the last 2 beats of the rhythm strip). Thus, there is some pathology involving the sinus mechanism (sick sinus, drug effects, ischemia, etc). Determining the origin of the ectopic bursts is a challenge. Options include a supraventricular versus a ventricular ectopic pacemaker. Ectopic beats of supraventricular origin would display a widened QRS owing to the bundle branch block (morphology consistent with sinus beats viewed from the same lead). Alternatively, an ectopic ventricular pacemaker arising in the right ventricle would produce a LBBB pattern in V. The clinical significance of the rhythm would drive therapy.

99. The first beat (obvious in leads I, II, III) is an ectopic beat of unknown origin. The remainder of the 12 leads reflect a sinus rhythm, rate approximately 78 per minute. The P-R interval measures 0.12 seconds. The QRS is widened, measuring 0.12 seconds, reflecting a bundle branch block. An inspection of the V leads reveals this is a left bundle branch block. The distortion of the ST segment is a characteristic of left bundle branch block.

100. Here we have evidence of an unhealthy patient! The rhythm is a sinus bradycardia (rate approximately 40) with first degree AV block (the P-R interval measures 0.28 seconds) and a bundle branch block (the QRS duration is 0.12 seconds). One would need to inspect a 12 lead EKG (the V leads) to determine right or left bundle branch block. Note: since this rhythm strip is from limb lead II, this is probably a left bundle branch block. A lone P.V.C is sandwiched (interpolated) between two normal beats. Owing to the slow rate, the P.V.C assists perfusion.

101. Here we have a 12 lead EKG with sinus rhythm (heart rate 94). The P-R interval measures slightly less than 0.16 seconds; the QRS measures 0.10 seconds. Marked ST depression (ischemic pattern) is noted in leads I, aVL and V$_1$, V$_2$, V$_3$, and there is slight ST depression in leads V$_{4-6}$. Tall, pronounced (hyperacute) T waves are evident in leads II, III and aVF. This EKG suggests current injury of the inferior myocardium with ischemia of the anteroseptal and lateral walls.

102. This EKG is a bit complicated, best identified by studying the lead II rhythm strip (bottom). Close observation of the P waves and measurement of the R-R intervals reveals that the pacemaker is wandering in the atria. Because the heart rate is rapid, this is a multifocal atrial tachycardia or, an atrial tachycardia with a wandering pacemaker. Commonly, wandering pacemakers are associated with pulmonary disease. Owing to the wandering pacemaker, the P-R interval varies slightly. The QRS measures 0.08 seconds.

103. This is a regular rhythm with a rate of 82 beats per minute. No atrial activity precedes the QRS. These leads do not assist the interpretation! The QRS is between 0.10–0.12. A precise measurement is difficult. It is unclear whether a retrograde P wave follows the QRS, though the last three beats in the top strip are highly suspect. This rhythm is either an accelerated junctional rhythm with a borderline bundle branch block or an accelerated idioventricular rhythm.

104. This rhythm strip can fool you. On first glance, one might think this is a coarse atrial fibrillation owing to the irregularity and appearance of the baseline. However, close inspection identifies a regular rhythm pattern with premature beats, all confounded by artifact. The first three beats are sinus beats, followed by a P.A.C. (the P wave of the P.A.C. rests on the T wave of the preceding beat). The P.A.C. is followed by a pause, then two sinus beats occur followed by another P.A.C. That pattern exists until the end of the strip, where the last four beats are sinus beats. The heart rate is approximately 115 per minute. The P-R interval measures 0.12 seconds. The QRS is widened, measuring 0.12 seconds indicating a block in one of the bundle branches. Since lead MCL$_1$ is a proxy for lead V$_1$, this is a right bundle branch block. So, this is a sinus tachycardia with right bundle branch block interrupted by frequent P.A.C.s, sometimes occurring in a trigeminal pattern.

105. This is a sinus rhythm with a rate of 75. The QRS measures 0.08 seconds. The pause is most likely a blocked P.A.C. In the lower tracing there does appear to be a P without a QRS.

106. The underlying rhythm is a sinus rhythm, rate approximately 70 beats per minute. The P-R measures 0.14 seconds and the QRS duration is approximately 0.10 seconds. Looking first at the limb and augmented leads, one finds ST depression in leads I and aVL. Leads II, III and aVF demonstrate ST elevation (injury) and prominent Q waves. This is an inferior STEMI. The ST depression in leads I and aVL represents reciprocal charges. There is normal R wave progression across the precordial (V) leads.

107. Another challenging strip worthy of debate! The rhythm is rapid, averaging 150 beats per minute. There is slight irregularity of the rhythm and P waves are occasionally visible. The QRS duration varies between 0.18 and 0.21 seconds. My first impression was ventricular tachycardia, despite the slight rhythm irregularity. I presumed the more narrow QRS complexes (see beats 4 and 10, in particular) were fusion beats. However, a colleague consultation suggests that the irregularity of the rhythm favors a supraventricular origin. The widened QRS may relate to an underlying bundle branch block or a rate-related bundle branch block. As always, a clear description is more helpful than a name! Also, remember to check your patient and treat accordingly!

108. The underlying rhythm is slow (slightly less than 40 beats per minute) and regular. The QRS measures 0.08 seconds. There are no P waves prior to the QRS, but an inverted P wave follows the QRS (most prominent in leads II, III and aVF). This is a slow junctional rhythm. Check your patient!

109. Here we have a rapid supraventricular tachycardia with a rate of 250 per minute. ST segment depression is evident throughout, likely due to the rapid rate. The genesis of this rapid rate dysrhythmia may be a re-entry mechanism.

110. This is a borderline sinus tachycardia, rate 100 per minute, with a right bundle branch block. The P-R interval measures 0.16 seconds. The QRS is wide, measuring 0.13 seconds. You will recall that secondary ST changes accompany bundle branch blocks!

111. This strip begins with 4 beats that appear to have P waves. But then the rhythm degenerates into coarse atrial fib with the QRS measuring slightly less than 0.12 seconds.

112. Leads II, III and aVF demonstrate marked ST elevation (injury) and pathologic Q waves indicating acute inferior STEMI. Reciprocal ST segment depression is noted in leads I and aVL. Normal R wave progression is noted in the V leads though ST segment depression (ischemia) is observed in leads V_2–V_6. The rhythm is a borderline sinus tachycardia (rate 100 per minute). The P-R interval measures 0.16 seconds. The QRS measures approximately 0.10 seconds.

113. Ugh! ST elevation is present in leads I and aVL (high lateral wall) and a pathologic Q wave is observed in lead I. Pathologic Q waves are also evident in leads II, III and aVF (interior wall). Unifocal P.V.C.s (most visible in the lead II rhythm strip) distort the precordial leads, though ST elevation (injury) is evident throughout. A pathologic Q wave is evident in lead V_4. Thus, this patient has injury of the anterior, septal and lateral surfaces of the left ventricle and an age-undetermined infarct of the inferior wall.

114. This is a great rhythm strip! The baseline is erratic suggesting either atrial fibrillation or artifact. No clear P waves are visible. The rhythm is regular at a rate of approximately 36 beats per minute. The QRS is widened, measuring 0.14 seconds. Atrial fibrillation is an irregularly, irregular rhythm. Given the regularity of this rhythm, the baseline is probably distorted by artifact. And, given the rate and width of QRSs, this is most likely an idioventricular rhythm.

115. Brain break! Here we have a *classic* atrial flutter (4:1 conduction pattern). The atrial rate is 300 per minute, and the ventricular rate is 75.

116. Hope this continuous rhythm strip did not block you! The rhythm begins (first two beats) as a borderline sinus tachycardia (rate 100, P-R interval 0.20 seconds, QRS 0.10 seconds). Then the rate increases to 115 beats per minute and the QRS complexes change in morphology. Beat 3 demonstrates a clear P wave, occurring on time though the following QRS is premature in relation to the previous beat. No further distinct P waves can be identified in this second rhythm pattern. The QRS is widened, measuring 0.14 seconds. In the middle of strip 2, the patient's own intrinsic rhythm resumes at a rate of 115 for four beats. A presumed P.V.C. is followed by a pause. A ventricular pacemaker (set rate of 75) appropriately kicks in following the pause for three paced beats. Then, the sinus rhythm (borderline sinus tachycardia) resumes at a rate of 100 beats per minute, again demonstrating upright P waves, and a P-R interval of 0.20 seconds. This is an example of appropriate pacing during increased activity. This patient is exercising, and the pacer increased rate to improve perfusion.

117. Here is another somewhat challenging rhythm, subject to debate! The rhythm is irregular, occurring at an approximate rate of 150 per minute. There is slight variation in the QRS duration (0.12 and 0.10). Though artifact partially obscures distinct P waves, varied presentation P waves can be observed throughout the rhythm strip. You will also note respiratory variation. Most likely, this is a multifocal atrial tachycardia (MAT) with ventricular aberration occurring secondary to the rapid rate. This type of dysrhythmia is often associated with C.O.P.D. or respiratory failure.

118. This is an example of second degree type II (Mobitz II) block. Note fixed PR interval of .20 with the fourth P wave not followed by a QRS.

119. This is an example of ventricular fibrillation. Note there are no discernable P, Q, R, S, or T waves. This rhythm requires immediate advanced cardiac life support.

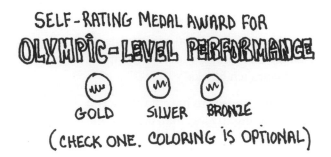

SELF-RATING MEDAL AWARD FOR
OLYMPIC-LEVEL PERFORMANCE

GOLD   SILVER   BRONZE

(CHECK ONE. COLORING IS OPTIONAL)

16

Notes

Index

C

frontal plane activity recording and, 4
Lead I recording, 4, 5, 9, 11
Lead II recording, 4, 5, 9, 11
Lead III recording, 4, 5, 9, 11
left arm/positive Lead I/negative Lead II, 5
left leg/positive pole, 5
left ventricular surfaces and, 9
myocardial activity, equidistant leads and, 5
QRS deflection and, 5
right arm/negative pole, 5
See also EKG; Leads
Starling's Law, 325
ST-elevation myocardial infarction (STEMI), 267,
    276–277, 283–284, 289–290, 310
    See also Acute coronary syndrome (ACS);
        Myocardial infarction
Stents, 311
Stimulants, 56
Stress tests, 309
Stroke, 73, 312
ST segment, 22, 23, 37
    atrial fibrillation and, 71
    children and, 356
    hypocalcemia and, 256
    hypokalemia, 251
    left bundle branch block and, 161
    myocardial infarction and, 277–278
    myocardial ischemia and, 271, 272, 273
Sudden cardiac death, 235
Supraventricular (SVT) rhythms, 63, 99, 100, 241–242
    causes of, 365
    children and, 365–366
    disease associations with, 365
    identifying features of, 365
    treatment for, 366
Swan-Ganz catheter, 320, 327, 328–329
S wave, 20, 21, 37
Sympathetic nervous system (SNS), 325
Synchronized cardioversion technique, 60, 69, 72, 73,
    100, 120, 192–193
Systemic vascular resistance (SVR), 326
Systole, 321, 322

T

Tachycardia. *See* Atrial tachycardia; Junctional
    tachycardia; Ventricular tachycardia
Temporary pacemaker codes, 211
Tension pneumothorax, 378
Three-lead monitoring systems, 10–11
Thrombus formation, 73, 273, 310, 376
Tobacco use, 51, 56, 108, 365
Toothbrush artifact, 177–178
Torsades de pointes (TdP), 123–124
    acquired long QT syndrome and, 124
    genetic mutation and, 124
    proarrhythmic effect of drugs and, 124

treatment of, 124
ventricular fibrillation and, 124
Transcutaneous electrical nerve stimulator (TENS), 183
Transcutaneous pacemaker (TCP), 95, 130, 131, 155,
    201, 360
Transesophageal echocardiogram (TEE), 73
Transient ischemia, 266
Transvenous pacemaker, 130, 154, 201
Trifascicular system, 156
Trigeminy pattern, 109
T wave, 16, 22, 23, 37
    artifacts and, 180
    atrial fibrillation and, 71
    cardiac cycle and, 192, 193
    children, 357
    first degree heart block and, 143
    hyperkalemia and, 253, 254
    hypocalcemia and, 256
    myocardial infarction and, 284, 297
    myocardial ischemia and, 271, 272, 273
    pacemakers and, 209
    premature atrial contractions and, 56
    premature ventricular contractions and, 109–110
    R on T phenomenon, 109–110, 121
2:1 AV conduction pattern, 148–149, 381–382

U

Urine output, 341
U wave, 22, 251

V

Vagal stimulation, 48, 60, 69, 129, 366
Vagal tone, 45, 60, 93, 362
Vagotonia, 139
Valsalva maneuver, 60, 69
Valve replacement, 311
Valvular regurgitation, 311
Vasodilators, 310
Ventricular contractions. *See* Premature ventricular
    contractions (P.V.C.s)
Ventricular electrical activation, 3, 4
Ventricular escape rhythms/beats, 128–131
    cardiac cycle and, 129, 131
    diagnosis of, 130–131
    hemodynamic disequillibrium and, 130
    idioventricular rhythm and, 129, 130
    potential pacemakers and, 128
    sinus pacemaker, failure of, 129, 130
    treatments for, 130
Ventricular fibrillation, 125–126, 134, 253, 254
    causes of, 125, 192, 377
    children and, 376–377
    defibrillation and, 193
    electrical activity, total irregularity of, 125, 377
    electrical defibrillation and, 125–126
    electrical shock and, 125, 192